Introduction to Psychological Theories and Psychotherapy

Introduction to Psychological Theories and Psychotherapy

Andrew Koffmann, PhD
Department of Psychology
University of Pittsburgh
Pittsburgh, PA

M. Grace Walters, MD
Department of Psychiatry
University of Pittsburgh School of Medicine
Pittsburgh, PA

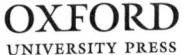

OXFORD
UNIVERSITY PRESS

Oxford University Press is a department of the University of Oxford.
It furthers the University's objective of excellence in research, scholarship,
and education by publishing worldwide.

Oxford   New York
Auckland   Cape Town   Dar es Salaam   Hong Kong   Karachi
Kuala Lumpur   Madrid   Melbourne   Mexico City   Nairobi
New Delhi   Shanghai   Taipei   Toronto

With offices in
Argentina   Austria   Brazil   Chile   Czech Republic   France   Greece
Guatemala   Hungary   Italy   Japan   Poland   Portugal   Singapore
South Korea   Switzerland   Thailand   Turkey   Ukraine   Vietnam

Oxford is a registered trademark of Oxford University Press
in the UK and certain other countries.

Published in the United States of America by
Oxford University Press
198 Madison Avenue, New York, NY 10016

© Oxford University Press 2014

All rights reserved. No part of this publication may be reproduced, stored in a
retrieval system, or transmitted, in any form or by any means, without the prior
permission in writing of Oxford University Press, or as expressly permitted by law,
by license, or under terms agreed with the appropriate reproduction rights organization.
Inquiries concerning reproduction outside the scope of the above should be sent to the
Rights Department, Oxford University Press, at the address above.

You must not circulate this work in any other form
and you must impose this same condition on any acquirer.

Library of Congress Cataloging-in-Publication Data
Koffmann, Andrew, author.
Introduction to psychological theories and psychotherapy / Andrew Koffmann,
M. Grace Walters.
   pages cm
Includes bibliographical references and index.
ISBN 978–0–19–991796–9 (alk. paper)
1. Psychotherapy. 2. Psychology. 3. Psychiatry. I. Walters, M. Grace, author.
II. Title.
[DNLM: 1. Psychological Theory. 2. Psychotherapy. BF 38]
RC480.K63 2014
616.89'14—dc23
                    2014008949

The science of medicine is a rapidly changing field. As new research and clinical experience broaden
our knowledge, changes in treatment and drug therapy occur. The author and publisher of this
work have checked with sources believed to be reliable in their efforts to provide information that
is accurate and complete, and in accordance with the standards accepted at the time of publication.
However, in light of the possibility of human error or changes in the practice of medicine, neither
the author, nor the publisher, nor any other party who has been involved in the preparation or
publication of this work warrants that the information contained herein is in every respect accurate
or complete. Readers are encouraged to confirm the information contained herein with other
reliable sources, and are strongly advised to check the product information sheet provided by the
pharmaceutical company for each drug they plan to administer.

9 8 7 6 5 4 3 2 1
Printed in the United States of America
on acid-free paper

Series Introduction

We stand on the threshold of a new Golden Age of clinical and behavioral neuroscience with psychiatry at its fore. With the Pittsburgh Pocket Psychiatry series, we intend to encompass the breadth and depth of our current understanding of human behavior in health and disease. Using the structure of resident didactic teaching, we will be able to ensure that each subject area relevant for both current and future practicing psychiatrists is detailed and described. New innovations in diagnosis and treatment will be reviewed and discussed in the context of existing knowledge, and each book in the series will propose new directions for scientific inquiry and discovery. The aim of the series as a whole is to integrate findings from all areas of medicine and neuroscience previously segregated as "mind" or "body," "psychological" or "biological." Thus, each book from the Pittsburgh Pocket Psychiatry series will stand alone as a standard text for anyone wishing to learn about a specific subject area. The series will be the most coherent and flexible learning resource available.

David J. Kupfer, MD
Michael J. Travis, MD
Michelle S. Horner, DO

Contents

1. Introduction — 1
2. Psychological Theories: Key Concepts — 7
3. Toward an Integrated Understanding of Psychotherapy: Useful Perspectives — 71
4. Learning Psychotherapy — 113
5. Current Psychotherapies — 137
6. Conclusions — 249

References 257
Glossary 273
Index 295

Detailed Contents

1 Introduction
Overview of the Book 4

2 Psychological Theories: Key Concepts
The Evolution of Psychodynamic Theory 10
   Introduction 10
   Freud's Life and the Origins of Psychodynamic Theory 11
   The Vienna Psychoanalytic Society 28
   Ego Psychology 37
   Object Relations Theory 43
   The Interpersonal School 46
   Psychodynamic Approaches to Character and the Self 48
   Child Analysis and Developmental Theory 52
   Current Trends in Psychodynamic Theory 54
The Evolution of Cognitive and Behavior Therapies 58
   Behaviorism: The First Wave 58
   Behaviorism: The Second Wave 63
   Behaviorism: The Third Wave 67
Recommended Reading 70

3 Toward an Integrated Understanding of Psychotherapy: Useful Perspectives
Neurobiological Correlates of Psychological Theory and Psychotherapy 74
   Neuroplasticity and Four Key Phenomena 74

Neurobiology and the Psychotherapy
   of Depression   78
Neurobiology and the Psychotherapy of PTSD   80
Summary   82
Research Findings in Psychology   84
   What Do We Know About the Rate of Recovery
      in Psychotherapy?   84
   In General, How Does Psychotherapy Work?   92
Research Findings from Treatment Studies   100
   Efficacy vs. Effectiveness   100
   Monotherapy vs. Combined Treatment   100
   Continuation and Maintenance Psychotherapy   103
   Bringing a Psychotherapeutic Understanding
      to Pharmacotherapy   105
Psychotherapy Within Psychiatry: Narrowing
   Indications and Broadening Options   108
Recommended Reading   112

4 Learning Psychotherapy

Introduction   114
Basic Skills   116
   Attending and Listening skills   116
   Restatements   117
   Questions   119
   Showing Empathy   120
   Challenges   122
Common Psychotherapeutic Techniques   124
Proposed Learning Sequence   130
Recommended Reading   136

5 **Current Psychotherapies**

Psychotherapy Training 140
Individual Psychodynamic Psychotherapies 142
   Psychoanalysis 142
   Psychodynamic Psychotherapy 150
   Transference-Focused Psychotherapy (TFP) 156
   Mentalization-Based Treatment (MBT) 161
   Supportive Psychotherapy
     (Including Psychoeducation) 165
   Play Therapy 168
Individual Behavior Therapies 174
   Cognitive-Behavioral Therapy (CBT) 174
   Exposure and Response Prevention (ERP) 192
   Brief Cognitive Therapy for Panic Disorder 196
   Prolonged Exposure for Posttraumatic Stress
     Disorder (PE-PTSD) 200
   Dialectical Behavior Therapy (DBT) 205
   Applied Behavior Analysis (ABA) 211
Other Individual Psychotherapies 214
   Interpersonal Psychotherapy (IPT) 214
   Motivational Interviewing (MI) 219
   Twelve-Step Facilitation 223
   Eye Movement Desensitization and
     Reprocessing (EMDR) 227
   Biofeedback for Mental Disorders 231
   Therapies from Complementary and
     Alternative Medicine 233
Psychotherapy for Multiple Patients 236

Group Psychotherapy 236
Mindfulness-Based Cognitive Therapy (MBCT) 240
Family Therapy 242
Recommended Reading 248

6 Conclusions

Psychiatry, Psychotherapy, and the Future 250
Anticipations in Neuroscience 252
Anticipations in Psychological Theory 254
Next Steps: Further Training and Self-Study 256

References 257
Glossary 273
Index 295

Introduction to Psychological Theories and Psychotherapy

Chapter 1

Introduction

Overview of the Book 4

Psychological Theories and Psychotherapy

In recent years there has been a resurgence within psychiatry of awareness regarding the value of psychotherapy in the treatment of individuals with mental disorders. A century ago psychotherapy was a new tool in the psychiatric armamentarium, and its practitioners believed that this treatment modality would bring relief to a large number of suffering people. Over time, however, it became evident that many patients did not respond adequately to "talk therapy," and the focus of interest within psychiatry shifted to somatic interventions (e.g., psychopharmacology, electroconvulsive therapy, emerging neuromodulation therapies, biofeedback, and phototherapy). More recently, as empirically supported psychotherapies have become widely available, psychiatrists have recognized that psychotherapy is often just as effective as a variety of somatic interventions for the treatment of mental disorders—and sometimes even more so. There is research evidence to support this view.

While today's practicing psychiatrist may or may not offer formal psychotherapy to patients, he or she does need to be knowledgeable about the range of psychotherapeutic interventions that are available and about the relative efficacy of each. Practicing psychiatrists should understand the means by which psychotherapy affects mental functioning, just as they need to understand how somatic treatments affect mental functioning. Both psychotherapy and somatic interventions appear to bring about changes in neurobiological as well as psychological functioning, accomplishing this by specific and not necessarily overlapping routes. The treatment provider who possesses a solid understanding of this information is able to develop a sophisticated understanding of the patient and can plan psychiatric treatment in a flexible and creative manner. Moreover, the knowledgeable clinician can provide clear and useful explanations to patients, with the effect of increasing the patient's cooperation and expectancy of a successful outcome. Research data clearly show that increased hope and better collaboration between treatment provider and patient lead to decreased symptomatology among individuals with mental disorders.

The current text is intended to provide psychiatric residents and practicing psychiatrists with a basic understanding of psychological theory and psychotherapy as well as an introduction to the range of psychotherapeutic treatment options. The text also contains useful information for other professionals who frequently work with patients who have mental disorders. Of course, virtually every healthcare provider comes in contact from time to time with patients who have emotional difficulties. In particular, primary care physicians, psychologists, social workers, licensed professional counselors, and nurses who work in the mental health field have daily contact with such patients. These professionals talk with patients about the treatment options that are available for mental disorders, they make referral decisions on a regular basis, and they themselves often provide first-line treatments. In light of the burgeoning knowledge base within psychiatry, these non-psychiatrist professionals need to have a solid understanding of both somatic and psychotherapeutic interventions and the relationship between these two approaches. This text delivers to all treatment providers not only a broad overview of psychotherapy but also sufficient detail to permit useful conceptualization and effective treatment planning.

The field of psychological theory is vast, and the number of psychotherapies currently used in various settings is seemingly infinite. In this text we focus on only the most important information that psychiatrists and other professionals need to know in order to make sense of the theoretical basis, practical implementation, and current research findings in psychotherapy. We have not attempted to cover the entire field of psychotherapy, however, and have limited our discussion to the kinds of psychotherapy that are appropriate for the mitigation of symptoms of mental disorders. Thus, we do not discuss models of psychotherapy that have as a goal the development of insight for insight's sake, nor do we provide information that is primarily useful in addressing the concerns of the "worried well." We provide very little information about psychotherapeutic interventions that lack empirical support. By contrast, we do discuss in detail all those psychotherapies about which psychiatric residents and primary care providers are expected to be knowledgeable.

Overview of the Book

We have presented the topics in this text in a particular sequence, and the reader is encouraged to proceed through the book chapter by chapter. Following this introduction, we begin our exploration of psychotherapy by reviewing in some depth the psychological theories that serve as foundations for the major models of psychotherapy. Without an understanding of these theories, it is almost impossible to make sense of psychotherapy as it is currently practiced, and one quickly becomes lost in any attempt to understand the details of each model of treatment. We present relevant psychological theory under two large rubrics: psychodynamic theory and behavioral theory. Many models of psychotherapy draw heavily from one or the other of these theories, and the reader is encouraged to think about the field as a whole from the perspective of these complementary approaches.

While psychodynamic and behavioral theory share the goal of understanding and ultimately changing human behavior, there are many contrasts between the two bodies of theory. One might suggest that psychodynamic theory is particularly well suited to *understanding* human experience and, in its therapeutic application, to guiding patients toward self-understanding, while behavioral theory is best suited to the development of treatments that are particularly effective in the rapid *amelioration of symptoms*, particularly in mood and anxiety disorders. However, each theory does provide both understanding and a technology for change.

Of note, psychodynamic and behavioral theory developed contemporaneously but more or less independently of one another. In recent years, however, there has been more cross-pollination between them, and as a consequence many models of psychotherapy now benefit from the ideas developed in both traditions. Still, the way that one conceives of patients and problems depends to a great degree on whether one relies on psychodynamic or behavioral theory. The two theories utilize different psychological constructs, they posit different change mechanisms, and the resulting models of psychotherapy contrast in many ways with one another. Even if the language and ideas of one theory differ substantially from the language and ideas of the other, the knowledgeable mental health professional needs to have an understanding of both. With a grounding in psychodynamic and behavioral theories the clinician has a far easier time than would otherwise be the case in making sense of almost any extant model of psychotherapy of relevance within psychiatry. Moreover, since a sophisticated conceptualization of the patient predicts to a better outcome in treatment, the knowledgeable professional is likely to have more success in the role of treatment provider.

In the current text we present psychodynamic and behavioral theory in historical context, because we believe that the large body of information contained within each theory is more easily grasped and remembered when the constituent ideas make both logical and historical sense. As well, it is much easier to remember the main points in this large corpus of knowledge when one can tie the two theories to the chronological sequence in which they unfolded. It is interesting to note that the history of psychodynamic theory closely tracks the histories of individual theorists, while the history of behavioral theory consists mostly of a history of theoretical concepts. In any event, we very much encourage the reader to spend time with this section of the book. Having read it, you will have much less difficulty making sense of what follows.

The professional who wishes to understand psychotherapy must also be aware of some information that is less theoretical in nature, reflecting the findings of research in a number of related areas. Following our review of psychological theories, we offer information from several useful perspectives. We begin with a discussion of the neurobiological correlates of psychological theory and psychotherapy. Although this information will be of particular interest to psychiatrists, it is likely to be very useful for non-psychiatrists as well. A grasp of the neurobiological correlates permits one to conceptualize, simultaneously and using similar language, the routes by which psychotherapy and various somatic treatments effect symptomatic change in individuals with mental disorders. Patients and providers are often perplexed about why one would wish to treat a mental disorder somatically and psychologically at the same time. Others may wonder which treatment is "correct" in a given situation. Our intention in the neurobiological section of the text is to provide insight for the reader into the roles played by "talk therapy" and somatic interventions in psychiatry, and we make the point that while these treatment modalities are not equivalent, they are usually complementary and may overlap more than one might imagine.

We continue our review of general research findings by summarizing what is known about whether and why psychotherapy actually works, this time from a psychological perspective. What is the evidence from research trials that psychotherapy works, and is one therapy more effective than another? The hypothesis that all psychotherapy is equally effective has been referred to as the Dodo bird hypothesis, with a nod to Lewis Carroll. The Dodo bird turns out to be partly true and partly false. We also discuss what is known about the trajectory of response to treatment, and we discuss the topics of sudden early gains and deterioration in treatment. While it is true that most psychotherapy depends in large measure on either psychodynamic theory, behavioral theory, or some combination of both, it is also true that all psychotherapy is substantially dependent on the interpersonal relationship between clinician and patient. Research in psychology has provided some important information about this relationship and has also elucidated patient factors and therapist factors that contribute to outcome in psychotherapy. We provide a summary of what is known on these topics.

Another useful perspective on psychotherapy comes from the findings of large psychiatric treatment studies. We begin our review of this area by discussing findings that suggest approximately equivalent efficacy of psychotherapy and psychotropic medications in the treatment of many mental disorders, and we summarize the literature regarding the efficacy of monotherapy, as compared with combined treatment. In particular, we discuss the issue of maintenance treatment, since relapse prevention becomes the most important goal following remission. In addition, we discuss evidence suggesting that, after all psychiatric treatment is discontinued, patients are less likely to experience relapse or recurrence if they have received psychotherapy in addition to or instead of pharmacotherapy.

Next, we offer some comments regarding issues that may arise when the same clinician simultaneously provides pharmacotherapy and psychotherapy. We end this section by suggesting ways for psychiatrists, in particular, to limit the range of psychotherapy indications to just those appropriate for the treatment of mental disorders while at the same time broadening options for treatment. In this connection, we discuss the issue of manualized treatments (i.e., therapies in which the provider's treatment follows a manual step by step), and we consider three therapeutic stances: dogmatic consistency, eclecticism, and pluralism.

Having considered all of this essential background, we begin the clinical applications section of our text with an outline of how one might go about learning psychotherapy. We focus on the development of basic skills, a list of basic techniques utilized in a wide range of psychotherapies, and a proposed learning sequence, with practical suggestions regarding the kinds of exercises to undertake and the training experiences to seek. We make the point that developing competence as a psychotherapist involves much more than simply learning a couple of theories and a list of techniques. Competent psychotherapists must develop and refine basic interpersonal skills that are of use in any model of psychotherapy. These skills are related to, but not the same as, the basic interpersonal skills clinicians use routinely in non-psychotherapeutic interactions with patients. The idea that all psychotherapy depends to some extent on competent execution of pantheoretical, core relationship skills is consistent with research findings that show empirically supported psychotherapies to be of roughly equivalent efficacy in many cases. This brings us back once again to the Dodo bird.

At this point in the text we are in a position to review each of the major models of psychotherapy that are of current significance within psychiatry. We divide our list of psychotherapies into several large groups, including individual psychotherapies, subdivided into those based primarily on psychodynamic concepts, those based primarily on behavioral principles, and those based on some other theory or concept, as well as group and family psychotherapy. Within each group, for each specific type of therapy, we describe the model of psychopathology, particular treatment strategies, and relevant research findings, after which we offer a case example, so that the reader has access to a full range of important information about each treatment model in one place.

In the final section of the book we offer some thoughts about the future of psychotherapy within psychiatry, with particular emphasis on anticipations in neuroscience and psychological theory, as well as a review of the next steps the reader may take to learn more about psychotherapy. The text ends with an extensive glossary of important names and terms.

Chapter 2

Psychological Theories: Key Concepts

The Evolution of Psychodynamic Theory *10*
   Introduction *10*
   Freud's Life and the Origins of Psychodynamic Theory *11*
   The Vienna Psychoanalytic Society *28*
   Ego Psychology *37*
   Object Relations Theory *43*
   The Interpersonal School *46*
   Psychodynamic Approaches to Character and the Self *48*
   Child Analysis and Developmental Theory *52*
   Current Trends in Psychodynamic Theory *54*
The Evolution of Cognitive and Behavior Therapies *58*
   Behaviorism: The First Wave *58*
   Behaviorism: The Second Wave *63*
   Behaviorism: The Third Wave *67*

8 Psychological Theories and Psychotherapy

In this chapter we provide an overview of the psychological theories that serve as foundations for almost all current psychotherapies. It is important to be familiar with this information, because without some understanding of the theoretical basis, you will have great difficulty making sense of why psychotherapy models are structured as they are, and it will be even more difficult to practice psychotherapy competently or to develop a thorough understanding of treatment options.

Our review is divided into two sections. We first discuss the theory that undergirds the psychodynamic psychotherapies, after which we examine the foundations of the behavioral psychotherapies. As it happens, these two bodies of knowledge developed more or less independently at about the same time in history. It is easiest to think of them as proceeding along parallel tracks, and that is how we present them. To make the theories easier to learn, we make reference along the way to the historical events that gave these theories their shape.

The Evolution of Psychodynamic Theory

Introduction

We begin our discussion of psychological theories with a tour of the theory and main treatment techniques that trace their lineage directly back to Sigmund Freud (1856–1939). These treatment techniques and all associated theory, while properly referred to as psychoanalytic, are often more generally referred to as *psychodynamic*, to distinguish them from formal *psychoanalysis*, a subset of rigorously Freudian techniques within the broader psychodynamic school. Actually, one might reasonably argue that all of modern psychotherapy, psychodynamic and otherwise, is dependent to a greater or lesser extent on Freudian thought. Indeed, many of the most useful concepts in psychotherapy were first carefully worked out by Freud, including transference, countertransference, unconscious, ego, resistance, defense, and many more. In this section, we explain such ideas (and quite a few others) in detail. We also explain how the ideas developed in the first place, in the expectation that if you know the historical context in which key psychodynamic ideas arose, you will have an easier time remembering and making sense of them.

So what are the main ideas to watch for on our tour? We will be talking about the notion of an *unconscious*, a concept that helps to make sense of the fact that people don't always act in a way that is consistent with their stated goals. Freud believed there is a psychic agent, the *ego*, that makes use of predictable and sometimes stereotyped strategies called *defenses* to prevent anxiety-inducing impulses from reaching conscious awareness. We will learn how later theorists in the field of *ego psychology* worked out these defenses in more detail. Freud made use of the idea of defense not only to understand the structure of the psyche but also in his examination of *resistance*, his term for all actions, including verbal communication, arising from the unconscious and serving to prevent unconscious material from reaching consciousness. For treatment providers of all types in all settings, this is a critical concept, as it offers one of the most important answers to a challenging question: Why do patients who wish to feel better fail to follow recommendations?

Freud underscored the importance of *subjective experience* in understanding why people act as they do. More specifically, he argued that our experiences in childhood lead us to view the world in an idiosyncratic manner. Freud insisted that if we wish to understand how an individual thinks, feels, and acts, we should focus less on the objective facts of the person's life and more on his or her particular history, beliefs, and perceptions. An important corollary of the primacy of early childhood experience states that the nature and quality of an individual's ego defenses are largely dependent on the details of interaction with caregivers early in life. Freud suggested that these all-important early interactions lead people to develop durable interpersonal templates with which they navigate their relationships. The idea that early interactions affect a person's defense structure and interpersonal perception is also a key concept in *object relations*, an important branch of psychodynamic theory that we will explore.

Freud suggested that our misperception of others based on early experience plays itself out in psychotherapy, as well. He used the term *transference* to describe the patient's failure to perceive the analyst clearly, and he came to view *analysis of the transference* and *analysis of resistance* as the cornerstones of psychoanalytic treatment. These techniques remain a central means to help psychodynamic psychotherapy patients obtain insight into their habitual defenses, providing an opportunity to learn to relate to those around them in a more fulfilling manner. Moreover, Freud suggested that the therapist also misperceives the patient based on the therapist's early experience. He called the latter phenomenon *countertransference*, and he warned that unmanaged countertransference might have grave implications for the patient.

On our psychodynamic tour we will repeatedly notice the tension between *one-person* and *two-person* psychology. Freud began his work with a view of the human psyche as a sort of machine that acts to decrease tensions. In effect, this is a one-person psychology. Later on, he and many others recognized that human beings are irreducibly social and that the really interesting psychology occurs *between* people rather than *within* a single person. This is two-person psychology.

Finally, as we review Freud's ideas and those of his followers, we will bump up against a range of answers to this question: What drives human development? The psychodynamic theorists we meet along the way readily agree that humans cope with uncomfortable thoughts and feelings by keeping them out of awareness through the use of various defenses, and they agree that an individual's predilection to use one defense rather than another depends to a great degree on early childhood experience. What these theorists disagree on is where the uncomfortable material comes from in the first place. Are we troubled by sexual impulses, by a sense of personal inferiority, by a failure to know ourselves, by an inability to experience ourselves subjectively, by anxiety, or by something else?

To help you keep the main psychodynamic theorists clearer in your head, we have depicted them all in Figure 2.1.

Freud's Life and the Origins of Psychodynamic Theory

Childhood and Family

Our tour of psychodynamic theory begins with a review of the events in Sigmund Freud's life that help to make sense of his theory. As we have suggested, the individual elements of psychodynamic theory frequently correspond directly to the individual theorist's life—which is not a surprise, in that the theoretical developments flowed largely from personal insights. In the case of Freud, much insight was achieved via his self-analysis and through his psychoanalytic practice. In this first section we illustrate the importance of subjective early experience, using Freud's life as our example, also locating within it the genesis of the many psychodynamic schisms of the twentieth century. In addition, we explore Freud's concept of the Oedipus complex and examine an application of psychoanalytic thought to a sociocultural phenomenon, religion. We end with an early reference to free association.

12 Psychological Theories and Psychotherapy

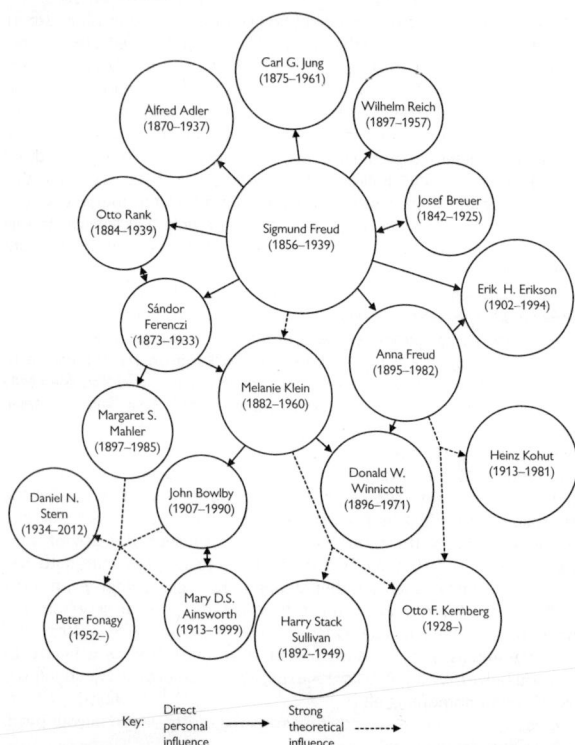

Figure 2.1. Schematic of major psychodynamic theorists mentioned in the text.

Freud was born in 1856 in the small Moravian town of Freiberg, now called Příbor, in the present-day Czech Republic. Although the local people in and around Freiberg spoke Czech, Freud was born into a German-speaking Jewish family. Reports from the time suggest that German-speaking Jewish families were always a bit the cultural outsiders, not only because of religion and occupations, but also because they identified with the German cultural elite rather than with the common local culture. They were reasonably well accepted by the Habsburg rulers in Vienna, at least in comparison to their treatment in previous centuries.

Freud's family situation was complicated. His father, Jakob Freud, was a wool merchant married to a woman 20 years his junior. The father had had two sons by an earlier marriage, and these sons were very close in age to Freud's mother. Indeed, the older of the two sons, Emanuel, had a son of his own, Johann, who was born in August 1855. Freud himself was born less than a year later.

As a very young child Freud played with his half-brother's son, Johann. Years later, in 1900, Freud wrote, "We lived together inseparably, loved each other, and at the same time . . . scuffled with and accused each other." As an adult, Freud maintained deeply ambivalent relationships with his colleagues, which set the stage for continuous conflict and ruptures among psychodynamic theorists and practitioners over the next century. In a continued reference to his early relationship with Johann, Freud wrote, "An intimate friend and a hated enemy have always been indispensable requirements for my emotional life; I have always been able to create them anew, and not infrequently my childish ideal has been so closely approached that friend and enemy coincided in the same person . . ."

Freud was the eldest of eight children of his mother and father. His next-younger sibling, Julius, was one and a half years his junior and died at the age of six months. Much later, in an 1897 letter to a friend Freud wrote, "I welcomed my one-year-younger brother . . . with ill wishes and real infantile jealousy, and his death left the germ of guilt in me." At about the time of Julius's death, a maternal uncle died, and these events plunged Freud's mother, again pregnant, into grief. As well, during this period the international economy slowed, and Jakob Freud's wool business began to fail. Ultimately, the entire Freud family left Freiberg. The older half-brothers emigrated to England, while young Sigmund, his siblings, and their parents relocated to Leipzig in 1859 and then moved again the following year, this time to Vienna. Freud's father never found full employment after that, and for a number of years the family lived in straitened circumstances. All this family trauma began when Freud was just two years old. And, soon enough, things became even more complicated.

Freud's surviving siblings included five sisters and a brother, who was born ten years after Freud. The children's mother doted on her first-born, to whom she referred as "my golden son" (Gay, 2006). She believed her son was destined to become a great man, at least in part because she subscribed to the folk belief that children were bound to accomplish much in life if they happened to be born with a portion of the birth membrane still on their head, as happened in Freud's case. Freud's mother certainly favored him over the other children, and from early on Freud exhibited notable ambition and even expressed his intention and expectation of becoming famous.

Years later, Freud's depression following the illness and death of his father in 1896 led him to conduct an experimental self-analysis. Through it he arrived at the insight that as a child he had wished to have his mother for himself, which would necessarily have meant getting rid of his father. For reasons we will subsequently address, Freud viewed this in sexual terms. He worked out what he referred to as the *Oedipus complex*, according to which a boy of three or four desires his mother sexually but fears castration by his father. The boy ultimately abandons his desire for his mother and comes to identify with the feared aggressor, his father, and in the process introjects his father's values. Freud later attempted to apply similar logic to female development but struggled with the details. Today the Oedipus complex is understood to encompass the complicated and conflicted feelings experienced by a child of three or four as he or she experiences rivalry with one parent while simultaneously experiencing erotic longing for the other. Freud concluded that his particular childhood experience of jealousy for his mother's affection was a universal phenomenon, and he insisted that the Oedipus complex be viewed as a cornerstone of psychoanalysis.

Freud's relationship with his father was difficult in another way, and this had to do with the issue of their shared Jewishness. It is reported that Freud was occasionally discriminated against due to his religion and culture. For example, he decided to study medicine because he expected that he would face less prejudice as a physician than in other fields. As well, in his last years in Vienna he risked imprisonment or worse because of his ethnicity, particularly after Austria was annexed into Germany following a *coup d'état* in March 1938. He eventually emigrated and, as we discuss a bit later in the text, spent the last 15 months of his life in London. His four sisters remained in Vienna, and they died in concentration camps during World War II.

For most of his life, however, Freud was little inconvenienced by being Jewish, and he always identified as an atheist. In the second half of the nineteenth century, it is known that many of the Jewish faith were turning away from religion, as the scientific worldview became more fashionable and some individuals decided to assimilate into the larger culture. In addition to the effect of the cultural trend and his own experience, Freud's views regarding religion were influenced by the example of his father. Jakob Freud's father and grandfather had been Hassidic rabbis, and both he and Freud's mother were *Ostjuden* ("Eastern Jews"), a group that was widely viewed as unsophisticated, superstitious, and little motivated to join the modern world. During much of his adulthood Jakob Freud was not interested in religion and was not at all pious or mystical, in sharp distinction to most Hassidic Jews. Later in life, however, he resumed reading the Torah every day.

Around the age of ten Freud was distressed to learn of an incident some years earlier in Freiberg, when his father was forced off the sidewalk by an anti-Semite who also knocked Jakob's hat into the mud. When Freud asked his father what happened next, Jakob replied that he had simply picked up his hat and walked away. One of Freud's biographers has suggested that Freud was devastated to learn that his father had behaved in what he viewed as a cowardly manner, and it further contributed to negative feelings about the older man and about Judaism generally (Gay, 2006).

Over the course of his life Freud recognized and accepted his Jewish cultural heritage, although early on he Germanized his Jewish name, such that Sigismund Schlomo became simply Sigmund. When it came time to name his own children, Freud gave none of them a typically Jewish name. Later in life he developed a lively interest in reinterpreting religion as an intrapsychic phenomenon. He believed one might understand religion as a defense against guilt over patricidal impulses. We worship an all-powerful but invisible "father figure" in order to atone for our wish to kill our actual father and also to reassure ourselves about facing life without the protection of a father. Indeed, Freud viewed the concept of "original sin" as mankind's collective guilt over patricidal impulses. Right at the end of his life Freud trained his sights on Judaism in particular, arguing that Moses was not Jewish but was an Egyptian prince who adapted a monotheistic Egyptian cult for

Jewish use. Of course, such an account of the genesis of Judaism destroys the revered foundational myth of Jewish history and might be viewed as a deeply antagonistic reaction to the piety of Freud's father in late life.

As a youngster Freud was rather interested in writing, and there is no doubt that as an adult he was possessed of consummate writing skills. At the age of 14 he was given a copy of a short essay by the German Jewish writer Ludwig Börne, published in 1840 and entitled *The Art of Becoming an Original Writer in Three Days*. In it Börne suggested that one "take a few sheets of paper and for three days in a row, without guile or hypocrisy, write down everything that goes through your head." He averred, "At the end of the three days you will be beside yourself with astonishment at the new and surprising thoughts you have had." Later in life Freud pioneered the technique of *free association*, according to which the patient is to tell the therapist whatever thoughts come up in the therapy session, without engaging in any censoring. It seems likely that the germ of this idea was planted when Freud read Börne's essay.

Medical Training and Early Career

In this section we discuss Freud's experiences during late adolescence and his twenties, when he completed his formal medical education, as a part of which he acquired certain ideas about the functioning of the central nervous system. He came in contact with an important early colleague, Josef Breuer, from whom he learned of the case of Anna O., and he became more knowledgeable about hypnosis during two trips to France, which set the stage for the later development of his ideas about the unconscious.

At the age of 17 Freud enrolled at the University of Vienna, and eight years later he completed his medical training, having also spent a year in the armed forces during this time. He continued to do basic research at the Vienna Institute of Physiology for a year after graduating from medical school and then embarked on what amounted to a three-year residency in neurology at the Vienna General Hospital, completing this in 1885. At the physiology lab Freud's supervisor convinced him that that the nervous system did not spontaneously produce any central activity but was essentially reactive. Freud came to believe that the central nervous system acted in such a way as to keep incoming stimuli to a minimum and that it remained at rest until stimulated by outside energies. Thus, he viewed the human central nervous system as a separate entity that acted only so as to decrease external input. From this reductionist perspective, he did not accept as first principle the idea that human beings strive toward goals. His later development of the theory of psychoanalysis relies heavily on such a non-teleological view of human behavior and is evident, for example, in his idea that religion is best understood as a reaction against the naturally occurring impulse to kill one's father.

During his residency at Vienna General Hospital in the early 1880s Freud completed some of the earliest studies on cocaine and for a few years was an enthusiastic supporter of the use of this drug. He suffered a career disappointment when a colleague received the scientific credit for demonstrating the anesthetic properties of cocaine. Moreover, before long it became evident that cocaine was highly addictive and had other serious side effects, particularly when injected. This proved to be something of a public embarrassment for Freud within the local medical community, given his enthusiasm. It is likely that this incident did not improve the reception of local physicians some years later when Freud came up with his next "revolutionary" idea, that of psychoanalysis.

During residency Freud became friendly with a somewhat older neurologist by the name of Josef Breuer (1842–1925), who told him of his patient "Anna O." One of only two surviving children, Anna O. had an older brother who was greatly valued by their parents. Anna O. herself was very bright but was never given more than a lady's education. When her father fell ill in 1880, Anna O., then 21 years old, had to look after him at night. She soon became unable to do so, because she developed contractures, loss of sensation in various parts of the body, visual disturbances, difficulty eating, and a distressing nervous cough. By November of that year she was taken to see Breuer, who began treating her for hysteria, a condition corresponding to more modern ideas of a conversion disorder. When her father died in April 1881, Anna O.'s symptoms became even more severe and now included difficulties with her speech, communication in alternating European languages, and two distinct personalities.

Breuer treated Anna O. daily, and very early in treatment the procedure involved having Anna O. talk about her life and symptoms while in a state of self-induced hypnosis. This capacity was familiar to Anna O., who had a longstanding habit of intense daydreaming, including spending time in her "private theater." Together, Breuer and Anna O. discovered that this process relieved her symptoms. It was Anna O. herself who described this cathartic approach as "the talking cure." Later on, Breuer hypnotized Anna O., with a similar symptom-relieving result, leading to the discovery that insight could be gained in this way about the origin of each symptom.

The story of Anna O. is important for several reasons. It demonstrated for Freud that mind and body are not separate. It demonstrated the power of hypnosis to afford relief but also illustrated the value of talking about symptoms and their origins as a means to resolve them. It pointed to a sexual component in the etiology of hysteria, a concept that Freud embraced more readily than Breuer. The origin of the word "hysteria" suggests its early association with women, as evidenced by the word's Greek origin, *hystera* ("uterus").

The differences between Freud and Breuer regarding this case were a factor in the falling out between the two shortly after they published *Studies on Hysteria* together in 1895. This was the first of many ruptures between Freud and his collaborators. At least in Freud's mind, this conflict replicated the pattern of his early relationship with Johann, the son of his half-brother.

Another very important point can be made here. The case history, as written by Breuer and published in *Studies on Hysteria,* is controversial because some of the details are known to be inconsistent with historically verifiable events, in particular the ultimate conclusion of the case. Throughout all of psychodynamic theory and most other psychological theories there are many case histories about patients in which the details have been altered in such a way as to make the stories more applicable to the theory and the inferences less ambiguous. It is important to understand that "teaching tales" of this sort are delivered within a particular context. The altering of details should not to be understood as frank mendacity but rather as an accepted way of presenting and illustrating theory. It is important to remember, when reading historical cases with colorfully embellished material, that this type of teaching tale was a culturally understood way of making a point in that time and place in history. The details of actual patients' lives are usually less perfectly consistent with theory.

Based in part on his discussions with Breuer, Freud undertook two trips to France to study hypnosis in the second half of the 1880s. At the end of his residency in 1885 Freud spent five months at La Salpêtrière Hospital in Paris, studying under the French neurologist Jean-Martin Charcot (1825-1893), who believed that hysteria was a legitimate central nervous system disease and not simple malingering. Like Breuer, Charcot believed that hysteria was inevitably related to sexual matters. Charcot was quite a famous man at that time—and rightly so. By inducing and removing paralysis through hypnosis, he was able to demonstrate more conclusively than anyone had done before that one's mind can influence the functioning of one's body.

Four years later Freud returned to France, this time to study hypnosis for three weeks in the city of Nancy. While there he observed French neurologist Hippolyte Bernheim (1840–1919) induce posthypnotic amnesia in a female patient. He was particularly struck that this woman was able to recall the forgotten incident when Bernheim firmly insisted that she do so. In another demonstration, Bernheim instructed a woman who had been hypnotized that when a certain number of minutes had passed after she awakened from the trance, she was to go to the corner of the room and open an umbrella she found there. When the woman subsequently opened the umbrella as instructed, Bernheim asked her why she had done so, to which she replied that she wished to determine if the umbrella were hers. From these demonstrations, Freud came away with two useful observations. First, he learned that memories can be repressed and then later recalled with effort. Second, he came to understand that people might act because of motivations of which they were unaware and subsequently offer incorrect explanations for their behavior.

Private Practice in Vienna

In 1886 Freud, now 30 years old, opened a private neurological practice with an initial specialty in treating hysteria, in the expectation that such a business model would afford him sufficient income to marry. Indeed, several months later he married his long-time sweetheart, Martha Bernays (1861–1951), a woman from Hamburg. The Freuds went on to have three sons and three daughters, of whom the youngest was Anna Freud, born in 1895. During the decade after his marriage, Freud continued to refine his ideas about the unconscious, and the idea of "working through" began to crystallize in his mind. In addition, his private practice patients afforded him an opportunity to experiment with the technique of free association.

In the late nineteenth century many educated people believed that an unconscious mind must exist, because manifestly rational people sometimes behaved in an unusual or self-defeating manner. By this point in his life Freud fully subscribed to the idea that people with mental problems might benefit from an investigation of their unconscious mind. Moreover, Freud now believed he had found a way to plumb the unconscious mind, based on his experiences with Breuer and while learning hypnosis in France. In time, Freud would have a great deal to say about the structure and function of the human unconscious.

Among Freud's early patients in his neurological practice were the pseudonymous Emmy von N. and Elisabeth von R. The first patient, Emmy von N., was a 40-year-old widow who presented with mild delirium, anxiety, various pains, and a speech disturbance. Freud treated her in 1889 and again the following year. Under hypnosis, he was able to address each of Emmy von N.'s symptoms, but the results were transitory, and a return of symptoms followed the end of treatment.

In the two years before the second patient, Elisabeth von R., began seeing Freud in the fall of 1892, she had suffered with leg pains and consequent difficulty standing and walking. Freud asked her to lie on a couch with her eyes closed. Instead of addressing her symptoms under hypnosis, he held his hand on her forehead and asked her to concentrate on the origin of each of her symptoms. Freud had learned from Anna O. the need to address psychological material repeatedly and in depth. He later wrote that this technique, which he called *working through*, permitted the therapist gradually to overcome the patient's resistance. For now, however, he simply understood that he needed to ask his patient questions, but Elisabeth von R. complained that he was asking too many questions and interrupting her train of thought. At another point she commented that she hadn't reported all her thoughts, explaining, "I didn't think it was what you wanted."

These events—and Freud's recall of Börne's essay on how to become an original writer in three days—appear to have contributed to the development of the free association technique. In time Freud concluded that hypnosis did not result in a lasting cure of hysteria, and he abandoned this treatment modality altogether.

The technique of *free association* is still applied in formal psychoanalysis and is relevant in other psychodynamic techniques, where free-flowing thought and spontaneity of speech deliver similarly useful material. In 1916–7 Freud described free association as follows: "We instruct the patient to put himself into a state of quiet, unreflecting self-observation, and to report to us whatever internal observations he is able to make." The patient is further exhorted not to "exclude any [observation], whether on the ground that it is too disagreeable or too indiscreet to say, or that it is too unimportant or irrelevant, or that it is nonsensical and need not be said."

Freud continued to work on making sense of the relationship between the symptoms of hysteria and sexual matters. For a short time he came to believe that his young female patients with hysteria had actually been sexually victimized. In 1896 he presented a paper at the local medical society in which he proposed the *sexual seduction hypothesis*. In the paper he described a series of 18 cases of hysteria, in which all patients reported having been sexually abused. The paper was not well received, and one and a half years later Freud modified his position, suggesting that these "seductions" were mostly imaginary and reflected the activity of the unconscious. He asserted that the normal early childhood sexual impulses of these female patients had led them at an unconscious level to respond as if they had actually been sexually abused, and they developed conversion symptoms because of that.

Although he backed away from his original hypothesis, even as doubts accrued, Freud never denied that some cases of hysteria stem from actual sexual abuse. Freud also never backed away from his belief in the sexual etiology of psychoneuroses, his term for mental conditions originating in childhood and caused by conflict or trauma. In any event, for the rest of his life Freud believed that the way a young child copes with sexual instincts was the prime mover in the development of personality, not only in cases of hysteria but in all human beings, including both those with and without psychopathology.

It was in the same year, 1896, that Freud's father, Jakob, became ill and died a few months later. Freud knew, of course, that his father would die, and he was surprised about how depressed he felt about this. He therefore set about to analyze himself, chiefly by dissecting his own dreams. From these he concluded that he felt guilty over a repressed wish that his father would die, and he went on to work out the importance of his Oedipal strivings. Freud was very excited to have discovered the "secret" of dreams, and he went on to write *The Interpretation of Dreams*, the first major work he would publish on his own. Although it was released in late 1899, the book's publication date was 1900. With this book Freud began to receive limited recognition of his ideas from the medical community, even if *The Interpretation of Dreams* sold only 600 copies in the first eight years after its publication.

At about this time Freud was also obsessively at work on a document posthumously published and dubbed "The Project" (Freud, 1895/1953). A neurologist by training, Freud hoped to develop a "psychology for neurologists." He quickly abandoned this idea—finding it untenable and utterly unworkable. Nevertheless, he used his knowledge of neurological structure as a basis for his psychological models, a fact reflected in some of the terminology he chose. Later in his life, Freud made occasional reference to his continued belief that ultimately psychological description would be based on our knowledge of organic substructure. In the end, Freud's "project" reflects his original intention to substantiate the biological basis of psychology, a stance with which many psychiatrists strongly identify.

Freud's Understanding of the Psyche

Over the quarter century that followed the publication of *The Interpretation of Dreams*, Freud continued to write extensively, and he gradually fleshed out theories of personality development and psychic structure, which later commentators have organized as five theories: the topographic theory, dynamic theory, economic theory, genetic theory, and structural theory. These theories should not be viewed as competing with one another. Freud seldom contradicted his earlier views—although this did occur on several occasions, such as when, in 1897, he repudiated the sexual seduction hypothesis of 1896. Rather, the five groupings of psychodynamic theory should be understood as Freud's alternative approaches to the same body of knowledge. Among these theories, the most important is structural theory, the well-known Freudian conception of the psyche as consisting of id, ego, and superego. However, to understand the developments that led to structural theory, it is important to follow Freud's evolving thought through the other theories.

Topographic Theory. While *The Interpretation of Dreams* lays out Freud's understanding of the meaning of dreams, the real significance of this book is that it contains Freud's first enunciation of certain enduring tenets of his evolving theory, such as the Oedipus complex and the features of the psyche as consisting of unconscious, preconscious, and conscious systems. Within these descriptions Freud also reveals his first version of his theory of instincts, later known as libido or sexual theory.

Freud's understanding of the *unconscious* was much more sophisticated and complex than the way in which the term was generally understood by educated people at the time. He viewed the unconscious as a storehouse of unacceptable desires, memories, thoughts, and feelings, all pushed out of conscious awareness by the defense of *repression*. He believed that introspection was insufficient to permit people access to the mental phenomena contained in the unconscious, whereas the feelings, thoughts, and impulses contained in the *conscious* were immediately available to awareness. Freud invented a new term, the *preconscious*, to describe the hypothesized "area" of the psyche that lies between the conscious and the unconscious. Material in the preconscious is available to awareness through effort (e.g., "Where did I leave my keys?"). The preconscious functions as a censor and *represses* threatening material that bubbles up from the unconscious, essentially pushing the material back into the unconscious.

The conscious and preconscious function on the basis of *secondary process* thinking, which is characterized by delay of instinctual discharge, binding of mental energy in accordance with external reality, and avoidance of unpleasure. By contrast, the unconscious functions on the basis of *primary process* thinking, which is alogical, lacks negatives but permits contradictions, has no time sense, and utilizes displacement, condensation, and symbolization.

Freud suggested that the unconscious was always trying to resolve conflicts, as a consequence of which upsetting thoughts, feelings, or impulses (e.g., "I want to murder my parent") in the unconscious seek conscious awareness. In response to this, a censor in the preconscious performs its function to "protect" the conscious and generally prevents such forbidden material from accessing conscious awareness.

However, when the individual is dreaming, the preconscious censor becomes less efficient, and if the unconscious material is so confused or distorted as to make it very difficult to decipher, it may be admitted to conscious awareness. Freud believed that dreams are "the royal road to the unconscious," and the usefulness of dream analysis as a method of gaining access to unconscious material remains an essential tool in psychoanalytic treatment. Although current theory extends our understanding of dreams beyond Freud's relatively simple wish-fulfillment scheme, dreams could be argued to allow us a glimpse into primary process thinking.

With regard to dreams, Freud concluded that the unconscious relies largely on two obfuscatory strategies, condensation and displacement, to prevent conscious awareness of the true subject of the dream, a wish-fulfillment fantasy. *Condensation* occurs when an aspect of the dream has more than one meaning, such as when a character in the dream represents more than one important person in the individual's life, such as boss, parent, and spouse at the same time. *Displacement* occurs when a threatening concept is replaced by something less threatening, such as when intercourse is symbolized by climbing a stairway. Freud also asserted that the conscious works to make sense of the disorganized welter of images arising from the unconscious by stringing together symbols in a way that yields a coherent story. This is referred to as *secondary elaboration*.

Dynamic Theory. An alternate approach used by Freud to understand mental life examines the ways in which unconscious factors affect *all* conscious mental life and behavior, including important thoughts, feelings, and actions, as well as dreams, jokes, slips of the tongue, choice of job, choice of spouse, and so on. This is the notion of *psychic determinism*, that every thought or act is caused by prior mental events, many not accessible to conscious awareness. Having rejected the sexual seduction hypothesis, Freud concluded that all humans have sexual instinctual drives that are repressed. He further believed that these sexual instinctual drives are the prime movers in shaping human development. Repressed drives manifest themselves in obscure ways, including symptoms and fantasies, sometimes called *drive derivatives*.

Just as Freud believed that condensation permitted a single dream element to carry multiple meanings, so too did he believe that symptoms, psychic events, and behavior may have more than one cause and may serve more than one purpose—that is, they are multidetermined. Furthermore, the idea that all conscious mental life is affected by unconscious factors necessarily means that in each of our behaviors it is possible to detect primary process thinking, with all of its lack of logic, self-contradiction, timelessness, and primitive distortions.

Multidetermination (or *overdetermination*, to use Freud's original term) reflects the idea that all psychic phenomena arise as a convergence or compromise among multiple factors or causes. The concept is important because it reminds us of the fact that, in a psychodynamic sense, there is no simple cause for any symptom or experience. We must look deeper and expect that any heavily reinforced psychological theme will have multiple origins, arising from any source—biological, psychological, or environmental. Because the mind is exquisitely adept at recognizing patterns, any point of similarity, including similar affective experience, can cause two elements to become associated.

Economic Theory. This view of mental life, which is sometimes referred to as the *energy transfer* or *hydraulic* theory, begins with Freud's assertion that the amount of psychic energy within the mind varies depending on circumstances. Freud believed that an increase in central stimulation occurs when the body makes a demand on the psyche, which is the definition of an instinctual drive. He explained that instincts have four characteristics. They correspond to a body deficiency of some kind (e.g., nutritional deficit), they aim to eliminate the deficiency (e.g., by satiating hunger), they seek an object that will accomplish this (e.g., food), and their magnitude depends on the degree of the body deficiency (e.g., how long since one last ate). When an instinctual drive arises, it creates a hypothetical central stimulation. This increases psychic energy and is referred to as *unpleasure*, as is consistent with Freud's view that the central nervous system functions to minimize incoming stimulation. The discharge of such psychic energy is said to be consistent with the *pleasure principle*.

Freud further indicated that one could localize the psychic energy that arises from drives, in the sense that the energy is *cathected* to a mental representation of a person or thing, called an *object*. Incidentally, *cathexis* is an awkward translation of Freud's use of the German word *Besetzung*, which means occupation or possession, particularly in the military sense. If the immediate discharge of the psychic energy, as would be consistent with the pleasure principle, might lead to some prohibited action, such as sexual impropriety or inappropriate aggression, then *countercathexis* (*Gegenbesetzung* or counter-possession) may be utilized to move the psychic energy elsewhere, perhaps using simple repression or displacement. Both cathexis and countercathexis require the investment of energy, which in turn means that energy must be withdrawn from other parts of the central nervous system. Freud believed that the need to cope with our instinctual drives weighs us down, because we expend energy for the resulting cathexes and countercathexes.

In 1905 Freud published *Three Essays on the Theory of Sexuality*, in which he drew together his ideas about sex and hysteria, on one hand, and sex and dreams, on the other hand. In this work he introduced the idea of *libido*, which is the term he used to describe the energy associated with the life-directed instinct, which he named *eros*. Of course, Freud viewed libido as mostly sexual in nature. For many years Freud wrote extensively about how libido is cathected or countercathected, and it wasn't until about 1920 that he began to write about aggressive instincts, which later became known as the death instinct, or *thanatos*.

Thus, the economic theory undergirds the idea that any human activity, no matter how refined or creative, ultimately results from the psyche's attempt to deal with instinctual drives, of which we are often unconscious. In Freud's view, the fundamental psychic activity of human beings is to achieve a state of equilibrium. It is the direction and redirection of instinctual drives that gives rise to art, culture, and all other human accomplishments.

A case in point relates to the phenomenon of *transference*, according to which people perceive one another in part based on interpersonal templates that are established early in life. It is self-evident that we do not respond *de novo* to each person in our daily lives but instead rely on habits and expectations based on early experience: male authority figures are like *this*, young females are like *that*, agitated people are likely to do *this*, and so on. However, most of the time we really believe that we are responding in a veridical fashion to our interlocutors, and we don't recognize the role played by habits and expectations, of which we are at best dimly aware. In treatment, Freud believed that by paying attention to transference distortions one might gain very useful information, insofar as such distortions signal the presence of earlier problems in relationships, which in turn might shed light on all kinds of personality problems. Moreover, Freud believed that transference distortions often point to the development of particular ego defenses and thus symptoms of psychopathology, a point to which will return.

Genetic Theory. In *Three Essays on the Theory of Sexuality* Freud first presented a theory of psychosexual development, which represents the fourth of Freud's approaches to mental life. The genetic theory builds on the economic theory by investigating developmental shifts in the cathexis of libido during childhood. Freud believed that during the first 18 months of life libidinal tensions are centered about the mouth, lips, and tongue, and unpleasure is discharged by sucking, biting, and chewing. This is the *oral* phase of development. Cathexis then moves to the *anal* zone, and unpleasure is discharged first by expelling feces and then by retaining them. Around the age of three cathexis moves to the genitalia, giving rise to the *phallic* or *Oedipal* phase of development, which we have already discussed. Following this period comes the relatively quiescent *latency* period, and concerns about sexual matters do not resurface until the *genital* stage, in which adolescents, according to Freud, rebel against parents and become amorously involved with peers as a means to avoid awareness of incestuous wishes vis-à-vis their parents.

Freud suggested that a person might move fairly comfortably through one or more of these stages, or there might be *fixation* or *regression*. Fixation involves frank developmental arrest, while regression involves a tendency to return to an earlier stage when under stress. Freud believed that both fixation and regression result from substantial frustration or, less often, from excessive gratification during the developmental tasks required in a given stage. Freud also discussed characteristic patterns of behavior that accompany fixation and regression at each developmental stage, but we will defer discussion of these characterological implications until we speak about one of Freud's psychoanalytic disciples, Wilhelm Reich.

By this time Freud had worked out a remarkably sophisticated theory of mental life, in which he related adult character structure to early childhood development and to responsive interaction by caregivers at crucial developmental stages, all driven by the individual's attempts to cope with the sexual instinct. It was Freud's view that when caregivers fail to meet a young child's shifting developmental needs, the child is likely to develop psychological difficulties characteristic of the particular developmental period that has gone awry.

Structural Theory. This version of theory was first presented in Freud's 1920 work, *Beyond the Pleasure Principle.* According to this last of the five theories, the mind is understood not as three systems (unconscious, preconscious, conscious) but as three agents (id, ego, superego).

The id doesn't differ too much in concept from the unconscious, and it contains all the sexual and aggressive instinctual drives, as well as all of the wishes reflecting memories of earlier gratifications. The id cannot tolerate tension, and when it experiences unresolved drives, it demands immediate gratification. It may accomplish this by *reflex action*, which is an automatic physical response to tension, like sneezing. Alternately, the id may seek gratification through *wish fulfillment*, in which it conjures up an image or hallucination of something that would satisfy the drive state. For example, the id imagines a breast in response to hunger. Thus, reflex action and wish fulfillment are the means by which the id seeks to decrease tension, and they are collectively referred to as *primary processes*.

While the id may not differ much from the unconscious, the ego is *not* equivalent to the conscious. In fact, the ego has both a conscious and an unconscious component. The ego includes all the mental elements that regulate the interaction between the id's instinctual drives and the demands of both the superego and the external world. The ego utilizes the *reality principle*, according to which it attempts to reduce tension in a manner that is as adaptive as possible to external reality. More emphasis is placed on the attainment of pleasure in the future than at present. If the id's operations reflect undirected passions, the ego's operations largely reflect good sense. Early on Freud believed that the ego was a small appendage of the id. Gradually, he began to view it as larger and more important. It was only at the end of Freud's life that he acknowledged the existence of more than a rudimentary ego at birth, having previously believed that the ego developed only as a consequence of the effect of the external world on the id's drives.

In an attempt to control and regulate the unacceptable material projected into it by the id, the ego makes use of various defense mechanisms. Freud described a number of such defense mechanisms, and more were subsequently worked out by other ego psychologists, particularly Freud's daughter, Anna. We will defer a description of the ego defenses until later on, focusing for now on only one, the fundamental defense mechanism described in some detail by Freud: *repression*. This involves preventing conscious awareness of threatening thoughts and feelings by either keeping them confined to the unconscious or by moving them from the conscious to the unconscious.

According to Freud, repression of dangerous impulses and painful memories occurs over the entire course of life. Of course, much of the material about which one is not currently conscious has not been repressed. For example, telephone numbers and appointment times are simply in the preconscious and are available to consciousness through effortful introspection. Freud believed that repressed material usually continues to have an effect on the conscious, in that such material might appear in distorted form, such as in dreams, anxiety, or other symptoms.

Freud believed that psychoanalytic patients require an adequately functioning *observing ego* in order to participate in treatment. He believed that most individuals are capable of observing their own psychological processes and can build an alliance with the therapist for this purpose, but he raised the question of whether a sufficiently strong observing ego is to be found in individuals with very severe personality disorders, psychoses, and other major disturbances. Thus, psychoanalysis and other forms of psychotherapeutic treatment often set as one goal of treatment the development of an observing ego.

Even when there is an adequate observing ego, one is still faced with an implicit contradiction. If in treatment one wishes to help the ego deal more effectively with id impulses, the observing ego must permit at least some conscious awareness of both the ego's defenses and the material against which it is defending itself. In other words, the ego has to permit awareness of that which it finds threatening. This is why *resistance* occurs in treatment. The ego is both invested in decreasing distress and, at the same time, fearful of taking the steps necessary to accomplish this, and progress therefore is slow. It is for this reason that *working through* is such an important aspect of treatment. Freud encouraged the therapist to focus on "whatever is present for the time being on the surface of the patient's mind," although work in depth is also required. The ego needs a relatively long time to drop its guard against material that it fears, and it will not permit the therapist to rush the process. Indeed, if the therapist pushes too hard, the resistance will become overwhelming and the patient may either flee treatment or, worse yet, decompensate.

The final agent in the structural theory is the superego, which is partly conscious and partly unconscious. The superego, which tends to be absolutistic and unforgiving, is thought to arise in connection with the resolution of the Oedipus complex, when the child takes on parental values and internalizes the risk of parental punishment. Although many psychoanalytic theorists and other commentators equate the superego with the conscience, in the *New Introductory Lectures* of 1933 Freud rejected the confusing idea that this structural agent is equivalent to one of its functions. The functions of the superego, according to Freud, are self-observation, conscience, and maintenance of the ego ideal.

Of note, the ego ideal is not a function of the superego but rather a counterpart function that is associated with the superego. Ultimately, in 1933 Freud declared that the ego ideal was contained within the superego. In the same 1933 paper, Freud described the ego ideal as "the precipitate of the old picture of the parents, the expression of admiration for the perfection which the child then attributed to them." Failure to meet the demands of the ego ideal produces the feeling of shame, in contrast to the feeling of guilt produced by failure to meet the demands of the superego.

Freud's Understanding of Psychopathology

In general, Freud viewed psychopathology as evidence that the ego has failed to mediate successfully among id impulses, superego demands, and the demands of external reality. In other words, he viewed each symptom as a defense against an unbearable experience. This might happen in three ways: an id impulse is opposed by the ego's awareness of reality contingencies (e.g., the fear of being fired if one yells at one's boss), or there may be conflict among psychic agents (e.g., the fear that speaking up for oneself will make one feel like a whiner), or the ego may defend against a dangerous, instinctually based wish (e.g., the impulse to pursue a potential sex partner who reminds one of a parent). Similarly, Freud believed that anxiety might come from three sources. He believed that external or "real" anxiety results from external danger, while neurotic anxiety reflects conflict between the id and the ego, and moral anxiety reflects conflict between the ego and the superego. Freud ultimately came to believe that anxiety was in effect a danger signal, leading the ego to mobilize its defenses against unpleasant consequences of some kind. He pointed out that people often view anxiety as external, but not infrequently such anxiety is due to internal conflict. For example, Freud viewed phobias as a reflection of conflict between ego and superego or—more commonly—between ego and id.

Psychosis was not well understood by Freud. This is not surprising since his theory encompasses an understanding of normal human development and psychoneurosis, his term for mental disorders arising in childhood from intrapsychic conflict, such as trauma or an inadequately resolved Oedipus complex. In short, there is not much in his theory that allows for a useful psychological understanding of psychotic thought processes.

Freud's Ideas About Psychoanalytic Treatment

Freud thought of psychoanalysis as a theory of personality, as a method of inquiry, and as a type of psychological treatment. He was quite direct in stating that he was less interested in psychoanalysis as a treatment technique than in the value of psychoanalysis as a method of inquiry leading in turn to a theory of personality. Nonetheless, he did offer a number of observations about treatment. In 1922 Freud wrote the following:

> The assumption that there are unconscious mental processes, the recognition of the theory of resistance and repression, the appreciation of the importance of sexuality and of the Oedipus complex—these constitute the principal subject matter of psychoanalysis and the foundations of its theory. No-one who cannot accept them all should count himself as a psychoanalyst.

Nine years earlier he had compared psychoanalysis to a chess game, and he wrote:

> Anyone who hopes to learn the noble game of chess from books will soon discover that only the openings and end-games admit of an exhaustive systematic presentation and that the infinite variety of moves which develop after the opening defy any such description.

In general, the goals of psychoanalysis include making the unconscious conscious, working through transference and resistance, and improving the functioning of ego, as a consequence of which, according to Freud (1933), "Where id was, there shall ego be." Of course, treatment requires that the patient have an *observing ego* that is sufficiently strong to be able to establish an alliance with the therapist. After a working relationship is established, patient and therapist focus primarily on the transference, because exploration of the associated distortions permits a better understanding of the patient's *defense structure*. With this greater understanding, the patient may be willing to try responding to formerly threatening unconscious impulses in a new way. Later commentators have pointed out that *analysis of the transference* also provides the patient an opportunity to learn to resolve differences in relationships, and they have noted that exploration of the transference has a particular advantage over discussion of the patient's relationships outside of therapy, in that the data are directly available and are not filtered through any misperceptions on the patient's part.

Freud urged that patient and therapist repeatedly *work through* whatever material comes up in the session, so that *resistance* gradually wears away. Finally, Freud warned that just as patients distort their perception of therapists based on early learning, so also do therapists distort their perception of patients based on early learning, a phenomenon he called *countertransference*. The therapist must utilize knowledge about the self to ensure that he or she doesn't misperceive the patient and thus proceed in treatment in a way that is based less on the patient than on the idiosyncrasies of the analyst's background. This self-knowledge is often most efficiently developed during a *training analysis* for individuals who are completing formal psychoanalytic education. Alternatively, such knowledge can come from psychotherapy that forms a part of a therapist's education or from case supervision.

Freud's Old Age

In this final portion of our thematic biography, we learn about the psychoanalytic diaspora and refer one last time to Freud's ideas about religion.

It was in 1923 when, at the age of 67, Freud was diagnosed with cancer of the palate. This was hardly a surprise, in view of his habit of smoking as many as 20 cigars per day throughout much of his adult life. Over the next 16 years Freud endured 33 surgical procedures. He had to wear a series of painful dental prostheses, and early on he secured a promise from his personal physician, Dr. Max Schur, to the effect that when he could no longer carry on, Dr. Schur would make available to him the means to end his life.

However, Freud did carry on. He continued to see patients and to publish extensively, and as his fame grew, he gained increasing acceptance from the medical establishment. In 1930 he was awarded the Goethe Prize for literature, the premier prize of its kind in German-speaking countries. To accept the prize he traveled to Frankfurt am Main, in Germany, but here his presence was protested by anti-Semitic organizations, whose members decried the receipt of this coveted prize by a Jewish scientist.

In January 1933 the National Socialists came to power in Germany, and four months later the first book burning took place in Berlin. One of the Nazis present at the book burning is reported to have shouted, "Against the soul-destroying overestimation of the sex life and on behalf of the nobility of the human soul I offer to the flames the writings of Sigmund Freud!" Upon learning of the incident, Freud deadpanned, "What progress we are making! In the Middle Ages they would have burned me; nowadays they are content with burning my books" (Jones, 1953).

Like many older Jews who minimized the significance of the Nazis' anti-Semitic rhetoric, Freud repeatedly delayed his flight from Central Europe. Hundreds of thousands of younger Jewish scientists, artists, and ordinary people left Central Europe during the mid-1930s, and many found refuge in English-speaking countries. In fact, this pattern of emigration had a profound influence on the history of psychoanalysis in the postwar years. But in the mid-1930s Freud was entering his ninth decade, and he felt unable to leave Vienna. He wrote to a friend, "Where should I go in my state of dependence and physical helplessness?" (Freud, 1970).

Freud's calculation began to change when in March 1938 the Germans marched into Vienna and officials of the new government began directly harassing the Freuds. After Freud's daughter Anna was picked up by the Gestapo for questioning and then subsequently released, Freud finally agreed to accept the assistance of his biographer, Ernest Jones, to find suitable arrangements in London. In June 1938 he left Vienna for London in the company of his wife, her sister, their daughter, and his personal physician, Dr. Schur. Jones took great pains to provide an appropriate setting for Freud in London, who continued to see patients, meeting with them in a consulting room that was designed as a replica of the one he left behind in Vienna.

Freud's final work, *Moses and Monotheism*, was published simultaneously in German and English in the summer of 1939. In it he took aim at the foundational story of Judaism, as we have previously described. In late September 1939, three weeks after the outbreak of World War II, Freud let Dr. Schur know that the time had come for him to die. Dr. Schur therefore administered increasing doses of morphine, and death followed within 24 hours.

The Vienna Psychoanalytic Society

We turn now to the theories of Freud's first acolytes, and we look in on some of the earliest disputes within psychoanalysis. In particular, we explore the logical consequences of building psychological theories that don't rely on sexual impulses as a foundational principle, and we learn of several attempts to make psychoanalysis briefer and more accessible. Perhaps most importantly, we learn about an early case in which erotic transference and countertransference went spectacularly wrong. A fundamental understanding that erotic transference is both real and common is extremely important for persons learning about psychotherapy. This story, featuring Carl Jung, is especially not to be missed.

In 1902 Freud began meeting with colleagues in his apartment after dinner on Wednesday evenings "to discuss interesting topics in psychology and neuropathology," as he wrote to an early invitee. By 1908 these meetings had developed into the Vienna Psychoanalytic Society and included such early luminaries as Alfred Adler, Carl Jung, Sándor Ferenczi, Otto Rank, and Ernest Jones, among others. Almost all of the early members eventually broke with Freud, and the tenor of the meetings was often rancorous. As we have noted, Freud had difficulty maintaining long-term collaboration with colleagues, particularly since he generally insisted that others subscribe unquestioningly to certain tenets of his theory, most importantly his theory of instincts, also known as libido or sexual theory. Unfortunately, this combination of rigid authoritarianism and a willingness to break ties continued to plague psychoanalysis for many years after Freud's death.

Here are some comments about four of the early members of the Vienna Psychoanalytic Society.

Alfred Adler (1870–1937)

The man who would become the first president of the Vienna Psychoanalytic Society grew up in a poor suburb of Vienna. Adler was the third of six children in a family of Hungarian Jews, a small child who suffered from rickets. Early on, Adler performed poorly in school, but by his teens he was earning better grades, and at the age of 18 he enrolled in the medical school at the University of Vienna. Upon graduating in 1895, he initially practiced as an ophthalmologist, but he soon transferred to general medicine. However, after several patients died of diabetes, he switched again, this time taking up psychiatry. Adler acquired a copy of *The Interpretation of Dreams* the year that it was published, and he wrote an article in its defense, which led to a meeting with Freud in 1902. The relationship between Freud and Adler lasted until 1911, having ended after Adler wrote a paper called *A critical review of the Freudian sexual theory of psychic life*.

Adler's convictions were very different from those of Freud, and the two men didn't actually have much in common. For example, Adler doubted that sexual factors played much of a role in development, believing instead that the fundamental organizing principle in human development was the wish to achieve superiority. In this connection, Adler reinterpreted the Oedipus complex as an attempt to assert power within the family. Adler paid little attention to repression and was not interested in the unconscious. He believed that human development was not much affected by instincts or drives but instead by the necessity to resolve cultural challenges. Thus,

Adler rejected every one of Freud's 1922 requirements for psychoanalysis. To the end of his life Freud remained unhappy about what he viewed as the apostasy of his first disciple. He said, "I have made a pygmy great" (Wittels, 1924).

Somewhat in contrast to Freud, Adler was greatly interested in issues of social welfare. He married a fiery Russian intellectual who had strong revolutionary convictions, and she later introduced him, with tragic consequences, to Leon Trotsky. This Russian revolutionary, whose real name was Lev Bronstein, had escaped en route to Siberian exile and was living with his family in Vienna during the years leading up to World War I. For quite a long time the Adlers and Bronsteins socialized together with their young families on Sunday afternoons in a Viennese park. It was during this period that Trotsky began publishing *Pravda*, and he also became interested in psychoanalysis, having subsequently championed this treatment technique in the newly formed USSR.

Years later, Adler's daughter, who was a committed Communist, decided to move with her husband to the USSR. However, Trotsky had since fallen out of favor, and Valentine Adler was ultimately arrested as a Trotskyite. Part of the evidence presented against her at trial referred to her social contacts with the Bronsteins from the time that she was ten years old. In the end, Adler's daughter was convicted and sent to a Soviet prison camp, where she died in 1942.

Given Adler's lifelong interest in issues of social justice and social welfare, one is not surprised to find a strong undercurrent of social utopianism in his theory. Indeed, when the Social Democrats came to power in Austria after the end of World War I, Adler consulted with them in attempts to improve the national educational system.

Adler's theory is referred to as Individual Psychology. His fundamental idea was that one's personality is shaped by an awareness of inadequacy. He began, in 1907, by focusing on *organ inferiority*, suggesting that humans naturally strive to compensate for their physical limitations by relying on strengths (Napoleon minimized the disadvantage of his height by cultivating his military skills) or by working hard to overcome weaknesses (Demosthenes overcame his stutter through practice speaking with pebbles in his mouth). By 1910, however, Adler suggested that it was not actual organ inferiority but, rather, our subjective *feelings of inferiority* that motivate us to seek aggression and power. Adler pointed out that human infants are weak and vulnerable, and he suggested that there is an innate drive to overcome this state. Still later, Adler suggested that people do not seek power or aggression but are innately programmed to seek superiority or perfection, and he viewed this *striving for superiority* as the fundamental fact of life. Finally, he revised his position again, adopting the view that people strive not so much for personal superiority as for a superior or perfect society.

Starting from the assumption that people strive to overcome inadequacy, Adler worked out a fairly sophisticated theory of personality. He developed ideas that are in some ways similar to Freudian concepts of character and specific defenses, but his theory embraces a teleological view of personality development (striving for superiority).

Adler adapted the German notion of *Weltanschauung*, or *worldview*, arguing that our early experiences cause us to adopt a certain view of the world. The child's worldview leads to the development of particular cognitive structures or goals, which Adler referred to as *fictional finalisms*, and these in turn lead to a specific *style of life*. Based on one's worldview one might develop any one of a number of fictional finalisms. For example, Person A might have the belief, "I should help other people," while Person B concludes, "You have to grab what you can get," and Person C decides, "Our only reward is in Heaven." Each fictional finalism leads to the choice of a particular *style of life*. Using our examples, Person A might become a social worker who volunteers frequently at food banks when not working, while Person B becomes an aggressive businessperson who later goes into politics, and Person C enters a religious community at a young age.

Note here the stark contrast to Freud. Adler believed it is one's goal in life, based on early childhood disappointments, that determines personality, rather than an attempt to bring about a ceasefire among psychic agencies at war over proscribed sexual impulses. Adler suggested that people are free to act on early influences and to combine them as they see fit. He argued that no two people are ever the same, even if the ingredients of their personalities are similar (Olson & Hergenhahn, 2011). Adler referred to this as the *creative self*.

Consistent with his political and philosophical beliefs, Adler argued that for one's style of life to be *effective*, it should be consistent with *social interest*, described as a desire to live in harmony and friendship with others. If one's style of life lacks social interest, it is considered *mistaken*. In contrast to the *socially useful* type of personality, Adler spoke about the *ruling-dominant* type, the *getting-leaning* type, and the *avoidant* type. He suggested that a mistaken style of life resulted from poor adjustment to physical inferiority or from a failure to develop social interest, the latter resulting from inadequate parenting. Adler was particularly interested in the effect of birth order, as he believed that one's position within the family affects one's sense of adequacy and view of the world. He placed particular emphasis on the mother–child relationship, which he insisted must be cooperative and not reflect primarily *authoritarian*, *neglectful*, or *pampering/spoiling* elements. He was direct in suggesting that parental spoiling behavior led to the development of the Oedipus complex, and he generally implied that Freud himself must have been pampered as a child.

Adler was a practical man who was particularly interested in developing short-term treatment methods. He experimented with group psychotherapy and utilized techniques in individual therapy that would now be thought of as cognitive and/or behavioral. He tried to make psychotherapy available to working-class people, and he openly acknowledged that their health and stability were affected by the social and economic milieu.

Carl G. Jung (1875–1961)

The elder of two surviving children of an unhappy couple, a minister and his wife, Jung was born in a small Swiss village along Lake Constance. Jung's father apparently found little solace in his religious beliefs, while Jung's mother was an irascible, powerful, sometimes psychiatrically ill woman, whose presentation was so variable from day to day that Jung began to think that she was really two persons in one body. In the same way that Jung saw his mother as two people, as a youngster Jung also viewed himself as two people—a schoolboy and a wise old man.

As a youngster, Jung was withdrawn and socially awkward. At the age of 11 he enrolled in an academic high school in Basel, about 100 miles from his home. Upon graduation from high school in 1895, he enrolled at the University of Basel, where he studied medicine. Throughout his childhood and adult life, Jung had experiences that he interpreted as occult phenomena. In fact, he wrote his dissertation on his view of the psychology and pathology of such phenomena. After gaining his medical degree in 1900, Jung entered the psychiatric residency program at the well-respected Burghölzli Hospital, the psychiatric facility associated with the University of Zurich. Several years into his residency, Jung married the daughter of a wealthy industrialist, and the couple went on to have five children.

At the Burghölzli, Jung trained under the supervision of Eugen Bleuler, a psychiatrist remembered for his seminal contributions to the diagnostic classification of mental disorders and for coining the terms schizophrenia and autism, among others. Bleuler and Jung had become interested in the work of Freud, and, as a consequence, Jung and a colleague undertook an experimental investigation of Freud's ideas about free association by conducting word association tests. They were in fact able to demonstrate a correlation between word associations and skin galvanometric responses. Of note, Bleuler subsequently collaborated more extensively with Freud but broke with him in 1911 over theoretical differences. These included concerns about what Bleuler viewed as excessive emphasis on sexuality, as well as his concern that the psychoanalytic movement was becoming something akin to a power-seeking political party.

Before he ever met Freud, Jung had begun treating a beautiful and highly intelligent Russian Jewish teenager, Sabina Spielrein, with Freud's techniques. She was admitted to the Burghölzli at the age of 19, in late 1904, with the diagnosis of "hysterical psychosis." Shortly after her discharge from the Burghölzli in mid-1905, Spielrein entered medical school in Zurich and started formal psychoanalysis with Jung.

By 1906 the dangers of naïvely conducting psychoanalysis were becoming manifest. Spielrein apparently fell in love with Jung rather quickly, a reflection of erotic transference. For his part, Jung did not manage his erotic countertransference. Indeed, Jung may not have even had any real understanding of countertransference, given the early date of the case. In 1906 Jung initiated correspondence with Freud and, in his first two letters, discussed this patient and the extensive problems that were arising. Although it is not entirely clear whether the erotic transference–countertransference relationship became an overtly sexual relationship, many scholars believe that it did. Spielrein's analysis with Jung ended abruptly in 1909, and she graduated from medical school two years later. After moving to Munich for a brief period, she settled in Vienna, where she began participating in the Wednesday-evening discussions at Freud's apartment. Her brilliance is evident in a paper she delivered there in 1911 on *thanatos*, the aggression or death instinct.

In Vienna Spielrein married another Russian Jewish physician. She worked for a number of years as a psychiatrist in Vienna before returning to the USSR in 1923, where she was one of the few trained psychoanalysts in a country that, thanks to Trotsky, had suddenly become very receptive to this treatment method. However, by 1924 Trotsky had begun to lose political power, and the next year the experimental nursery at which Spielrein briefly worked was closed under a cloud of scandal. This nursery, operated on psychoanalytic principles, was attended by the children of important Soviet figures, including the son of Joseph Stalin. Over time psychoanalysis itself was viewed with increasing skepticism by the Communist government, and in 1930 the Russian Psychoanalytic Association was dissolved altogether. Spielrein had long since returned to her native Rostov-on-Don, where she continued to work as a psychiatrist until 1936. Her extended family suffered grievously during Stalin's purges in the mid-1930s, and she and her children were ultimately murdered by a German mobile killing squad in Rostov-on-Don in 1942.

Transference and countertransference received increasing theoretical attention from Freud and his colleagues in the early decades of the twentieth century. Freud and Jung both published papers on transference, as did others. Jung was notably the first analyst to suggest that all psychoanalysts have a training analysis as a prerequisite to seeing patients. He had come to believe that the first step to helping patients effectively is the development of self-knowledge on the part of the analyst.

In early 1906 Jung sent Freud the paper he had published on word association tests, and late in the following winter Freud invited Jung to visit him in Vienna. The first encounter between Jung and Freud was a highly engaged conversation that went on for fully 13 hours. On that evening the two men discovered that they had several interests in common, including the unusual hobby of collecting objects of antiquity, not to mention their equally matched energy for intense theoretical discussion.

In 1907 Jung published a paper on the psychology of schizophrenia, and his theory essentially supported many of Freud's views. As discussed earlier, Freud's theory was organized around other phenomena and didn't satisfactorily explain psychosis. Jung, who had more experience with psychotic patients, felt that adjustments to Freud's ideas did explain certain aspects of psychosis.

Freud's relationship with Jung is arguably the most famous, or infamous, of all of Freud's relatively short-lived collegial relationships, and their breakup led to the creation of a Jungian branch of psychoanalysis, called Analytical Psychology. The intense relationship was marked by points of agreement, but from early on Jung expressed doubts about elements of Freud's theory, especially the universal primacy of sexual libido over other instincts.

Freud and Jung frequently discussed their relationship with one another. In a letter to Freud in early 1908, Jung suggested that he and Freud avoid a future split, given Freud's pattern of separating himself from equals, by agreeing that Freud would act in the role of father and Jung in the role of son, thereby establishing "distance" to "enable two hard-headed people to exist alongside one another." The father–son concept was readily embraced by both parties. Freud was more than eager to have a non-Jewish "heir" to promote and secure the future of psychoanalysis. At that time he openly worried about the fact that most psychoanalysts were Jewish and the possibility that his movement might be viewed as a sort of Jewish sect. This led Freud to support Jung's career by deliberately placing him in positions of authority within what was now an international psychoanalytic movement. The collaboration with Freud didn't last, however, and their association ended in 1913, when theoretical differences adversely affected their personal relationship.

The lead-up to the development of Jung's own psychoanalytic theory reminds us eerily of Freud's experience in creating psychoanalysis. Having lost a father figure in Freud, Jung suffered a severe psychological crisis, leading him to develop new techniques of self-analysis as a means of understanding and manipulating his severely disturbing experiences. During the seven years after his break with Freud just before World War I, Jung was unable to do any meaningful outside work. He resigned from all of his academic and psychoanalytic organization appointments, focused on his self-analysis, and slept at night with a gun by his bed in case he could no longer bear his "confrontation with the unconscious."

Jung also spent time trying to understand Freud and analyzing the differences between Adler and Freud, having later published papers explicating his ideas about this. When he ultimately resumed treating patients more actively, he consciously chose between his own techniques and the techniques of Freud and Adler, based on patient characteristics.

After those seven long years, Jung resumed a more normal life. What he had created was a record of his self-analysis that became the basis for his body of theory. The technique of active imagination, as Jungian analysis is called, is active and creative for both the patient and the analyst, who work in collaboration and engage in activities that may involve drawing or building things, as Jung did, or activities such as dancing, with the goal of fearlessly confronting and integrating previously unconscious material. In the 1920s, an early translator of Taoist texts pointed out the convergence between Taoist philosophy, on one hand, and the drawings from Jung's self-analysis and his personality integration techniques, on the other. This led Jung to examine Eastern philosophy and techniques and to publish several books on related topics in subsequent years.

One might argue that, just as Freud took his self-analysis as far as he needed to in order to gain insight into his own difficulties, so too did Jung take his own analysis and theory far enough to understand himself. Both men concluded that symptoms serve a psychological purpose, but Jung believed they worked to restore balance. Jung proposed a creative process called *individuation* that he believed explained personal development and offered a means to treat mental disorders.

Jung was and remains a controversial figure. His theories are as much spiritual as psychological. Beyond that, there has been debate regarding a series of events that began when the National Socialists came to power in Germany in 1933. Very soon thereafter the Jews were ejected from the General Medical Society of Psychotherapy as national society members, and Jung acceded to a request that he become the Society's president. To his credit, he very quickly used his authority to reorganize the society as an international association, which had the effect of permitting German Jewish analysts to rejoin as individuals. In his position as president Jung also edited the Society's journal. There was an incident in which some material he had written some 20 years earlier on the topic of Germanic and Jewish psychology was published, evidently without his knowledge. The material in question was actually rather similar to other essays Jung wrote about the collective psychology of national or racial groups, in which he argued that each group had specific combinations of features, and in every case there was an imperative to move forward toward balance (to become what is missing). Some have argued that Jung should have been more circumspect in dealing with the Nazis. However, he stated repeatedly that in accepting the presidency he hoped to be able to help Jewish analysts. Moreover, he later resigned the Society presidency and published a series of essays that were highly critical of Germany. He also attempted to help some Jewish colleagues at the time of their flight from Germany in the late 1930s, including Sigmund Freud, but the latter rebuffed his offers.

It has been suggested that no other Western theorist has proposed such a complicated and detailed personality structure as did Jung. He is particularly known for the distinction he made between the *personal unconscious* and *collective unconscious*, the former reflecting only one's personal history and the latter containing universals shared by all humans. In fact, the idea of a collective unconscious was not novel, inasmuch as Freud had referred to something like a collective unconscious as well. However, Jung developed the idea well beyond Freud's thoughts on the matter, and it is generally agreed that the collective unconscious is fundamentally a Jungian concept.

Jung worked out how a collective unconscious might function. He posited that mental activity is organized around *complexes*, which he described as groups of ideas with a particular emotional tone. The outer shell of the complex is related to immediate personal experiences and associations, while the nuclear element contains *archetypes*, that is, the transpersonal structures for such experiences, which come from the collective unconscious. He described the *persona* as a complex mediating between the ego and the external world, a sort of mask worn by people in their everyday lives, while the *shadow* is an alter ego image, filled with repressed or primitive feelings. He also discussed the *animus* and the *anima*, part-personality complexes with respectively male or female characteristics that permit the ego to connect to the inner world or objects in the outer world. The *self* is the archetype that provides unity, organization, and stability in personality functioning.

Jung developed a theory of personality types along three orthogonal axes: extraversion–introversion, sensation–intuition, and thinking–feeling. In this way he derived $2 \times 2 \times 2 = 8$ personality types (Fig. 2.2), although he apparently didn't believe that these were categorical but simply represented extremes along the various axes. Jung believed that in each person one function (e.g., intuition) was dominant. The "opposite" function (in this case, sensation) is the least developed function, while the other two functions (in this case, thinking and feeling) are a little more developed, as they support the dominant function. Thus, each person has a dominant function and also a dominant attitude (introversion or extraversion). Jung (1921/1976) described each of the resulting eight personality types in detail.

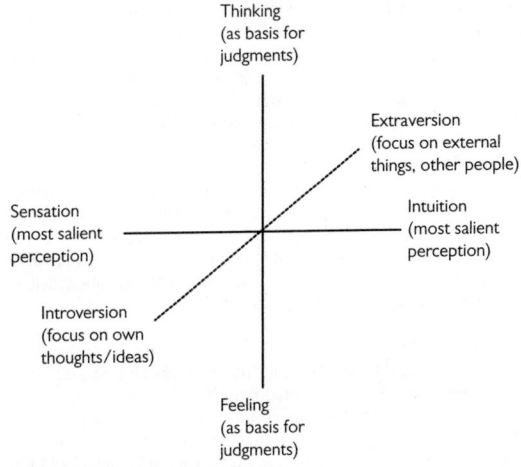

Figure 2.2. Jung's theory of personality types.

Jung believed that decreased psychopathology would result from the development of better balance among one's functions and attitudes. He believed that the *self* is the archetype responsible for this process. Jung argued that the goal of life is to achieve *self-realization*, and he suggested that psychopathology results from complexes that are out of balance or markedly opposed to one another. Thus, Jung rejected as prime movers in personality development both Freud's instinctual vicissitudes and Adler's striving for superiority, although he acknowledged that in some situations one or the other of these theories might offer the best explanation. More fundamentally, he said, we are driven to know ourselves, both personally and collectively, and when we fail to do so, psychopathology results. Further, in contrast to the theories of Freud and Adler, Jung's developmental theory covers not only childhood but the entire lifespan. He was generally of the view that one is influenced not only by one's experience but also by one's goals, thus integrating both causality and teleology into his theory.

Sándor Ferenczi (1873–1933)

Born near Budapest, Hungary, Ferenczi was the son of Polish Jews. He was a middle child among 11 or 12 surviving children, and his father died when he was 15 years old, plunging the mother into a deep depression. Ferenczi, like Jung, was interested in spiritualism but decided to study psychiatry. He completed medical training in Vienna in 1894, after which he returned to Budapest before meeting Freud in 1908. In subsequent years Freud and Ferenczi maintained a voluminous correspondence with one another, and he may have been personally closer to Freud than any other disciple, even if Ferenczi was ultimately banished by Freud in 1932 due to disagreement over the details of analytic technique.

Ferenczi (1934) published a *tour de force* in which he described parallels between sexual ontogeny and phylogeny (e.g., comparing intrauterine life with the oceanic existence of earlier life forms), and this was consistent with Freud's frequent speculation that ontogeny mimics phylogeny. However, Ferenczi's main contribution to psychoanalysis has to do with technique rather than theory. Early on, he wrote extensively about how the analyst might take a more active stance, either by confronting the patient directly or by permitting the patient greater freedom. He urged that psychoanalysis be shortened. He was also very interested in the issue of countertransference. In contrast to Freud, Ferenczi maintained that some countertransference was appropriate, perhaps inevitable, in psychoanalysis. He permitted patients to kiss him, and this brought about a negative reaction from Freud, who worried that such behavior might lead to more intimate activities and thereby sully the good name of psychoanalysis.

Otto Rank (1884–1939)

Originally called Otto Rosenfeld, this future psychoanalyst was born into a family of modest means in Vienna, having worked for a time as a locksmith before being introduced to Freud in 1906 by his family physician, Alfred Adler. Rank became Freud's protégé, and the older man helped Rank finish high school and obtain a doctorate in philosophy in 1912 from the University of Vienna. Rank became the first non-medical analyst. He was long in Freud's inner circle but began to break with him in 1924, at the time that Rank first visited the United States, a country for which Freud had little use. By 1926 the break was complete, and Rank moved to Paris, where he remained for eight years before emigrating to the United States in 1934.

In terms of psychoanalytic theory, Rank was interested in how people move from union to separation. He went so far as to argue that all developmental crises are based on the terror of leaving the womb and the wish to return to a state of primal bliss. He suggested that only through *will* can people develop and move from union to separation. Rank rejected Freud, Adler, and Jung when he averred that human development is driven not by attempts to cope with sexual instincts, not by a drive to overcome inferiority, and not by the need to individuate. Rather, Rank asserted that we can understand a person psychologically by examining his or her success in negotiating the tension between union and separation. If Freud was mostly focused on the father–child relationship, Rank was much more interested in the mother–child relationship, as would be consistent with his ideas about the importance of the birth trauma.

Rank was another member of Freud's inner circle who found himself in trouble after he recommended changes in analytic technique, primarily with a view toward shortening the process and avoiding a strong focus on the past. In 1925 he and Ferenczi wrote a book together in which they described a model for brief therapy. In treatment Rank did not take on the role of expert but instead comported himself as a nonjudgmental helper, thus foreshadowing the work of the American psychologist Carl Rogers. Rank was much more focused on the present, on the real relationship with the therapist, and on psychology than was Freud, who focused on the past, on transference, and on biology.

In the short term Rank had limited influence on psychoanalytic practice, and it wasn't until the 1950s, when Carl Rogers worked out the details of client-centered therapy, that Rank's ideas became more widely known, albeit often without attribution. Some have suggested that Rank's lack of influence within psychoanalysis may have resulted from the fact that few came to his defense in the late 1920s when he began arguing more directly with Freud over technique. In particular, Ferenczi kept himself above the fray, even though just a few years earlier he and Rank had worked closely on issues of technique. It has been suggested that Ferenczi failed to support Rank for fear of offending Freud.

Ego Psychology

We now discuss some basic ideas in ego psychology and focus on the contributions of two important theorists in this area: Anna Freud and Erik H. Erikson.

In the 1930s the center of psychoanalytic thinking began to move westward. Central Europe was becoming more and more dangerous for Jews, who still constituted the vast majority of psychoanalytic theorists and practitioners. Many fled to England and to the United States, and at the end of World War II they did not return to their earlier homes, choosing instead to remain in their adopted countries. In particular, London became a hotbed of psychoanalytic thinking, and it is there that ego psychology and the object relations school both developed. True to form, the theorists and practitioners of these two schools did not tolerate one another gracefully.

Now, over the course of his life Freud had gradually shifted his view regarding the importance of the ego. Early on, he believed that the ego was a small appendage to the id and was not present at birth. By the end of his life, however, Freud acknowledged that a rudimentary ego existed at birth, and he had come to appreciate the centrality of the ego in regulating mental life. Still, classical psychoanalysis is aptly characterized as *id psychology*.

By contrast, in ego psychology the various defenses employed by the ego are no longer seen just as obstacles that obscure one's view of the unconscious. Rather, ego defenses are thought to be useful coping strategies that help us to live in the world. Thus, the ego is no longer reactive but becomes proactive, at least in part. Yes, the ego has to deal with the id, but its coherent organization is important in and of itself. Correspondingly, we understand mental phenomena in terms of optimal ego functioning, rather than as the efficiency with which id impulses are dispatched or neutralized.

Anna Freud (1895–1982)

It was Freud's youngest child who laid the groundwork for *ego psychology*. She never earned a university degree but did work for a time as a schoolteacher. In her mid-twenties she was psychoanalyzed by her father at about the time that he was first diagnosed with cancer. After Freud's diagnosis, he and Anna gradually grew closer to one another, and eventually Anna supplanted her mother as Freud's chief confidant, particularly inasmuch as Freud could not discuss psychoanalysis with his wife, who considered it to be something like pornography (Gay, 2006).

Anna Freud was one of the first people to think carefully about the application of psychoanalysis to the treatment of children. In brief, she argued against major changes in technique, although she acknowledged that children's superegos are less well developed than in the case of adults. In line with her early work as a teacher, she also utilized educational methods with children.

However, Anna Freud's most important contribution has to do with her work on understanding ego defenses. Building on her work and the work of others, we review below the main ego defenses cited by psychoanalysts, although it should be noted that there are multiple lists of analytic defenses, and certain defenses appear on some lists but not on others. Understanding and recognizing ego defense mechanisms improves our ability to understand the underlying motivation for behaviors that may otherwise seem counterproductive. It is expected that psychiatry residents understand and learn to recognize ego defenses in working with patients. Indeed, specific ego defense mechanisms are thought to be associated with particular psychiatric illnesses (e.g., undoing and reaction formation are thought to correspond to obsessive-compulsive disorder).

Repression: We have already discussed *repression*, Freud's fundamental defense mechanism, which involves moving threatening thoughts and feelings from the conscious into the unconscious. Repression may be reflected in memory lapses, naïveté, or a failure to understand one's situation. Repression is sometimes apparent when an individual is aware of an emotion but not the associated thoughts.

Suppression: By contrast, *suppression* involves the displacement of threatening thoughts and feelings from the conscious into the preconscious. Thus, while repressed material is unavailable to conscious awareness, suppressed material can be accessed later on.

Displacement: *Displacement* involves shifting an emotion from its real target to a target that is less threatening. The classic example is the worker who comes home after an unpleasant interaction with the boss, becomes upset when the dog barks, and then yells at the dog.

Sublimation: Closely related to displacement is the defense of *sublimation*, which is the basis of civilization. In sublimation sexual or aggressive impulses are transformed into more socially acceptable actions, behavior, or emotions. Thus, one might author a work of fiction in response to feelings of murderous rage toward another person.

Conversion: *Conversion* is the expression of proscribed impulses in the form of physical symptoms, such as the paralysis of a limb, certain pain phenomena, blindness, or deafness.

Regression: *Regression* refers to the phenomenon in which one may begin functioning in a manner consistent with an earlier developmental level, instead of dealing in a mature way with a threatening situation. Many people behave in a regressive manner when they become angry.

Identification: *Identification* involves improving one's self-esteem by affiliating with those who have more power. This, of course, is how fashion develops. More specifically, Anna Freud wrote about *identification with the aggressor*, which involves the adoption of the values and mannerisms of a feared person. This is thought to be the means by which the superego develops. Anna Freud also proposed the defense of *altruistic surrender*, in which one obtains vicarious satisfaction of one's own ambitions by identifying with the satisfactions and frustrations of another person.

Rationalization: *Rationalization* involves the use of faulty logic or reasoning to overcome guilt regarding past actions. Parents who harshly punish their children may later explain that they are only doing so because their children require a firm response to misbehavior.

Undoing: *Undoing* involves ritualistic activities that atone for unacceptable thoughts or actions. Lady Macbeth's hand washing after Duncan's murder is an example.

Denial: *Denial* is the frank refusal to accept external reality because it is too threatening. This can take the form of arguing that an anxiety-provoking stimulus doesn't exist or simply not perceiving the more threatening aspects of a given situation. Of course, it is thought that people with addictions are likely to engage in denial regarding their addiction.

Projection: In *projection* a person shifts unacceptable thoughts, feelings, and impulses to someone else. Thus, the troubling material can be expressed, which is a relief, but one doesn't assume any responsibility for it. Some examples of projection include the inappropriate attribution of aggressive impulses to significant others, marked prejudice, or unreasonable jealousy.

Reaction formation: *Reaction formation* involves converting worrisome unconscious impulses into their opposites. For example, one might experience strongly solicitous feelings toward someone for whom one harbors unconscious hostility.

Splitting: *Splitting* occurs when an individual fails to integrate the negative and positive aspects of other people or the self. For example, one might view some people as entirely good and others as entirely bad, or one might view one's own behavior as sometimes completely healthy but at other times mysteriously disturbed.

Isolation of affect/dissociation: More particularly, *isolation of affect* involves separating the feelings from one's thoughts and actions. Thus, one might describe a tragic event in an entirely neutral manner. *Dissociation* is a more extreme version of isolation of affect. When this defense is operative, one part of conscious ego operates more or less independently from the rest of conscious ego. The separation is so extreme that the individual cannot simultaneously attend both to the separated processes and to the other integrated functions. Dissociation may be operative when individuals act and speak in a way that is quite inconsistent with their usual presentation and have little or no access to their habitual thoughts, feelings, and memories.

Erik H. Erikson (1902–1994)

We now turn to the most accessible of the ego psychologists. For reasons that will quickly become clear, Erikson had a particular interest in a concept he referred to as the *identity crisis*.

Erikson's mother was born into the Jewish community in Denmark, while Erikson himself was born and spent his childhood near Frankfurt am Main, Germany. He was the product of a relationship his mother had while she was separated from her first husband. When Erikson was three years old, his mother took him to see a pediatrician, Dr. Homburger, whom she subsequently married. Until adolescence Erikson believed that Dr. Homburger was his father, and in fact it wasn't until the age of 37 that he changed his name from Erik Homburger to Erik H. Erikson.

Dr. Homburger wished his adoptive son to study medicine. However, after finishing high school Erikson briefly trained as an artist and then floated about in Italy and elsewhere, until in the mid-1920s he landed in Vienna, where he taught in a progressive school to which many of Freud's patients and friends sent their children. Here he met Anna Freud just as she was completing analysis with her father, and she suggested that Erikson become her training analysand. Erikson attended seminars in Vienna, and when he completed analytic training, he was given full membership in the Vienna Psychoanalytic Society.

When the political situation in Europe began to heat up in 1933, Erikson attempted to obtain Danish citizenship by capitalizing on his mother's nationality. However, Denmark did not agree to naturalize him. He married an American, and later in the year he was able to emigrate to the United States, where he remained after that, having variously worked in Massachusetts, Connecticut, California, and Pennsylvania.

Erikson's tripartite model of human development differs from Freud's, and it includes somatic, ego, and cultural-historical aspects. His primary interest was in the development of the ego, and he made the point that ego development is dependent on somatic experiences (feeding, elimination, etc.) and family responses to any crisis that might develop. Of particular note, Erikson expanded Freud's stages of development. He believed that people pass through eight stages of ego development, and the conflict implicit in each stage reaches a crisis point at a specific time in one's life. He proposed that human culture provides *ritualizations* that promote both adaptation to social conditions and the successful completion of specific developmental stages. He went on to suggest that when ritualizations are exaggerated (e.g., conformity to rules becomes legalistic), problematic *ritualisms* result. Thus, Erikson was able to tie together physical maturation, family/cultural influences, and ego development. Here are the eight stages, each focused on a specific conflict, each influenced by a particular ritualization (or ritualism), and each leading, if all goes well, to a specific virtue. These eight stages are also summarized in Table 2.1.

Erikson stated that in *infancy*, his first stage (corresponding fairly closely to the Freudian oral stage), the individual works out a balance between trust and mistrust. Through interaction with caregivers, the infant may develop the feeling of *basic trust*, or *basic mistrust* may develop. If, as a result of experience, the infant is more trusting than mistrusting, he or she develops the virtue of *hope* and is able to focus on the future rather than always to worry about the satisfaction of present needs. Erikson stated that ritualized parent–child interactions (which he referred to as *numinous*) provide the necessary support to negotiate this developmental stage and lead the infant to develop reverence and respect for the parent. However, if this is exaggerated, *idolism* results, and later on the child may be inclined to blind hero worship.

In *early childhood* the conflict is between autonomy, on one hand, and shame and doubt, on the other. This is similar in some ways to Freud's anal age. According to Erikson, the child learns to exercise will while still conforming to social expectations. If the child develops more *autonomy* than *shame* and *doubt*, the virtue of *will* emerges, which Erikson (1964) describes as a "determination to exercise free choice as well as self-restraint, in spite

Table 2.1 Erikson's eight stages of development correlate ego development with physical maturation and family/cultural influences. At each stage, relatively successful resolution of the conflict strengthens the ego's capacity to adapt, because the resulting virtue becomes available to it. Culture contributes either positively (through ritualizations) or negatively (through ritualisms) to successful resolution at each stage.

Stage	Approx. age range	Basic conflict	Resulting virtue	Cultural component		Approx. Freudian equivalent
				Ritualization	Ritualism	
infancy	0–15 mos	basic trust vs. mistrust	hope	numinous	idolism	oral
early childhood	15 mos–3 yrs	autonomy vs. shame and doubt	will	judiciousness	legalism	anal
preschool	3–6 yrs	initiative vs. guilt	purpose	authenticity	impersonation	phallic
school age	6–12 yrs	industry vs. inferiority	competence	formality	formalism	latency
adolescence	12–20 yrs	identity vs. role confusion	fidelity	ideology	totalism	genital
young adulthood	20–24 yrs	intimacy vs. isolation	love	affiliation	elitism	(none)
adulthood	24–64 yrs	generativity vs. stagnation	care	generationalism	authoritism	(none)
old age	65 yrs–	integrity vs. despair	wisdom	integralism	sapientism	(none)

of the unavoidable experience of shame and doubt in infancy" (p. 119). In this stage the ritualization of *judiciousness* is required for children to learn social rules and expectations. If exaggerated, the ritualism of *legalism* becomes operative, and the child becomes more concerned about punishment of transgressors than about the intent of rules in the first place.

During the *preschool* period, which overlaps with Freud's phallic period, when the Oedipus complex plays out, the child works through the conflict between initiative and guilt, which permits the child to initiate ideas and actions and to plan future events. If parents support children in this stage, children develop a sense of *initiative* and do not feel *guilt* in response to the impulse to plan for the future. The virtue of *purpose* thus develops. During this period children frequently engage in play-acting and so try on new roles in order to work out who they really are. If this ritualization of *authenticity* is exaggerated, however, it becomes *impersonation*, and the child is unable to distinguish between role playing and his or her actual identity.

The *school-age* child struggles with industry versus inferiority and learns to work cooperatively with others. This is very similar to Freud's latency period. If the child comes to appreciate the value of attending and persevering, then *industry* results. Otherwise, the child is plagued by feelings of *inferiority*, and the virtue of *competence* does not develop strongly. *Formality*, the ritualization required for this stage, involves learning how to do tasks at home, at school, and with peers. If formality is exaggerated, it becomes *formalism*, which involves a myopic focus on technique without appreciating the meaning of the task at hand.

During *adolescence* (Freud's genital stage) the conflict is between identity and role confusion. In this period the young person moves from childhood toward adulthood and commits to a particular strategy for life. This is the period in which the *identity crisis* occurs, the desirable outcome of which is that the young adult develops a sense of *identity*, rather than *role confusion* (moving from one identity to another, without keeping any strategy for long) or perhaps a *negative identity* (adopting a parentally proscribed identity). The virtue that results from a positive balance between identity and role confusion is *fidelity*, according to which the individual is able to sustain loyalties despite contradictions in value systems. The ritualization required in this period involves finding and adapting to an *ideology*—but doing so without losing sight of one's individuality, an adverse influence that Erikson refers to as *totalism*.

Erikson's last three stages do not have direct equivalents in Freud's system. The task of *young adulthood* is to resolve the conflict between intimacy and isolation. This period, which occurs between the ages of about 20 and 24, requires that the individual establish a pattern of love and work, as Freud suggested in another context. If one can't establish this pattern, one recedes into *isolation* and doesn't develop the virtue of *love*. Erikson describes this stage's ritualization of *affiliation* as supporting one's involvement with like-minded others. However, if affiliation becomes extreme, it becomes *elitism*, in which the individual becomes isolated from anyone who does not share a similar, narrowly defined identity.

Erikson believed that during *adulthood*, which lasts from about 25 to 64 years of age, the individual struggles to work out the conflict between generativity and stagnation. The individual must try to support the next generation, either through social interaction or in other contributions to society. If one doesn't develop a pattern of generativity, one is instead troubled by *stagnation*, and one doesn't develop the virtue of *care*, which Erikson (1964) described as "the widening concern for what has been generated by love, necessity or accident" (p. 131). The ritualization associated with this stage is *generationalism*, by which one transmits cultural values to younger people. If this is too exaggerated, however, it becomes *authoritism*, which leads more mature adults to dominate the younger generation.

Finally, in *old age* the conflict is between ego integrity and despair. This period, which lasts from age 65 to death, may permit one to feel fulfilled by the accomplishments of life and to anticipate death with little fear, or one may be filled with *despair* over lost opportunities. The virtue that arises from this stage is *wisdom*. The ritualization associated with this stage is *integralism*, from which one comes to see one's role in learning, adhering to, and passing along cultural rules over the course of one's life. If exaggerated, however, integralism becomes *sapientism*, and one imagines one has all the answers now, notwithstanding the constant evolution of human culture.

Object Relations Theory

A second important neo-analytic movement that developed primarily in London is the school of object relations. The theories in this school are somewhat complicated; we focus here on two exponents of object relations, Melanie Klein and Donald W. Winnicott.

We begin our exploration of object relations by returning briefly to the basic Freudian idea that early childhood interactions with caregivers cause us to rely to a greater or lesser extent on particular ego defenses and to misperceive those around us based on the development of idiosyncratic interpersonal templates. In object relations language, we refer to a person, a part of a person, or a mental representation of the same as an *object*. We distinguish between those objects that are *internal* (mental representations) and those that are real. The *self* is an internal image of one's own person, not to be confused with the actual physical self or the psychological sense of "self." *Object relations* are the structural and dynamic interactions between *self* and *internal objects*. We are interested here in understanding how people relate mental representations of the self to mental representations of others. Of course, we have to remember that object relations theorists are particularly interested in relationships that are formed between self and objects very early in life, which means that we are discussing foundational perceptions and resulting intrapsychic representations that are constructed by very immature brains.

Melanie Klein (1882–1960)

This important figure in the object relations school was born in Vienna. Klein began medical studies at the age of 15 but left the course when she married at the age of 21, after which she took up the study of art and history at the university. She never completed a university degree, at least in part because she moved frequently with her husband for his job. She was unhappy in her marriage, and she felt increasingly depressed following the death of two older siblings, her father, and in 1914 her mother, who had lived with Klein during the mother's final illness. Significantly, much of Klein's later psychoanalytic work focused on depression and melancholia.

Klein first came in contact with Freud's work after she and her husband moved to Budapest in 1910, and in about 1917 she took up analysis with Sándor Ferenczi, who encouraged her to raise her three-year-old child according to psychoanalytic principles. In 1919 she delivered a paper at the Hungarian Society of Psychoanalysis and was subsequently accepted as a member. The following year she was introduced to Freud's disciple, the German psychiatrist Karl Abraham (1877–1925). Abraham invited Klein to Berlin, where he was working. Klein accepted, and she separated from her husband.

Once in Berlin, Klein analyzed several children, including Rita, whose analysis she undertook in 1923. Then 33 months old, Rita manifested an obsessional fear that something would come in the night to bite her. Abraham wrote to Freud that Klein's analysis of Rita provided "clear evidence of the original melancholia . . . [and] of oral eroticism." The analysis also played a role in Klein's subsequent recommendations regarding treatment techniques with children, such as that treatment occur in an appropriate setting (not at home) and with certain toys.

After Abraham died of a lung infection in late 1925, Klein accepted the invitation of Ernest Jones to come to London. She continued to undertake the analysis of young children, and she responded to increasingly virulent attacks by Anna Freud (then still in Vienna), who argued with her about developmental issues and felt that educational techniques were required in the treatment of these patients. Eventually Freud himself joined the fray when he wrote to Ernest Jones to complain about Klein's attacks on his daughter.

Klein remained in Britain for the rest of her life, and she continued to expand on her theories related to the development of young children. She tried to adapt psychoanalysis directly to children by analyzing their play. She talked about developmental *positions*, rather than stages, making the sensible point often overlooked in developmental theories that stages don't necessarily follow one another in strict succession. As well, she stated that one might return to an earlier "position" as a consequence of certain stresses in life, a phenomenon Freud also acknowledged in the phenomenon of *regression*.

Consistent with her view that psychoanalysis could be applied directly to infants, Klein at one point argued that infants have strong cognitive skills, in part because these are not yet clouded by repression. She moved up the timetable for the development of the superego from after the resolution of the Oedipus complex to around the age of three months, which became one of the points of contention with Anna Freud and her partisans.

Klein had an active interest in the death instinct and believed that aggressive impulses were an important part of development. Indeed, she suggested that anxiety or psychic conflict was always a reflection of conflict between libido and thanatos within the id, rather than conflict between the ego and the id, superego, or reality considerations. She believed that it was this conflict between libido and thanatos that roused the ego to action and that the ego learned to cope with these instincts through the interaction between self and internalized objects.

As part of her investigation of the relationship between self and internal objects, Klein worked out a detailed theory linking the defenses of splitting, projective identification, introjection, and projection to developmental stages in early infancy. In particular, she described the *paranoid-schizoid* position as a period in the first three months of life during which the infant is fearful regarding self-preservation. This stage is marked especially by the defenses of splitting and projection. For example, the infant becomes convinced that there is a "good breast" and a "bad breast." If the infant is dominated by positive fantasies, it can project the negative instincts outward and maintain some degree of stability. By contrast, if the negative fantasies predominate, the infant becomes overwhelmed by anxiety and adopts psychotic defenses, such as the rejection of all real experience.

The *depressive* position, according to Klein, occurs in the second three months of life and reflects the infant's fear that aggressive or greedy impulses will destroy external objects. Klein believed that it was at this point in development that the infant begins to combine good and bad objects, which concomitantly permits the ego to become better integrated. Klein believed that rudimentary development of the superego might occur in the depressive position. More ominously, the infant might regress to the paranoid-schizoid position or experience a swing into a manic state. Klein believed that individuals continue throughout their lives to work through aspects of the paranoid-schizoid and depressive positions.

Some commentators have applied Klein's ideas regarding early development to attempts to understand psychosis in adults, particularly inasmuch as she described infants whose cognition seemed similar to that of psychotic adults. As a group, Kleinian therapists offer very "deep" interpretations and are able to find primary process and transference distortion in virtually all patient verbalizations and actions. For example, in 1924 Klein wrote that a child's experience at school was strongly affected by sexual matters. Among other ideas, she suggested that while studying division the child might make an association to violent coitus, while the study of music might remind the child of the sounds of parental intercourse.

Klein had strong opinions; like Sigmund Freud before her, she demanded absolute loyalty from others. Her legendary battles with Anna Freud (leading to the so-called "controversial discussions" in the British Psychoanalytic Society during World War II) continued until at last the British Psychoanalytic Society elected to split itself into three factions (Kleinians, Freudians, and Independents); this split has persisted for over 60 years.

Donald W. Winnicott (1896–1971)

Winnicott was born in England into a prosperous and overtly happy family. However, his mother was at least mildly depressed, and years later Winnicott spoke of working to assuage his mother's distress so that she would remain "alive." Winnicott attended medical school after participating in the Navy during World War I. Working as a pediatrician, he began a training analysis in the mid-1920s. While he received early psychoanalytic supervision from Melanie Klein, he gradually distanced himself from her thinking, and he was in fact a member of the Independents in the British Psychoanalytic Society.

Winnicott asserted that it was the nature of the *actual* relationship between child and caregiver that leads either to appropriate development or to psychopathology. This marks a departure from Klein's idea that the infant's *perception* is all that matters. Winnicott's idea was that children require certain experiences with caregivers in order to develop a *true self*, which enables them to feel fully alive, with complete access to their feelings. The caregiver must respond in a welcoming, reassuring manner to the child's behavior while at the same time protecting the child from a frightening awareness of its helplessness in the world. If, by contrast, the caregiver is not appropriately responsive, the child might conclude that the world is not a safe place and would then develop a *false self*, a façade designed to please others, such that the child does not experience spontaneity or the sense of being fully alive. The child with a false self comes to believe that by meeting others' needs, he or she gains a measure of safety in the world. Winnicott stated fairly directly that this was his experience in his relationship with his own mother.

Winnicott suggested that a *primary maternal preoccupation* occurs during the last trimester of pregnancy and in the ensuing first few months of life, and the mother responds empathically to the baby's excitatory state and also to periods of quiescence. Later, the mother begins to withdraw and thus helps the baby begin to separate. Winnicott called this pattern of behavior *good-enough mothering*, and he made the point that perfect attunement between mother and child is not required. He said that as a mother it is enough to be "ordinarily devoted." He suggested that it was in fact the mother who was the primary player in the developmental scheme, although he noted that after a period in which the mother engages in *holding* and then interaction with the infant, the infant begins to interact with both parents and learns to negotiate more complicated relationships.

Winnicott also introduced the notion of *transitional object* (a teddy bear or special blanket, for example), which he suggested helps the baby to move from self as center of the universe to self among many selves in the universe. This represents a shift from *subjectivity* to *objectivity* while also supporting the development of fantasy operations.

In terms of treatment, Winnicott urged that the therapist adopt a spontaneous, playful attitude with the patient, because it is only through play, he said, that people feel fully alive and interested in what they are doing. He argued against the analyst taking an authoritarian position (as Melanie Klein was doing), because he felt this might reinforce maintenance of the patient's false self. As therapist he aimed to supply missing parental provisions and to fulfill early developmental needs.

The Interpersonal School

In this section we briefly discuss the life and theory of American psychiatrist Harry Stack Sullivan (1892–1949). In some ways, Sullivan might be viewed as an object relations theorist, but he takes object relations a step further by insisting that psychopathology exists entirely within the interpersonal realm.

Born near Norwich, New York, Sullivan was the only child of Irish immigrants in an area described as strongly anti-Catholic. His father was withdrawn, while his mother, a bitter, complaining woman, was hospitalized for depression when Sullivan was two and a half years old. Sullivan had difficulty fitting in with other boys when he was young. During this period he did establish a close relationship with a boy who was five years his senior, and later in life he speculated that such a relationship might help to transform an immature preadolescent into a healthy adult.

Sullivan did well in school but then flunked out of Cornell University during his second semester as a physics major. He may have had a psychiatric hospitalization after that, and in 1911 he entered the Chicago College of Medicine and graduated just as the school closed in 1917. Notwithstanding his lack of training in psychiatry, in 1923 Sullivan was somehow able to obtain a psychiatric position at St. Elizabeth Hospital, in Washington, DC, and for some years after that he worked extensively with patients with schizophrenia, having been the first to experiment extensively with the therapeutic milieu.

Sullivan had numerous social difficulties. He was reportedly a heavy drinker, was cold and standoffish, declared bankruptcy twice, and at the age of 35 began residing with a 15-year-old patient; they continued to live together for the remaining 22 years of Sullivan's life. Although he told associates that the patient was his adopted son, some report their relationship was romantic. Once again we observe the specter of unmanaged countertransference.

Sullivan took the position that "personality" does not exist, other than in the context of a relationship. In other words, one's personality is entirely dependent on interactions with others. Thus, Sullivan adopted an extreme position in advocating for a two-person psychology. In his attempt to explain human development, he took as his starting point the universal drive to overcome anxiety. He suggested that the infant acquires anxiety when it is transmitted through an empathic linkage between mother and child. He averred that anxiety is not evidence of internal conflict, as Freud would have argued; instead, he said that anxiety represents a failure to obtain a comforting response ("tenderness") from a parent figure, perhaps because of the parent's own anxiety. Sullivan described specific patterns of behavior, which he called *self-dynamisms*, that protect against anxiety. These include dissociation and selective inattention, among others.

Like the object relations theorists, Sullivan believed that one's understanding of other people and of the self is strongly dependent on early interpersonal experience, primarily with caretakers (Sullivan, 1940). He described development, from infancy through adulthood, in seven stages, and he tied the appearance of "symptoms" to the failure of important interpersonal relationships at various stages of development (e.g., relationships with parents, with same-sex friends, and with romantic partners).

Based in part on his work with patients with schizophrenia, Sullivan described three modes of experiencing. The *prototaxic* mode, which is asymbolic and prelinguistic, is the way in which infants apprehend the world. However, adults may have momentary experiences that they cannot communicate verbally, thus briefly returning to the prototaxic mode. The *parataxic* mode uses private symbols, and it involves experience on a moment-by-moment basis, without any connection between the moments. Finally, the *syntaxic* mode involves spoken language that is understood by others, thus permitting one to symbolize.

Given his view that personality is irreducibly interpersonal, Sullivan made the point that psychotherapy occurs in a two-person field, and the therapist is in fact an active *participant-observer*. While developing a relationship with the patient, the therapist observes the patient's recurring patterns and ultimately sets about to help in clearing up parataxic distortions, improving relationships generally, and learning to solve problems more efficiently. As the patient moves into more consistently syntaxic experiencing, therapy comes to an end.

Psychodynamic Approaches to Character and the Self

Beginning with Freud, psychodynamic theorists have had a lot to say about character structure, personality disorders, and self-representation. Freud believed that when people use one or just a few ego defenses, to the exclusion of other coping strategies, a *character disorder* results. He believed that character disorders are linked to fixation at a psychosexual stage.

More specifically, Freud believed that individuals fixated at the oral stage make heavy use of the defenses of denial and introjection. They also project responsibility for anxiety onto others. Freud suggested that oral characters are conflicted about dependency issues and are therefore fundamentally indifferent to the reality of other people. Oral incorporative characters will "swallow anything" and tend to be overindulged, optimistic, gullible, and passive, while oral aggressive characters are frustrated, pessimistic, suspicious, and manipulative. The anal character engages in intellectualization, reaction formation, and undoing. They can be anal retentive (controlled, frustrated, stingy, orderly, meticulous, and precise) or anal expulsive (expressive, overindulged, overly generous, messy, dirty, and vague). According to Freud, anal characters are conflicted about aggression, and they have difficulty distinguishing love from hate. Individuals fixated at the phallic stage engage in repression, according to Freud. They vacillate between the poles of vanity/self-hatred, pride/humility, gregariousness/isolation, and promiscuity/chastity. These people are conflicted about sex and sexual identity. Finally, the genital character is fully able to love and to work. These individuals make use of the defense of sublimation.

Three other theorists have contributed heavily to either the psychodynamic understanding of character structure or to our understanding of how to work with individuals with character disorders. These theorists are Wilhelm Reich, Otto F. Kernberg, and Heinz Kohut, and we review them each in turn.

Wilhelm Reich (1897–1957)

This energetic, iconoclastic, and ultimately rather disturbed man was the elder of two surviving sons of German Jewish stock born in small farming community in southeastern Poland. Reich discovered around the time of puberty that his mother was carrying on an affair with Reich's tutor. Although closer to his mother than to his brutal and jealous father, Reich nonetheless told his father about the affair, after which his mother ingested bleach and died several days later. Five years thereafter, when Reich was 17 years old, his father died of pneumonia after purchasing a life insurance policy and then standing for four hours in a cold pond. Reich was obliged to take over the family farm, but the following year it was destroyed by advancing Russian troops at the beginning of World War I. He joined the Austro-Hungarian Army and served on the Italian front as a lieutenant. At the end of the war he entered the University of Vienna, from which, under a program for war veterans, he graduated four years later with a degree in medicine.

As early as 1919 Reich became a member of Freud's circle, and the latter quickly permitted Reich to begin seeing analytic patients, although he was only 22 years old at the time and had not yet graduated. Very early on Reich began sleeping with one of his patients, and in November 1920 she died of sepsis, perhaps following a botched abortion by Reich. This was the first of a series of affairs with patients. Two months later Reich began treating a friend of his deceased patient, and he initiated an affair with her as well, ultimately marrying her under pressure in March 1922, five months before he graduated from medical school. Reich then undertook a residency in psychiatry at the University Hospital, and he worked in one of Freud's outpatient clinics at night.

Reich wished to integrate psychoanalysis with Marxism, and he developed the idea that mental health depended on the ability to abandon oneself completely to orgasmic release. He was a prolific writer, and among other titles he authored *The Function of the Orgasm* in 1927 and, two years later, *Dialectical Materialism and Psychoanalysis*. Altogether, this was not a winning combination, and in time Reich found himself shunned both by the psychoanalytic establishment (which feared scandal) and by the Communist Party (which did not approve of Reich's promotion of adolescent free love). In 1930 he left Austria, spent some time in Germany, settled in Norway for several years, and then came to the United States in 1939. In this country he developed notions about cancer, cosmic radiation, cloud seeding, and flying saucers, and he was eventually convicted of violating an injunction against interstate transportation of "orgone accumulators," which the government viewed as fraudulent medical devices. He succumbed to myocardial insufficiency in the Lewisburg Penitentiary approximately halfway through his two-year sentence.

For all of the difficulties in his life, Reich had at least two ideas worth remembering. The first idea was that psychoanalytic treatment should take into account the socioenvironmental circumstances of patients. In this regard he went even further than Adler. For example, while still in relatively good graces in Vienna he organized mobile sex clinics, in which patients could obtain psychoanalytic counseling, Marxist advice, and contraceptives on the spot. He had a genuine regard for the working class and was particularly interested in applying the techniques of psychoanalysis to improve the lives of laborers, farmers, and students.

Reich's second interesting idea had to do with his observations regarding character disturbances. He concluded that people develop a characteristic muscular tone (*body armor*) to prevent themselves from behaving in a proscribed manner, such as urinating in public. He made the point that each character style has a physical manifestation, and in this connection he fleshed out a theory of characters, with particular emphasis on the somatic concomitants of each. For example, he believed that "hysterics" are soft and rolling, while "compulsives" are tense and restrained, and "narcissists" are cold, reserved, and bristly, with strong erectile functions among men. Reich's classic 1949 text on this topic, *Character Analysis*, continues to warrant study and consideration.

The idea that character structure is reflected in one's muscle tone led Reich to conclude that one might need only to loosen up muscle knots in order to provide psychological relief, and he therefore encouraged the use of deep massage as a way to release dammed-up energy, in the expectation such treatment might lead to the strong expression of feelings or perhaps to sexual excitation. A number of current mental health practitioners agree that muscle tension and psychopathology might have a reciprocal relationship; however, few concur with Reich's insistence that sexual functioning mediates the relationship.

Otto F. Kernberg (1928–)

Sometimes referred to as a mixed-model theorist, Kernberg attempted to understand narcissistic pathology and borderline personality organization by combining ego psychology with object relations theory. Kernberg was born in Vienna but in the late 1930s fled with his family to Chile, where he lived until he came to the United States on a fellowship in 1959. For many years he worked at various institutions in New York, including the New York State Psychiatry Institute, Columbia University, and Cornell Medical Center.

Kernberg started from the position that, contrary to the ideas of Freud and others, libidinal and aggressive drives are not innate but develop based on the infant's experience of pleasure and pain. He believed that the relationship between self and object develops over a series of stages, in which the infant first learns to distinguish self from object and then learns to integrate "good" and "bad" objects. In other words, the infant learns to integrate libidinally invested objects with aggressively invested objects and to understand that these two drives can coexist. Similarly, the infant learns to integrate "good" and "bad" aspects of the internal representation of self. Kernberg asserted that in psychosis one cannot clearly distinguish self from object, while individuals with borderline personality organization engage in *splitting* and cannot integrate "good" and "bad" objects or, correspondingly, the "good" and "bad" aspects of self.

Kernberg also utilized his developmental scheme to understand narcissistic pathology, of which he believed there are three variants. At the least pathological extreme, individuals may experience positive self-esteem by behaving in such a way as to meet their infantile needs. At the most pathological extreme, individuals maintain self-esteem by behaving in a way that reflects their pathological ego and superego structures, for which development has gone awry as a consequence of early, poorly organized self and object images. Kernberg also posited the existence of a third variant of narcissistic pathology, in which individuals identify with a representation of the infantile self that is projected onto an object, so that the functions of self and object are reversed.

Based on his understanding of the organization of borderline personality, Kernberg developed a psychoanalytic technique called *transference-focused psychotherapy*. Specifically designed for individuals with borderline personality disorder, this intensive but time-limited treatment has shown some promise. We review it in the individual psychodynamic psychotherapies section of Chapter 5.

2 PSYCHOLOGICAL THEORIES: KEY CONCEPTS

Heinz Kohut (1913–1981)

Kohut was born into the Jewish community in Vienna and was the only child of a war veteran turned businessman and a shopkeeper. Kohut's mother largely isolated him from interaction with others until he started the fifth grade. Eventually, he attended medical school at the University of Vienna but did not graduate until shortly after German troops marched into Vienna in March 1938. Kohut soon fled to England and then came to the United States in 1940, where he eventually settled in Chicago. He is viewed by many to have founded a new psychodynamic school, called *self psychology*, as distinguished from other branches of psychodynamic thought: classical Freudian theory, ego psychology, and object relations.

Through his experiences and work with a number of patients diagnosed with what he referred to as narcissistic personality disturbance, Kohut became interested early on in the development of the self. He came to view the creation of a coherent self as the goal of psychological development. Kohut believed that the self is basically interpersonal, and there can be no self, even in adulthood, without an interpersonal context. Furthermore, Kohut believed that each individual has a narcissistic line of development and that it is possible for this trajectory to become arrested. In more detail, Kohut believed that the self has four major components: the nuclear self (which is biologically present at birth), the virtual self (the parents' view of their baby), the grandiose self (the baby's view of self as the center of the universe), and the cohesive self (which effectively combines the nuclear and virtual selves). Kohut stated that when the child's *blissful union* with his or her mother is ruptured, the child introjects perfection or assigns it to the parent, with divergent consequences for later development. It is the responsibility of adult caregivers, Kohut felt, to help the child work through these developmental stages, and failure to do so leads to developmental arrest and problems later in life. However, Kohut made the point that small empathic failures between parent and child permit the child gradually to develop a sense of separation from the parent, a necessary step in the development of a sense of self.

Thus, Kohut believed that actual relationships create self-cohesion and self-esteem. He developed the idea of *selfobjects*, the functions that other people perform, such as mirroring and idealizing, to help the child to develop appropriately. Selfobjects are distinguished from other objects, in that selfobjects are experienced by the individual as part of the self. Selfobjects are to be found in a wide range of things and experiences, including the transference phenomenon, relatives, and physical objects. They give cohesion and harmony to the adult self and may include transitional objects, artists, sports figures, and politicians. Two selfobjects of particular interest are *mirroring selfobjects*, which confirm one's innate sense of vigor and perfection, and the *idealized parent imago*, into which one hopes to merge as an image of calmness, infallibility, and omnipotence. A third selfobject is that of *alter-ego/twinship*, which permits a more general identification with other people.

Kohut asserted that psychopathology results from a failure to develop strong selfobjects. He said that psychosis results from a complete lack of idealized selfobjects, while borderline disorder results from a fractured self, presumably due to inadequate selfobjects early in life, He said that narcissism results from the failure to integrate the grandiose self and idealized selfobject into the rest of self, resulting in loss of self-esteem.

With regard to treatment, Kohut defined a technique for conducting psychoanalysis with persons with narcissistic personality disturbance. This was important since Freud and later theorists, especially the ego psychologists, considered significantly narcissistic individuals to be unanalyzable (because they are presumably unable to develop a transference). Kohut suggested a focus on the fractured relationships between self and selfobjects, in the expectation that through strong (but inevitably imperfect) empathy the therapist can help the patient strengthen the self. The empathic therapist, according to Kohut, must engage in *vicarious introspection* and not focus on the therapist's position in the relationship. Kohut asserted that when therapists behave in a way that slightly lacks empathy (which he referred to as *optimal frustration*), the patient develops the ability to self-soothe.

Of interest, Kohut and Kernberg differ substantially in their understanding of pathological development, and their treatment recommendations also diverge. For example, Kohut views idealizing transference as a useful phenomenon, while Kernberg believes it is pathological. Thus, Kohut encourages the therapist to support the development of narcissistic impulses in the transference, while Kernberg confronts narcissistic themes in the hope of helping patients to integrate their fractured object relations.

Child Analysis and Developmental Theory

Earlier discussion in this text featured ego psychologist Anna Freud and object relations theorist Melanie Klein. Aside from their contributions to overall psychodynamic theory, it is appropriate to note that these two women pioneered the use of analytic techniques with children. We will not repeat their theoretical contributions here, as this has already been covered in detail. In the individual psychodynamic psychotherapies section of Chapter 5 we will say more about Anna Freud's and Melanie Klein's contributions to the treatment of children via play therapy.

A number of psychoanalysts have concluded that children's early attachment experiences are likely to have a crucial influence on later development. These workers have investigated the effects of successful and unsuccessful attachment early in life, and they have linked attachment to one's willingness to explore the world of objects and people. They have also connected it to the development of a sense of self. We briefly review the work of four theorists in this area.

Margaret S. Mahler (1897–1985)
Mahler was a Hungarian pediatrician who trained as a psychoanalyst in Vienna in the 1920s and 1930s. She eventually immigrated to Britain and then came to the United States in 1938, where she practiced for many years in New York. Mahler was particularly interested in developing a theory of *separation-individuation*. She concluded that children learn to view themselves as autonomous beings over the course of several phases of development between birth and the age of two. Of particular interest is the relationship between caregiver and child when the infant learns to crawl and begins to explore the physical world. As the child recognizes that he or she

is separate from the caregiver, anxiety ensues. At this point the caregiver must remain physically and emotionally available to the infant so that he or she does not fear abandonment. If the process goes well, the infant alternates between emotional closeness and independent exploration. Over the course of about a year, the child adapts to being separate from and yet emotionally connected to the caregiver. If the process goes awry, however, the child's anxiety may become more pervasive, and he or she may fail to internalize an image of the caregiver when they are separated.

John Bowlby (1907–1990)

An English physician whose psychoanalytic training was supervised by Melanie Klein, Bowlby devoted his career to the study of maternal deprivation and human attachment. While he recognized that both humans and infrahuman species demonstrate attachment behavior, probably as a survival tactic to protect them from predators, he was particularly interested to be able to show that successful human attachment predicts effective social behavior later in life, and unsuccessful attachment is likely to have an adverse effect on subsequent emotional and cognitive development. Bowlby believed that infants need *a secure base* from which to explore the world, and absent this, normal social and emotional development does not occur.

Mary D. S. Ainsworth (1913–1999)

Ainsworth was a developmental psychologist who was born in the United States but grew up in Canada and then subsequently worked in England and in the United States. A colleague of John Bowlby, Ainsworth completed important cross-cultural work in Africa as well. Ainsworth developed an experimental measure of attachment called the *strange situation*, in which a young child is observed playing in a room for about 20 minutes, during which time the child's caregiver and a stranger variously enter and leave the room. Ainsworth and others concluded from their work that children develop persistent attachment styles. If the child is *securely attached*, he or she obviously enjoys interacting with the caregiver, is eager to explore when the caregiver is present, and engages with the stranger when the caregiver is present but is otherwise wary of the stranger. The *anxious-resistant* child is reluctant to explore or to interact with the stranger and responds ambivalently when the caregiver returns. The *anxious-avoidant* child is also reluctant to explore and seems to make little distinction between the caregiver and the stranger. Finally, a child who demonstrates *disorganized attachment* may become anxious when the caregiver leaves but then either avoids the returning caregiver or alternately approaches and retreats from the caregiver.

Daniel N. Stern (1934–2012)

Stern was an American psychiatrist and psychoanalytic theorist who worked primarily in New York. He carefully tied the infant's developing sense of self to its interaction with the caregiver. Stern believed that when the infant is very young, the caregiver helps to regulate the infant's sense of self, which permits the baby to develop a sense of *core self*. This is followed by a sense of *core-self-with-another*, after which, when the infant reaches the age of about seven months, the caregiver begins to engage in *purposeful misattunements*, a phenomenon we discussed in connection with Kohut's self-psychology. These misattunements permit gradual estrangement from the caregiver, such that the infant develops a sense of *subjective self* without feeling painfully abandoned by the caregiver. Finally, with the onset of language around the age of 15 months, the child begins to develop a sense of *verbal self*, which enables the construction of a narrative about the self.

Current Trends in Psychodynamic Theory

Psychoanalysis has seen the passage of its first century, and it continues to evolve. Questions and insights from the object relations school, in particular, continue to fuel development in the field, and psychodynamic theorists continue to struggle to understand the concept of *self*, about which Freud had very little to say but subsequent writers, including particularly Kohut, have thought and written more extensively. There is continuing tension between *one-person* and *two-person* psychology, and the field has yet to agree upon the fundamental causes of psychological development. In this section we briefly explore the topics of intersubjectivity, relational approaches, and mentalization, newer iterations in psychodynamic thinking—and theories that address all of these unresolved issues.

Psychodynamic theorists have begun to focus on the individual's ability to understand self and others in terms of intentional mental states, such as needs, desires, and feelings. It is the view of these theorists that successful psychological functioning requires a minimum level of *psychological-mindedness*, which is defined as the recognition and efficient modulation of one's internal mental state. These theorists have suggested that awareness and acceptance of one's internal state is invariably correlated with empathy for the internal states of others. Moreover, they believe that certain early childhood experiences play a crucial role in the individual's ability to view self and others as full psychological beings.

Psychodynamic theorists who subscribe to the *intersubjective* perspective reject the tenets of *one-person psychology*, that human development results primarily from the organism's reaction to internal or external events. Instead, adherents of intersubjectivity firmly subscribe to a *two-person psychology*, according to which psychological functioning must be understood as an interaction between people or, equivalently, between different experiential worlds. Psychopathology is thought to occur when an individual has difficulty accurately understanding or representing a psychological self and other.

Another perspective on two-person psychology is *relational psychoanalysis*, a recent psychodynamic movement that draws on intersubjectivity theory and incorporates the ideas of Sándor Ferenczi, Harry Stack Sullivan, and Heinz Kohut, among others. Relational psychoanalysis focuses on the co-created nature, between analyst and patient, of the psychoanalytic experience and the data that arise within it. This approach, therefore, emphasizes the active role of countertransference as it contributes to this co-creation.

The development of an ability to understand self and others has been shown to depend in part on early *attachment* experiences. Human beings (and members of many other species) seek safety in social interactions, particularly during childhood, and they develop fairly consistent interpersonal relationship styles over the course of life. In the past several decades there has arisen a relatively new psychodynamic psychotherapy, called *mentalization-based treatment*, which takes as its premise the idea that psychological functioning must be understood interpersonally, that mental health rests upon the ability to understand empathically the intentional mental states of self and other, and that such empathy requires successful resolution of the attachment process.

Mentalization-based treatment was developed in large part by a Hungarian psychologist and psychoanalyst called Peter Fonagy (1952–), who has lived for many years in Britain. This treatment sets as its goal the enhancement of the patient's capacity to represent mentally the psychological states of self and other. It is thought that enhanced mentalization strengthens and stabilizes the patient's sense of self and improves relationship skills. This approach has been offered to individuals with borderline personality disorder, although there has also been some interest in applying mentalization theory to other populations, including individuals with posttraumatic stress disorder, eating disorders, and depression. We provide further detail about mentalization-based treatment for individuals with borderline personality disorder in the individual psychodynamic psychotherapies section of Chapter 5.

Summary

1. The structural theory is Freud's most important model. In it he described the mind as composed of three agents (id, ego, superego). Previously, in his topographic theory, he had posited that the mind consists of three systems (unconscious, preconscious, conscious).

2. Transference and countertransference are among the most important Freudian concepts. They are always present in psychotherapy because they are present in all human relationships. Analysis of the transference is an important psychodynamic technique.

3. Resistance is the psyche's tendency toward maintenance of the status quo. It is universally present and, therefore, an important factor all therapeutic interactions.

4. Anna Freud enumerated varieties of defense mechanisms. All are rooted in childhood and operate unconsciously. Defense analysis is a key technique for promoting insight in psychodynamic psychotherapy.

5. Object relations theory posits that psychological development depends heavily on the various mental relationships between one's image of oneself and one's image of significant others.

6. In Kohut's self psychology, psychological development is said to depend on the construction of a coherent self, which is largely accomplished with the use of selfobjects, functions other people perform to help the child develop appropriately.

7. Attachment theory describes an infant's need for a secure bond with the mother. Mary D. S. Ainsworth described four persistent attachment styles: secure, anxious-resistant, anxious-avoidant, and disorganized.

Psychological Theories and Psychotherapy

High-Yield Psychodynamic Topics

If this text is being used to prepare for standardized exams, the following psychodynamic topics represent particularly important material. The reader should review the listed content within the chapter.

1. Freudian terminology (italicized in text)
2. Freud's structural theory (id, ego, superego)
3. Defense mechanisms (listed and defined in text)
4. Erik H. Erikson's eight stages of development
5. Donald W. Winnicott's theory
6. Attachment theory, including Mary D. S. Ainsworth's attachment styles

The Evolution of Cognitive and Behavior Therapies

We now embark on a tour through the history of behavioral approaches to the treatment of mental illness. This history occurs in the same timeframe and runs parallel to the development of psychoanalysis, even though for many years there was such a difference in the language and ethos of behaviorism and psychoanalysis as to cause researchers and practitioners in the two schools largely to ignore one another. Now, after more than a century of development, behavioral interventions demonstrate increasing and rather dramatic effectiveness in helping psychiatric patients, as is best known in the case of cognitive-behavior therapy, initially developed by Aaron T. Beck (e.g., Beck, 1979). However, as important as cognitive-behavior therapy may be, there are many other successful variants of behavioral treatment, and we touch on them briefly in this section, returning in the individual behavior therapies section of Chapter 5 to examine them in more detail.

The history of behaviorism is often viewed as occurring in three waves. This may be a particularly apt metaphor, in that each new wave arises out of the last one. To help you keep track of the people mentioned in the text, we have listed them in Table 2.2.

Behaviorism: The First Wave

Researchers began laying the groundwork for the first wave of behavioral treatments for mental illness just before 1900, the year in which Freud published *The Interpretation of Dreams*. However, while psychoanalysis was always focused on understanding the unique experience of human beings, early behavior theory was mostly directed toward understanding how animals learned. In the 1890s the future Nobel Prize winner Russian physiologist Ivan P. Pavlov (1849–1936) discovered while researching canine digestion that over time dogs began to salivate in response to a previously neutral stimulus, such as a bell, that the animal had come to associate with food.

At about the same time the American psychologist Edward L. Thorndike (1874–1949) compiled detailed observations on how cats learned to escape from "puzzle boxes," small cages that required the animal to press a bar or pull a lever in order to escape. He determined that the pattern by which each cat learned to "solve" the puzzle box depended on the animal's particular sequence of successes and failures, and one cat didn't seem to benefit from watching another cat learn to escape from a similar puzzle box. Thorndike concluded that cats (and presumably humans) increased the frequency with which they performed behaviors that led to some kind of satisfaction, and they decreased the frequency of behaviors that led to dissatisfaction. He believed that cognitive mediation of learning (e.g., behavior change after observing the successes and failures of someone else) was not particularly important.

The experiments with Pavlov's dogs and Thorndike's cats gave rise to two important concepts in behavior theory: classical and operant conditioning. Any hungry dog will salivate in response to the smell of food. The unconditional response of salivating is more or less hardwired to the

Table 2.2 Prominent behavioral theorists and psychotherapists mentioned in the text.

First wave
Teodoro J. Ayllon (1929–)
Nathan H. Azrin (1930–2013)
O.H. Mowrer (1907–1982)
W.M. Mowrer (1907–1979)
Ivan P. Pavlov (1849–1936)
B.F. Skinner (1904–1990)
Edward L. Thorndike (1874–1949)
J.B. Watson (1878–1958)
Joseph Wolpe (1915–1997)

Second wave
Albert Bandura (1925–)
Aaron T. Beck (1921–)
Thomas J. D'Zurilla (1938–)
Albert Ellis (1913–2007)
Marvin R. Goldfried (1936–)
George Kelly (1905–1967)
Donald H. Meichenbaum (1940–)
Julian B. Rotter (1916–2014)
George Spivack (1927–)

Third wave
Steven C. Hayes (1948–)
Jon Kabat-Zinn (1944–)
Marsha M. Linehan (1943–)

unconditional stimulus of food aroma. However, when a neutral ("conditional") stimulus, like a bell, is consistently associated with the unconditional stimulus, after a while the dog begins to salivate in response to the bell. It is then said that the conditional stimulus (the bell) elicits a conditional response (salivation). Because a specific response has been conditioned, this is referred to as respondent conditioning—but its better-known name is *classical conditioning*.

Pavlov demonstrated the power of classical conditioning by, for example, chaining conditional stimuli together. Thus, he elicited a canine conditional response (salivation) to a black square after it had been consistently paired with the sound of a ticking metronome, which had itself been previously associated with the unconditional stimulus of food aroma. Such chained conditional stimuli were theoretically important, because they permitted behaviorists to understand how language might work. In essence, early behaviorists argued that people responded to words as conditional stimuli.

Operant conditioning differs from classical conditioning in that it has to do with the relationship between a behavior that acts (or "operates") on the environment and its associated reinforcement schedule. Thus, the frequency with which Thorndike's cats pressed bars or pulled levers in the puzzle box depended on their previous experience with the consequences of those behaviors. Later on, American psychologist B. F. Skinner (1904–1990) spent years working out the details of operant conditioning, experimenting extensively with animals such as rats and pigeons. In an attempt to extrapolate his findings to human beings, Skinner wrote *Walden Two* in 1948. In this book he sketched out how the principles of operant conditioning might be applied to human society, specifically arguing against the concept of free will. This created quite a stir at the time.

Importantly, the theories of classical and operant conditioning place little or no emphasis on an organism's awareness or understanding of the associated contingencies. Indeed, consistent with his belief that learning principles apply equally to humans and infrahuman species, Skinner derided the notion of "mentalism," the idea that one's behavior is guided by thoughts, perceptions, and emotions. Skinner viewed such unobserved experiences and motivations as epiphenomenal. Such a fervent rejection of cognitive mediation in understanding human behavior was typical of most first-wave behaviorists, going right back to Pavlov. The prominent early American behaviorist, psychologist J. B. Watson (1878–1958), went so far as to argue that such human attributes as personality, morality, and career choice are entirely due to one's environmental conditioning, and heredity plays no role. Such a position is referred to as *radical environmentalism*.

Before long the ideas of classical and operant conditioning were applied to the treatment of human behavior problems. In the mid-1930s a young married couple, the American psychologists O. H. Mowrer (1907–1982) and W. M. Mowrer (1907–1979), developed a classical conditioning scheme to treat nocturnal enuresis. A special pad was placed in the bed of an enuretic child. If the pad became wet, an alarm sounded and the child awakened. The unconditional stimulus (alarm) led to an unconditional response (awakening). Because the unconditional stimulus was closely associated with a conditional stimulus (sensation of a full bladder), soon the sensation of fullness began to trigger the conditional response of awakening *before* the alarm sounded, and the child was able to get to the bathroom in time.

A somewhat more sophisticated variant of classical conditioning, called *counterconditioning*, became a mainstay in the treatment of phobias. Systematic desensitization was developed by a South African psychiatrist called Joseph Wolpe (1915–1997). In it phobic individuals are taught to achieve a deep state of relaxation; they then pair this state with increasingly disturbing mental images of the phobic object—or, better yet, with decreasing physical distance from the phobic object itself. Counterconditioning is said to occur when patients learn a new conditional response (calmness) to the phobic object. Anxiety dissipates, and the phobia resolves.

By the 1960s psychologists Teodoro J. Ayllon (1929–) and Nathan H. Azrin (1930–2013) were applying operant conditioning principles in the treatment of regressed individuals living in institutions for the mentally ill and intellectually disabled. On selected wards they instituted carefully designed schedules to reinforce residents' grooming behaviors and their participation in various hospital "jobs." Wishing to make such a system practical on a hospital ward, they established a token economy, in which residents earned points for preferred behaviors and were later permitted to "cash in" their points for desirable items, ward privileges, and the like. This operant conditioning scheme was quite successful in modifying behavior in the hospital, but the improved behavior didn't generalize to environments with different reinforcement contingencies. Moreover, the researchers discovered that residents were most likely to modify their behavior in response to operant reinforcers when they were told ahead of time what the rules for dispensing the reinforcers would be.

Classical and operant conditioning were the primary constructs of behavior therapy well into the early 1970s. Often referred to as the first wave of behavior therapy, this approach to the treatment of mental disturbance largely ignored any cognitive mediation of behavior. Behaviorists in the first wave distrusted anything they couldn't easily count, and this led them to view the mind as a black box. They often ignored cognition and, like Skinner, believed that human suffering could be understood and treated solely by relying on observable behaviors. Some behaviorists went so far as to suggest that cognition itself actually reflected observable behaviors. For example, J. B. Watson, the American behaviorist (and later executive at the J. Walter Thompson advertising agency), believed that "thoughts" were actually a kind of subvocalization (i.e., essentially inaudible movements of the vocal cords; Watson, 1930). In its heyday even systematic desensitization was not thought to require any awareness or understanding of the effect of conditioning; cognition was considered to be entirely incidental to its success.

Behavior therapists in the first wave attempted to manage behaviors through positive reinforcement, negative reinforcement, extinction, and punishment (Fig. 2.3). *Positive reinforcement* increases the frequency of a target behavior by following it with a desirable consequence, such as was used in the token economy of Ayllon and Azrin. When ward residents groomed themselves or went to work off the ward, they received tokens that permitted them access to desirable items or ward privileges. *Negative reinforcement* (not to be confused with *punishment*) increases the frequency of a target behavior because the expected punishment does *not* occur. This mechanism underlies the behavioral treatment of obsessive-compulsive disorder, which is called exposure and response prevention; we discuss this in more detail in the individual behavior therapies section in Chapter 5. Briefly, the individual with obsessions or compulsions is encouraged to tolerate the feared thought or situation without engaging in mental or physical rituals meant to "neutralize" the threat. After doing this many times over, the individual comes to learn that the expected and greatly feared negative consequence does not occur, even in the absence of the neutralizing ritual. This leads to an increase in the frequency with which the feared thoughts and situations are simply tolerated.

Extinction works to decrease the frequency of a target behavior by withholding an expected positive reinforcer. For example, parents often ignore children when they misbehave, in the expectation that a child will decrease such misbehavior in order to avoid being deprived of the pleasure of parental attention and social interaction. However, careful observers have noticed that at some point following extinction trials the conditional stimulus may regain its ability to elicit the conditional response. This is referred

	Consequence delivered?	
	Yes	No
Positive (Valence of consequence)	Positive reinforcement: increases behavior frequency	Extinction: decreases behavior frequency
Negative (Valence of consequence)	Punishment: decreases behavior frequency	Negative reinforcement: increases behavior frequency

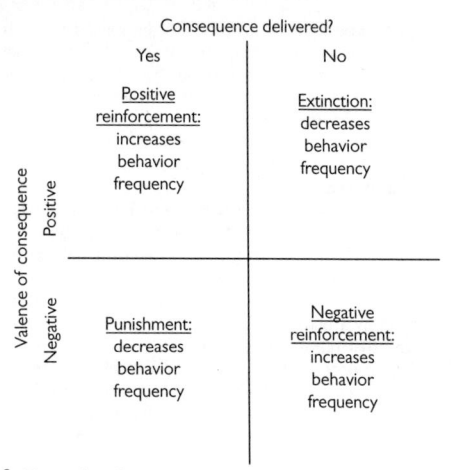

Figure 2.3. Types of reinforcement.

to as *spontaneous recovery*. Pavlov, for one, concluded that extinction only suppresses but does not eliminate conditional responses. However, most behavior therapists view extinction as a potent means to decrease the frequency of objectionable behavior. Finally, *punishment* decreases the frequency of a target behavior by following that behavior with an aversive consequence. While punishment as a psychotherapeutic mechanism is subject to ethical concerns, there is a history of employing it in the treatment of certain sexual behaviors and other addictions.

Behaviorists also discovered that some *reinforcement schedules* are more effective than others, even when utilized with the same class of reinforcement. A *fixed-interval* reinforcement schedule is one in which the individual receives a reinforcement after performing the target behavior only if a certain amount of time has passed since the last reinforcement was delivered. This is not a very efficient strategy, because the individual soon learns that nothing will happen as a result of emitting the target behavior until the time interval has passed. Spotty behavior change results. By contrast, a *variable-interval* or *intermittent reinforcement* schedule is one in which the individual is reinforced at varying time intervals for performing a target behavior. Sometimes the reinforcement is given and sometimes it isn't, and it is impossible to predict whether a reinforcement will occur the next time the behavior is emitted. This leads to very durable behavior change, because the individual does not interpret the absence of a reinforcer as evidence that the rules have changed; instead, the individual continues to emit the target behavior in anticipation of an eventual reinforcer.

There are other reinforcement schedules that have still other effects on behavior. In the *fixed-ratio* reinforcement schedule, the behavior is reinforced only after it is performed a fixed number of times. This may be what explains the persistence of nagging in some families. In the *variable-ratio* reinforcement schedule, the behavior is reinforced only after it is performed a certain number of times, but the number of required repetitions varies over time; the behavior might be reinforced the second time it is emitted, then the fifth time after that, then the third time, and so forth. Slot machines utilize variable-ratio reinforcement schedules and can be quite addictive.

Behaviorists select from among these types and schedules of reinforcement in order to increase or decrease the frequency of target behaviors. They may utilize *shaping* to increase the frequency of a complex behavior by reinforcing successive approximations of the behavior in question, moving in small steps from a behavior already in the individual's repertoire to the target behavior. Such shaping forms the basis for learning to play a musical instrument, for example, and it plays a major role in Applied Behavior Analysis, a therapeutic technique we review in the individual psychotherapies section of Chapter 5.

A final important behavioral concept focuses on the extent to which a newly acquired response *generalizes* to multiple stimuli or remains bound to a particular stimulus, as a consequence of *discrimination*. Behaviorists wish to ensure that specific behaviors are emitted only in appropriate settings and not at other times, and this requires that the organism discriminate correctly between target and non-target stimuli, so that the newly acquired response generalizes to one set of stimuli and not to another. To maintain the desired balance between discrimination and generalization, the behaviorist may reinforce the target response when it is emitted in response to many related stimuli, which decreases discrimination, or may reinforce only when it is emitted in response to very few, precisely defined stimuli, which increases discrimination.

In strong contrast to the psychodynamic theorists we discussed earlier, first-wave behaviorists didn't place emphasis on the development of a "theory of personality." They were content simply to discover the rules that control the acquisition, modification, and extinction of observable behaviors. Even so, most of the behavioral concepts we have described up to now have been presented in a way that implies awareness on the part of the individual regarding the contingency between stimulus and response. Although first-wave behaviorists took the position that such awareness was unnecessary, certainly human beings are acutely aware of their thoughts, and they work hard to figure out their environments. Most people subscribe to the proposition that their actions are strongly influenced by their aspirations, memories, and beliefs about the world.

The task of the second wave of behavior therapy was to incorporate mental phenomena into behavior therapy while maintaining its "scientific" ethos of measurement, replication, and falsifiability. This became possible only after researchers learned to measure cognitive phenomena in a reliable and useful way.

Behaviorism: The Second Wave

The science of cognitive measurement advanced, and over the course of several decades after World War II learning theorists began to add manifestly cognitive variables to learning theory. The Canadian psychologist Albert Bandura (1925–) developed *social-cognitive* theory, in which he argued that human beings, unlike Thorndike's solipsistic cats, frequently learn by observing others. He delineated four processes (attention, retention, motor reproduction, and motivation) that he believed were required for observational learning. Of course, the observer must pay *attention* to the model, and the level of attention might well depend on the observer's emotional connection to the model. Further, the observer must remember the modeled behavior, and such *retention* might occur in either imaginal or verbal form, each form having particular advantages and disadvantages. Bandura emphasized the quality of the observer's *motor reproduction processes*, and he made the sensible point that an observer can't demonstrate a new behavior without specific motor skills. Finally, Bandura emphasized the importance of the observer's *motivation*, which he thought was due to reinforcement contingencies. However, he made the point that in addition to *external* reinforcement, one might be *vicariously* reinforced, which occurs when the observer expects to be reinforced in the same way that the model was. Bandura also suggested that observers engage in *self-reinforcement* for learning new behaviors when they conclude that the new behavior will help them reach a standard or goal they have set for themselves.

Bandura thought that human beings strive to maximize *self-efficacy*, the belief that they can cope effectively with problems. For example, Bandura designed studies appearing to show that systematic desensitization worked by changing an individual's belief about his or her ability to deal effectively with the phobia. He thus suggested that systematic desensitization changes a person's willingness to touch a snake less through simple conditioning than through cognitive mediation ("I guess I can do it, after all").

At about the same time, American psychologist Julian B. Rotter (1916–2014) proposed a general theory of learning that included a different cognitive variable. According to Rotter, the probability that an individual will emit a target behavior in a given situation depends on the individual's subjective belief—a cognitive variable—about the consequences of the behavior and the desirability of those consequences. Thus, the likelihood that a person will touch a snake in the lab depends on the *expectancy* that certain consequences will occur and the reinforcement value of those consequences. In turn, the expectancy regarding relevant reinforcements depends on previous experience regarding the linkage between the behavior and the reinforcements in similar situations, which leads back to the idea of classical conditioning. Rotter's idea was that if one wishes to predict current behavior, it is more pertinent (and practical) to measure current expectancy rather than to assess an individual's past reinforcement history.

Bandura, Rotter, and other early cognitive theorists viewed cognitions as private behaviors that could nonetheless be reliably examined, counted, and manipulated. They believed that lawful relationships could be established between these covert behaviors and more easily observable overt behaviors. In other words, they set about to treat the mind as something other than a black box. However, it wasn't until the 1960s and 1970s that behavior therapists like Albert Ellis (1913–2007) and Aaron T. Beck (1921–) identified which cognitions had to be modified in order to alleviate emotional distress, and they began to develop methods to modify those cognitions. Their approaches to psychotherapy became known as cognitive-behavioral therapies, because they advocated the examination and modification of not only overt behaviors but also cognitions.

The American psychologist Albert Ellis developed an approach to psychotherapy that he eventually called rational-emotive behavior therapy (REBT). In common with virtually all second-wave behaviorists, Ellis believed that cognitions intervened between external situations and emotional consequences. He offered an A-B-C model of emotional disturbance: *activating* events trigger *beliefs* about those events, resulting in emotional *consequences*. Actually, the A-B-C model was not inconsistent with his earlier training in psychoanalysis. Ellis concluded that when people rigidly adhere to certain kinds of beliefs, called "demands," they suffer adverse emotional consequences. Demands are extreme ideas about how the world should or must be. For example, a person might believe that others should always treat the person in a certain way, that the person's life ought to follow a certain course, or that he or she must never feel anxious or upset. Rigid adherence to beliefs in the face of an activating event that is inconsistent with the beliefs (e.g., a bad grade in school) will feel extremely uncomfortable and the person will have a hard time responding effectively because of an unwillingness to acknowledge the event in the first place ("I *can't* have earned a bad grade. There must be a mistake!").

From within a relatively small universe of irrational beliefs the REBT therapist chooses one or two that seem to cause the patient the most trouble. The therapist then sets out to help the patient modify the irrational beliefs, either by adopting more useful beliefs or by learning to hold the irrational beliefs more tentatively. In working to modify irrational beliefs, Ellis utilized a variety of methods, including direct disputation, emotional release, and behavioral tasks, such as decreasing avoidance of certain situations. Unfortunately, few studies demonstrating the effectiveness of REBT are well designed and/or part of an ongoing program of research, and this has limited the popularity of REBT. Indeed, REBT has been somewhat overshadowed by the next second-wave theory we discuss, the cognitive-behavior therapy of Aaron T. Beck. In contrast to REBT, Beck's cognitive-behavior therapy has generated very many well-designed research studies.

Beck is an American psychiatrist who during childhood experienced an episode of depressed mood. Years later, after he completed psychoanalytic training, Beck set out to prove the Freudian hypothesis that depression results from anger turned inward. Rather to his surprise, he was unable to find consistent evidence for this in the dreams and free association of depressed patients. Instead, he began to notice that depressed patients had streams of barely recognized *automatic negative thoughts* about themselves, the world, and their future. Beck concluded that these automatic negative thoughts lacked accuracy or utility—or both. He further noticed that when patients stopped interpreting their experience based on the automatic negative thoughts and began to view the world in a less biased manner, their depressive symptoms remitted. He recognized that this was consistent with his own experience in overcoming depressed mood in his youth.

Like Ellis, Beck concluded that symptoms of mental disturbance come about as a result of people's ineffective or incorrect beliefs about the meaning of their experiences, and he proposed to modify such problematic cognitions directly, in the expectation that this would lead to symptom relief. Unlike Ellis, Beck recommended starting treatment at the more superficial level of automatic negative thoughts, rather than to proceed directly to the underlying core beliefs. Over time, he identified a variety of cognitive and behavioral approaches to help patients respond more effectively to their experiences. Beck recommended that, working together, therapists and patients isolate specific problematic thoughts and the underlying substructure of beliefs, and he offered a structured way to change them. He also urged patients to conduct *behavioral experiments* in their everyday lives to help them evaluate the accuracy and utility of their beliefs. Moreover, he encouraged patients to behave in a manner that was inconsistent with the continuation of their emotional disturbance. For example, he urged passive, depressed individuals to become more physically active. Beck and his collaborators modified some of the details of his theory in order to apply it to conditions other than depression, and at present there are cognitive therapy approaches to many psychiatric disturbances, including various mood disorders, anxiety disorders, psychoses, eating disorders, substance abuse, and personality disorders, among other conditions. Indeed, Beck's theoretical net of constructs aimed at understanding the development and maintenance of psychopathology is sufficiently complex that it permits the description and explanation of most symptoms of mental disturbance. Beck and his followers have produced a large corpus of sophisticated research to support his theory of psychopathology and psychotherapeutic treatment, and at present his approach to psychotherapy is widely practiced.

While Ellis and Beck are by far the most important second-wave behavior theorists, there were other individuals of note during this period. American psychologist Donald H. Meichenbaum (1940–) concluded that some individuals demonstrated disordered behaviors because they hadn't learned to "talk themselves through" complex behavioral sequences. He developed a way of teaching people to utilize self-talk to implement more effective behaviors, with goals like decreasing impulsivity and aggression, managing mood, and learning to deal with chronic pain. Several American psychologists, including particularly George Spivack (1927–), Marvin R. Goldfried (1936–), and Thomas J. D'Zurilla (1938–), have developed ways of teaching children and adults to solve problems more efficiently, in the expectation that this would decrease symptoms of emotional distress.

Finally, American psychologist George Kelly (1905–1967) proposed a novel theory of psychopathology, called Personal Construct Theory, of which the central postulate is that a person's psychological organization depends on how he or she anticipates the future. Kelly's idea of *constructive alternativism* was that people construct their views of the world from among a number of choices. He believed that psychopathology always resulted from the persistent use of specific constructs despite their consistent invalidation in the world. For example, an individual might view normal self-assertion as a personally unacceptable form of aggression toward others. However, over time this same individual might become aware of feeling helpless to prevent inconsiderate treatment in many kinds of relationships. Kelly offered the view that the two main goals of psychotherapy are to help patients to understand the particular constructs on which they rely and to provide them assistance in modifying ineffective or outmoded constructs, so as to permit more effective functioning in the world. Kelly suggested specific techniques to help patients apply particular constructs either more or less broadly in their lives, and he encouraged therapists to modify constructs by adding or withdrawing certain features from them. Among other techniques, he suggested that the psychotherapist clarify the patient's expectations or beliefs about the world and then offer a set of modified beliefs with the encouragement that the patient try behaving for a couple of weeks as if he or she subscribed to the altered belief system. Of course, the patient must find the new beliefs to be plausible—they cannot reflect a completely new way of looking at the world. Kelly expected that if patients are reinforced in daily life for behaving in a new way, they will be likely to alter the fundamental constructs they use to guide their behavior in the world.

In recent decades behavioral treatments in the second wave have proven to be very successful in providing relief for a broad range of psychopathology. In large studies these treatments have often shown themselves to be as effective as somatic interventions in the treatment of disorders like anxiety and depression. They have even helped to ameliorate symptoms of bipolar disorder and schizophrenia as an adjunct to psychotropic medications.

However, some have argued that second-wave behavior therapy is limited by its focus on modifying cognitions. In certain conditions, such as some anxiety disorders, it is not particularly helpful to dispute and modify every single worry, in the expectation that this will permit one to cope more effectively with reality. Rather, it may be more useful to work toward a change in how one views the meaning and very nature of one's thoughts. A more helpful approach to treatment might be to teach patients that thoughts are transient mental phenomena, and some of them have little to do with external reality. This is the idea that if one simply doesn't become engaged with certain thoughts, the thoughts will naturally dissipate. Such a philosophy forms the foundation of the third wave of behavior therapy.

Behaviorism: The Third Wave

In recent decades Buddhist and other meditation practices have become increasingly popular in the West, leading to its ultimate incorporation into medical care by healthcare providers. Meditation practice can lead to two key insights. First, mental phenomena (like all phenomena) are fundamentally transient. Second, one can learn in a systematic way to control the direction of one's attention. The third wave of behavior therapy capitalizes on these insights, and it is certainly no coincidence that virtually all of the major theorists in behavior therapy's third wave have had extensive meditation experience. Nor is one surprised to find that meditation practice is a component of many third-wave treatments, even if there are some recent data to suggest that meditation practice itself might be an incidental component of third-wave treatments (e.g., Vettese, Toneatto, Stea, Nguyen, & Wang, 2009; but cf. Williams et al., 2014).

Patients in third-wave behavioral treatments are helped to establish a new relationship with mental phenomena. While some symptoms need to be changed or relieved, in other cases it may be more helpful to learn to think differently about one's symptoms, to wait them out, or to stop reacting to them as one has in the past. For example, one might suggest to an individual with chronic, relapsing depression that sad thoughts come and go, and one has the choice of engaging with the thoughts (and feeling worse) or simply letting them pass. Some people grasp this idea directly, but others remain skeptical, and meditation practice can provide immediate evidence that mental phenomena do really behave in this way. As well, meditators learn to control the direction of their thoughts and are thus better able to choose how and what to think. Moreover, through meditation practice one decreases one's autonomic arousal quickly and efficiently.

Third-wave behavioral treatments are proliferating rapidly. We mention below several well-known variants and will discuss a few of them at greater length in Chapter 5, in the sections on individual behavior therapies and psychotherapy for multiple patients.

American psychologist Marsha M. Linehan (1943–) has developed an intensive, multimodal approach to the treatment of self-injury in borderline personality disorder. Linehan's dialectical behavior therapy (DBT) combines a wide range of standard cognitive-behavioral strategies with techniques to help individuals develop better awareness of their thoughts and feelings, in the hope that they can learn to become less reactive to their shifting and often contradictory impulses. In certain situations patients are encouraged to experience and accept emotional upheaval, to recognize that it will pass, and to divert their attention elsewhere, rather than to analyze each thought, correct logical errors, and develop a coherent plan of action. As well, patients are encouraged to abandon "either-or" views, so that they develop a more integrated view of self, including both emotion and rationality, and they come to accept themselves in the present while acknowledging the need to change, reflecting the *dialectical* part of DBT. In early versions of DBT Linehan asked patients to engage in formal meditation practice, but this was not successful, and the current version of DBT attempts to teach the "wisdom" of meditation without expecting patients to practice meditation on a regular basis.

Another American psychologist, Jon Kabat-Zinn (1944–), has developed a manualized, group-based, time-limited psychotherapeutic treatment called mindfulness-based stress reduction. Designed specifically to help people learn to cope with chronic pain, this treatment combines extensive meditation practice with discussion of stress and coping techniques. The goal is to teach participants to observe themselves in an alert, nonjudgmental way. Early studies suggest that the treatment may also help individuals who have anxiety-spectrum or mood disorders. A very similar treatment package, called mindfulness-based cognitive therapy (MBCT), was developed by some British and Canadian psychologists to treat recurrent depression. MBCT is also a manualized, group-based, time-limited psychotherapeutic treatment that combines extensive meditation practice with encouragement to learn to view one's thoughts and feelings in a decentered manner. For example, participants are encouraged to think about depressive thoughts as *thoughts*, rather than as a reflection of reality. MBCT also includes discussion of how to prevent relapse and recurrence. There have been solid research findings showing that MBCT plus treatment as usual is more effective in preventing depression relapse than treatment as usual alone, but this is only the case for individuals who have had at least three previous episodes of major depression; the finding doesn't appear to extend to those who have had just one or two previous episodes. We discuss MBCT in more detail near the end of Chapter 5.

Another important third-wave treatment is called acceptance and commitment therapy (ACT). Developed by American psychologist Steven C. Hayes (1948–), ACT aims to teach patients to view their thoughts in a "defused" manner. For example, rather than responding to anxiety-inducing thoughts as evidence of potential danger, patients are encouraged to think, "I'm having the thought that I'm anxious." Patients are encouraged to clarify their goals and values in life and to act in furtherance of them, rather than to respond to thoughts that may get in the way. This focus on goals and values is one way in which ACT differs from many other psychotherapeutic techniques. At the end of successful treatment, the ACT patient *accepts* troubling thoughts and feelings as transient mental phenomena while remaining *committed* to pursuing the goals and values that make life worthwhile. Like DBT, ACT de-emphasizes formal meditation practice but aims to teach patients some of the lessons of meditation, including the ability to direct one's attention as one wishes and the fact that thoughts are just thoughts and don't necessarily reflect some sort of external reality.

Summary

1. The first-wave behaviorists ignored cognition and focused primarily on how observable behavior can be learned or unlearned. They identified types of conditioning (classical, operant) and reinforcement schedules, and they developed such treatment techniques as the token economy and systematic desensitization. Therapeutic targets of change during this period include only observable behaviors.

2. Second-wave behaviorists incorporated a cognitive variable, which ultimately gave rise to various "cognitive" therapies, such as rational emotive behavior therapy, cognitive-behavior therapy, and various problem-solving techniques. Therapeutic targets of change during this period include observable behaviors and discrete cognitions.

3. Third-wave behaviorists are interested in the use of attention to manage symptoms. This has led to the development of such treatments as dialectical behavior therapy, mindfulness-based stress reduction, mindfulness-based cognitive therapy, and acceptance and commitment therapy. Therapeutic targets of change during this period include observable behaviors, discrete cognitions, and the patient's *relationship* with symptoms.

Recommended Reading

Akhtar, S. (2009). *Comprehensive dictionary of psychoanalysis*. London, England: Karnac Books.
Craske, M.G. (2010). *Cognitive behavioral therapy (Theories of psychotherapy)*. Washington, DC: American Psychological Association.
Freud, S., & Gay, P. (1995). *The Freud reader*. New York: W.W. Norton & Co.
Gay, P. (2006). *Freud: A life for our time*. New York: W.W. Norton & Co.

Chapter 3

Toward an Integrated Understanding of Psychotherapy: Useful Perspectives

Neurobiological Correlates of Psychological Theory
 and Psychotherapy 74
  Neuroplasticity and Four Key Phenomena 74
  Neurobiology and the Psychotherapy of Depression 78
  Neurobiology and the Psychotherapy of PTSD 80
  Summary 82
Research Findings in Psychology 84
  What Do We Know About the Rate of Recovery in
    Psychotherapy? 84
  In General, How Does Psychotherapy Work? 92
Research Findings from Treatment Studies 100
  Efficacy vs. Effectiveness 100
  Monotherapy vs. Combined Treatment 100
  Continuation and Maintenance Psychotherapy 103
  Bringing a Psychotherapeutic Understanding to
    Pharmacotherapy 105
Psychotherapy Within Psychiatry: Narrowing Indications and
  Broadening Options 108

Psychological Theories and Psychotherapy

In the previous chapter we reviewed the psychological theories that serve as foundations for much of psychotherapy. We now summarize three areas of research that offer alternative perspectives contributing to our understanding of psychotherapy. We discuss here the neurobiological correlates of psychological theory and psychotherapy, relevant research findings from psychology, and some of the results of treatment studies. We close this chapter by offering a few thoughts on how psychiatrists and therapists might sort through this welter of information to develop a holistic understanding of psychotherapy.

3 TOWARD INTEGRATION: USEFUL PERSPECTIVES

Neurobiological Correlates of Psychological Theory and Psychotherapy

Some individuals conceptualize the mind and brain as separate entities, as if there were a fundamental separation between them. However, neuroscience research demonstrates that the brain changes as a consequence of both somatic treatment and psychotherapies. In this section of the book we briefly direct our attention to the neurobiology of psychotherapy. We begin our exploration of this topic by making reference to the concept of neuroplasticity. We then consider four psychological variables of interest: memory, attention, learning, and attachment. Finally, we review some neurobiological features of two common mental disorders, depression and posttraumatic stress disorder (PTSD), and we offer some suggestions about how to view the psychotherapy of each condition from a neurobiological perspective. As you read through this information, consider how the development and formation of learning, memory, attention, and attachment affect theoretical observations and the practice of psychotherapy.

Neuroplasticity and Four Key Phenomena

The concept of neuroplasticity serves as a bridge between the fields of neurobiology and psychotherapy. It has long been understood that humans and infrahuman species depend on synaptic and nonsynaptic plasticity to permit them to respond to changed environmental circumstances. Without the ability to modulate both neuronal potentiation and the probability of synaptic transmission, no living thing could respond to environmental changes.

However, it is only in the past four decades that there has been increasing awareness that neurogenesis and cortical mapping can occur following the critical period of human development. At present, there is general agreement that cortical remapping can occur following brain injury at any time in a person's life and that the formation of new neurons occurs across the lifespan in particular subcortical areas of the brain, including the hippocampus, the olfactory bulb, and probably the cerebellum. At some point we may learn that neurogenesis occurs in other subcortical areas as well. The important point is that neuroplasticity is a frequent and natural phenomenon, and it occurs in response to routine human activity, quite apart from somatic interventions in response to illness. In particular, it occurs as a consequence of participation in psychotherapy.

Having identified the bridging concept of neuroplasticity, we are now in a position to consider the psychotherapeutic implications of four psychological constructs: learning, memory, attention, and attachment.

Learning

We have previously discussed *learning* at some length. Of course, learning involves the acquisition, modification, or strengthening of thoughts, feelings, and behavior. Inasmuch as problematic thoughts, feelings, and behaviors are the stuff of psychotherapy, this treatment technique involves a great deal of learning. For example, clinicians provide patients information about their conditions, they teach them new skills (e.g., self-assertion and problem-solving techniques), and they expose patients to circumstances that are designed to help them *unlearn* previous associations (e.g., phobic responses in anxiety disorders). At the neurobiological level learning occurs as a direct result of neuroplasticity, usually but not always in the form of synaptic plasticity. Psychotherapeutic interventions are designed to maximize the likelihood of such neuroplasticity, including through the establishment of an optimal atmosphere for learning, a point to which we will return.

Memory
We think of *memory* as the process of encoding, storing, and retrieving information. Since there can be no memory without learning and no learning without memory, these two concepts cannot be fully disambiguated. There is some dispute about the taxonomy of memory. In addition to the categorization of memory by duration (how long one has held a memory) and modality (whether it is in the auditory, visual, or some other domain), a particularly important distinction has to do with whether one is aware of a memory. We refer to *explicit memory*, also called declarative memory, as the kind of memory that can be called into awareness with effort. Explicit memory includes the recall of personal experiences and memory for general facts and concepts. *Implicit memory* refers to traces of previous experience of which one is not aware, even though the traces affect one's performance on a task. Implicit memory may involve *priming*, in which one is more likely to act in a certain way based on previous experience, even though one is not now (and may never have been) conscious of the earlier event. Priming is the reason you choose a particular brand at the store after seeing an ad for it, even though you have no recall of having ever seen the ad. Another kind of implicit memory is *procedural memory*, which supports the skills one can accomplish without thinking about them, such as taking a shower or riding a bicycle.

Memory plays a central role in the development of many psychiatric disorders—and, correspondingly, in their treatment. Decontextualized memory of trauma (i.e., a faulty explicit memory) sets the stage for the development of PTSD. Implicit memory is a key component in the development of mood, anxiety, and personality disorders, among other conditions. Individuals with these disorders hold assumptions that lack utility, such as that the world is a dangerous place, that one won't be able to respond effectively to an unexpected challenge, that other people are uncaring or can't be trusted, that one's efforts will accomplish little, and on and on. Such assumptions can be viewed as implicit memories, and much of the work of psychotherapy consists of modifying these implicit memories, with the goal that patients think and act differently in response to new procedural memories and priming—or in response to now-explicit memories. In psychotherapy implicit memories are often changed by bringing them into awareness and then examining them, thus creating explicit memories. Alternatively, in some models of psychotherapy therapists simply challenge patients by pointing to evidence that is inconsistent with the patient's ineffective beliefs about the world.

Newly acquired information is initially held in *working memory* for up to 30 seconds, either in a phonological loop, on a visual-spatial sketchpad, or in an episodic buffer. It is thought that working memory is largely dependent on a circuit involving the prefrontal and parietal cortices (Baddeley, 2000). Acute or chronic stress is known to lead to reduced activation of the prefrontal cortex and decreased functional connectivity, with negative consequences for working memory—and learning, which crucially depends on working memory.

After leaving working memory, newly forming explicit memories undergo *synaptic consolidation* in the hippocampus, for which the best understood underlying process is long-term potentiation, a neuroplastic phenomenon of enhanced signal transmission between neurons resulting from repeated simultaneous stimulation. The precise sequence of chemical events giving rise to long-term potentiation depends to some extent on where it occurs in the brain. It can become well established within minutes to under an hour, while synaptic consolidation is generally thought to be complete within several hours. Of particular significance is the fact that since the basolateral region of the amygdala projects into the hippocampus, stress hormones affecting the amygdala may increase or decrease the strength of a memory. The presence of abnormal concentrations of neurotransmitters in the synaptic cleft may also affect synaptic consolidation.

For about a week after synaptic consolidation, recall of an explicit memory depends entirely on the presence of an intact hippocampus. However, we mentioned earlier that the hippocampus is one brain region in which neurogenesis is known to occur throughout life. It demonstrates a very high level of neuroplasticity and is therefore particularly well suited for *encoding* new memories, but it is not necessarily as well suited for *retaining* memories. Through the phenomenon of *systems consolidation* many memories are ultimately stored elsewhere in the brain, thus "freeing up" capacity in the hippocampus for new memory encoding. Systems consolidation, which occurs over years or decades, moves explicit memories from the hippocampus to the cortex. The hippocampus is thought to facilitate the process by which partial representations of a specific memory retained at modality-appropriate locations in the cortex are gradually connected with increasing strength to one another. Over time, the various representations of a memory in cortex become so strongly connected that recall becomes possible without mediation by the hippocampus. However, some have argued that memory of personal experiences always requires hippocampus involvement, while memory for general facts and concepts does not.

The details of implicit memory consolidation are less well understood. These memories do not appear to be consolidated in the hippocampus, as would be consistent with the fact that amnestic individuals can learn new motor tasks and are susceptible to priming. Consolidation of procedural memories, in particular, may occur in the extrapyramidal motor system (Squire, 1986); Levin (2011) suggests that implicit memory consolidates in the cerebellum, basal ganglia, and amygdala.

A final aspect of memory that has relevance for psychotherapy is the concept of *memory reconsolidation*. This is the phenomenon by which well-established memories can be strengthened or altered after they are called up. It is thought that the recall of a memory decreases its stability, and in the reconsolidation process it may be changed somewhat. This may be the mechanism by which memories change over time. Reconsolidation is thought to be a process that is distinct from consolidation and also from processes such as extinction, which we previously described as occurring when an expected consequence does not follow a stimulus, thus weakening the link between stimulus and consequence.

Attention

It is difficult to offer a comprehensive definition of the concept of *attention*. As we use the term here, we refer to the ability to sustain one's focus on the target of one's choice. When individuals are able to attend well, they have the capacity to select a target on which to focus, notwithstanding the high salience of other targets, they can martial their resources to focus on only that target, and they are able to maintain their focus without becoming unduly distracted by internal or external stimuli. If we think of disordered attention as an inability to sustain one's focus as one wishes, it becomes evident that attention plays a major role in the development and maintenance of psychopathology. Conditions that are associated with disordered attention include attention-deficit/hyperactivity disorder, obsessive-compulsive disorder, various anxiety and mood disorders that involve rumination, and many others.

As defined above, attention requires intact executive processes in the brain, thus implicating the dorsolateral prefrontal cortex, the anterior cingulate cortex, and the orbitofrontal cortex. A variety of subcortical areas are also involved in the function of attention, as has been demonstrated in imaging studies with individuals who have sustained closed head injuries. Another source of neurobiological data regarding attention comes from studies of meditation training. Meditation training, of particular interest to third-wave behaviorists, consists of the practice of sustaining one's attention in either a focused or open manner. In their review of five mindfulness meditation studies comprising 57 participants, Chiesa, Brambilla, and Serretti (2010) showed that such "open" meditation training corresponded to fMRI evidence of increased prefrontal cortex and anterior cingulate cortex activation.

Attachment

We discuss the concept of attachment on several occasions in this text. As we will describe in more detail in a subsequent section, *attachment* in adults can be thought of as a plane described by the orthogonal axes of seeking/avoiding intimacy and expecting acceptance/rejection by others. Securely attached individuals are those who usually seek intimacy and expect acceptance. Attachment patterns are thought to be established in early childhood, and they are felt to be predictors of behavior over the course of life.

In a review of the literature Mikulincer and Shaver (2007) concluded that insecure attachment is associated with the full range of mental disorders, including mood and anxiety disorders, personality disorders, and many others. However, they cautioned that insecure attachment might not be a sufficient explanation for most psychiatric disturbances, which also depend on other factors, such as genetic predisposition and life experiences unrelated to early attachment.

There is evidence from brain imaging studies that individuals with disordered attachment patterns (fear of rejection, avoidance of intimacy, or both) demonstrate atypical prefrontal cortex activation in response to social or emotional arousal (Lenzi et al., 2013; Vrtička, Bondolfi, Sander, & Vuilleumier, 2012; Warren et al., 2010). By contrast three recent studies have demonstrated that the introduction of attachment cues increases prefrontal activation and/or cortico-limbic integration among healthy children, adolescents, and adults (Eisenberger et al., 2011; Karremans, Heslenfeld, van Dillen, & Van Lange, 2011; Tottenham, Shapiro, Telzer, & Humphreys, 2012).

There are several findings regarding the relationship between attachment and psychotherapy. We explain in a later section of the text that insecurely attached patients establish weaker therapeutic alliances than securely attached patients, and anxious attachment (i.e., the expectation of rejection) predicts to poor outcome from treatment. Moreover, in a large study comparing the relative effects of cognitive-behavior therapy (CBT), interpersonal therapy, imipramine, and case management in the treatment of depression, patients' appraisals early in treatment of therapists as sensitive and supportive predicted positively to outcome at the end of treatment and at 18-month follow-up, regardless of treatment type, patient characteristics, or severity of depression (Zuroff & Blatt, 2006). As well, Buchheim and colleagues (2012) demonstrated decreased cortico-limbic reactivity to attachment-related cues following 15 months of psychodynamic psychotherapy with depressed outpatients.

Thus, we see that disordered attachment patterns are correlated with the presence of psychopathology, and they predict negatively to several variables of interest in psychotherapy. Disordered attachment is also associated with inefficient prefrontal cortex response to social and emotional challenges, while attachment cuing among healthy people increases prefrontal activation and/or cortico-limbic integration. Brain correlates of poor attachment improve following a course of psychodynamic psychotherapy. One final correlate of interest is the suggestion by several researchers (e.g., Kandel, 1999) that attachment failures decrease learning and memory in humans and other species due to inefficient long-term potentiation. Taken together, these inferences provide a basis for the suggestion that more secure attachment in the course of psychotherapy might be correlated with increased cortico-limbic integration and, as a result, improved learning and memory.

Neurobiology and the Psychotherapy of Depression

The concepts of neuroplasticity, learning, memory, attention, and attachment permit us to make more sense of what is known about the treatment of depression from a neurobiological perspective. A series of papers have identified abnormalities in cortico-limbic pathways among individuals who are depressed. In a 2012 meta-analysis of ten brain imaging studies Sacher and colleagues found that, relative to normal controls, individuals with unipolar depression have decreased gray matter volume in the amygdala, dorsomedial frontal cortex, and right paracingulate cortex, together with increased resting glucose metabolism in the right subgenual and pregenual anterior cingulate cortices.

Other studies have shown corresponding changes as a consequence of successful pharmacological or psychotherapeutic treatment for depression. In the most rigorous such study to date, Kennedy and colleagues (2007) investigated the response to treatment of 24 individuals diagnosed with major depressive disorder. Study participants were randomly assigned to 16 weeks of treatment with either CBT or venlafaxine. PET scan changes in the group of 7 participants who responded to CBT were compared with changes in the group of 9 individuals who responded to venlafaxine. In short, PET scan changes following successful depression treatment demonstrated similarities but also some differences between CBT and venlafaxine treatment. More specifically, between pretreatment and posttreatment both groups demonstrated decreased metabolism in the left and right orbital frontal cortex and the left dorsomedial prefrontal cortex, together with increased metabolism in the right inferior occipital cortex. However, venlafaxine responders had increased metabolism in the posterior cingulate, while CBT responders showed decreased metabolism in that area. In the left inferior temporal cortex venlafaxine responders showed decreased metabolism, while CBT responders showed increased metabolism. CBT responders showed decreased metabolism in the thalamus and increased metabolism in a region encompassing the anterior portion of the subgenual cingulate/ventromedial frontal cortex and in the right occipital-temporal cortex. Venlafaxine responders showed decreased metabolism in the right nucleus accumbens and in a posterior portion of the subgenual cingulate.

This study and others have demonstrated fairly consistent modulation of cortico-limbic pathways following CBT applied to depression, while changes following psychopharmacological treatment of depression appear to depend somewhat on the particular drug used. Clark and Beck (2010) proposed that CBT applied to depression causes "top-down" effects, in the sense that increased executive control inhibits limbic reactivity, and they contrasted this with "bottom-up" control of the limbic system itself. As we have noted, Chiesa and colleagues (2010) showed that meditation training may also increase cortical control over the limbic system. As well, in the previously cited psychodynamic treatment study by Buchheim and colleagues (2012), depressed outpatients demonstrated decreased cortico-limbic reactivity in response to attachment cuing following 15 months of treatment, while healthy, untreated controls did not show such changes over the same time course.

Why might previously depressed individuals experience an increase in prefrontal control over the limbic system following a course of psychotherapy? Virtually all models of psychotherapy involve teaching patients, directly or indirectly, new ways to manage depressive affect. Treatment inevitably involves paying careful attention to thoughts and feelings, which requires that patients sharpen their attentional skills, and psychotherapists strive to relate to patients in a warm, supportive, encouraging manner. As well, we will review in a later section the finding that psychotherapy appears to have a better outcome if there are at least minor ruptures over the course of treatment, assuming that these are skillfully addressed by the therapist. Many depressed patients, particularly those who are insecurely attached, have had few experiences working through relationship conflicts in a satisfying way, and the experience of doing so in psychotherapy might well decrease attachment anxiety and avoidance. As we have suggested, when patients feel a strong sense of attachment to the therapist, they are more likely to be able to learn efficiently. Moreover, the reduction of stress is likely to optimize working memory, which permits greater learning and, ultimately, memory. Finally, psychotherapy often involves a shift of troubling material from implicit to explicit memory. This permits patients to act in the world with greater intention and not to be so much in the thrall of ineffective ideas and beliefs.

In short, psychotherapy for depression establishes optimal conditions for patients to learn how to attend appropriately and to respond more effectively to painful affect, all of which strengthens prefrontal functioning. On its face, such a route to improved mood would seem to differ from the effect of psychopharmacological treatment. It is therefore not surprising that there are differences in brain imaging studies of depressed patients following successful treatment with either psychotherapy or psychotropic drugs. However, some commentators have pointed out that the rather limited neurobiological data now available are insufficient to permit firm conclusions regarding the contrasting effects of psychotherapy and pharmacotherapy. For example, Zellner (2012) points out that varying levels of activity within particular brain regions might reflect either generation or suppression of negative affect and/or cognitions. Thus, while there appears to be some overlap in the brain regions affected by psychotherapy and pharmacotherapy, it isn't yet clear whether research data will consistently support the elegant model that psychotherapy operates primarily on "top-down" processes by increasing the efficacy of prefrontal cortex in suppressing limbic reactivity, while pharmacotherapy operates primarily on "bottom-up" processes by directly decreasing limbic reactivity.

Neurobiology and the Psychotherapy of PTSD

In this section we review some studies relevant to the treatment of PTSD and attempt to make sense of the neurobiological findings from the perspective of neuroplasticity and related concepts. However, we note at the outset that all the studies we cite relied on DSM-IV diagnostic criteria, and the diagnosis of PTSD changed in the transition from DSM-IV to DSM-5. The diagnosis no longer requires that the person's response to the trauma have involved "intense fear, helplessness, or horror," and it excludes trauma due to unexpected deaths from natural causes. Some of the other criteria have been reorganized, and additional symptoms have been identified. Finally, changes have been made in the way that PTSD can be diagnosed in children and adolescents. It is possible that the findings of studies we cite in this section might have been different if the newer criteria had been used.

Brain imaging studies have consistently demonstrated decreased hippocampal volume in individuals diagnosed with PTSD. There is evidence that exposure to trauma accounts for some of this volume reduction. However, depending on brain scan methodology, either right or left hippocampal volume is decreased in individuals with PTSD when compared with the hippocampal volume in individuals exposed to trauma who did not develop PTSD (Kühn & Gallinat, 2013; Woon, Sood, & Hedges, 2010). Additionally, Gulf War veterans currently diagnosed with PTSD had smaller hippocampi than veterans with remitted PTSD (Apfel et al., 2011). It is unclear whether smaller hippocampal volume results from trauma exposure and/or PTSD or whether it is a risk marker for the development of PTSD in the first place, as at least one twin study has suggested (Gilbertson et al., 2002).

Other neurobiological correlates of PTSD include elevated activity in the amygdala and hippocampus and decreased activity in the medial prefrontal regions (Patel, Spreng, Shin, & Girard, 2012). However, increased activity of the amygdala, like decreased volume in the hippocampus, may reflect exposure to trauma, rather than the development of PTSD per se.

There is evidence that individuals with PTSD have more difficulty encoding traumatic scenes and rely more on gist memory (i.e., fuzzy memories vs. verbatim memories) than do those without PTSD. Hayes and colleagues (2011) found that among trauma-exposed combat veterans, those with PTSD were more likely than those without the diagnosis to err in believing that they had seen specific trauma-related pictures a week after they were exposed to similar pictures. These false-alarm errors were correlated with increased activity in the bilateral precuneus. As well, initial list learning among veterans with PTSD was correlated with decreased amygdala and hippocampus activity in comparison with list learning among veterans without PTSD.

Among healthy people suppression of neutral material results in decreased hippocampus activity and is known to be a fairly effective strategy. However, suppression of distressing memories is not as effective and does not lead to decreased hippocampus activity. In a paired associate word list paradigm Butler and James (2010) found that healthy individuals demonstrated *increased* activation of several brain regions (amygdala, insula, anterior cingulate, and fusiform gyrus) when asked to suppress negative words (e.g., agony, rape) in comparison with activation in these areas when they were asked to suppress neutral words (e.g., tower, bowl). Avoidance strategies are frequently utilized by individuals with PTSD. They are more likely to experience stress-induced analgesia than are those who do not have PTSD, as evidenced by studies of pain responsiveness in this population, both by oral report and in terms of brain changes (Diener et al., 2012; Mickleborough et al., 2011). Brain imaging data suggest that individuals become aroused in response to subliminally presented fearful faces, but they are able to suppress awareness of fearful faces when these are presented more slowly and conscious awareness is possible. In one study dissociative individuals with PTSD demonstrated increased prefrontal activity in response to fearful faces presented for 500 ms, but when fearful faces were presented for 16.7 ms, followed by neutral masking, they demonstrated increased activity in the amygdala, insula, and left thalamus (Felmingham et al., 2008).

Based on all these findings, it seems likely that individuals with PTSD fail to encode the initiating trauma accurately, and the combination of smaller hippocampi and prefrontal hypoactivity makes it harder for them to achieve extinction later. Instead, they may re-experience the trauma and fail to learn that it is no longer threatening. Due to faulty reconsolidation, their memory of the trauma shifts over time, such that it becomes vaguer or contains new, inaccurate details. Individuals with PTSD, like those with depression, demonstrate decreased cortico-limbic integration. They may have difficulty solving problems effectively, they find it difficult to modulate emotions, and they are particularly likely to utilize avoidance strategies. While individuals with PTSD find conscious avoidance to be an effective strategy, unconscious avoidance is not effective for them, and it actually leads to increased emotional arousal, which presumably fuels further attempts to avoid.

How are these problems addressed in psychotherapy? The behavioral treatment of PTSD, for example, is based on imaginal exposure to the trauma and in vivo exposure to other feared situations (such as environmental cues), in the expectation that with repeated exposures avoidance will decrease. The therapist asks the patient to recount the trauma in detail and helps the patient to recall forgotten details, thus increasing accurate recall of the trauma. Such repeated exposure occurs in an optimal learning environment, in which the therapist encourages attachment on the part of the patient. As a result, the patient's stress level decreases, at least during the session, and this improves working memory and leads to less emotional interference in the laying down of new memories. Extinction is also more likely to occur in this circumstance. Prefrontal cortex activation is presumably encouraged by the effort the patient must put forth to pay attention during exposure. Further, the therapist provides the patient general strategies to manage emotional arousal, which presumably enables the patient to exert better control over limbic reactivity and to improve mood, as was the case in the treatment of depression.

Summary

We have offered a few examples of how one might think about psychotherapy from a neurobiological perspective. The key principle in the crosswalk from psychology to biology is the concept of neuroplasticity, a phenomenon that permits us to understand psychological change in physical terms. As neuroimaging techniques continue to proliferate in psychiatric research and treatment, we can expect a continued cross-pollination between the psychology and biology of mental functioning. One expects that in the not-too-distant future it will become possible to make rational selections among mental health interventions, not just on the basis of proven efficacy, but also in consideration of the most efficient approach to specific symptoms, considered from the bridging perspective of neuroplasticity.

Section Summary

1. The concept of neuroplasticity informs one's understanding of important psychological variables (learning, memory, attention, attachment) that underlie mental disorders.

2. The use of psychotherapy in the treatment of depression has been shown to be correlated with imaging changes throughout the brain. Prefrontal cortex changes may be more common following psychotherapy than following psychopharmacological treatment.

3. Decreased hippocampal size and prefrontal hypoactivity are known to be associated with posttraumatic stress disorder (PTSD), although causality is unclear. Psychotherapeutic techniques are likely to target these areas of the brain, among others.

Research Findings in Psychology

Casual observers of psychotherapy often come away with two conflicting impressions. On one hand, brief snippets of the therapy session may appear similar to any other normal, unremarkable human interaction. The entire enterprise may seem to rest primarily on the therapist's fundamental kindness and common sense. On the other hand, therapist behaviors are occasionally surprising and seem to be inappropriate for normal human interactions. When the observer inquires why the therapist has said or done such an eccentric thing, the answer may be something like, "The experts recommend it, and my experience shows that it works." Our casual observer may be forgiven for suspecting that psychotherapy is more like an art or religion than it is like a science.

In fact, there is plenty of psychological research that supports the activities of psychotherapy. In the following section we briefly review studies that address several topics of central importance for psychotherapy, including the overall effectiveness of psychotherapy, dose-response issues, the relative efficacy of one model of psychotherapy over another, the existence of certain empirically supported treatment models, issues of deterioration in psychotherapy, issues related to the therapeutic alliance, patient characteristics that predict to outcome, and therapist factors that predict to outcome.

What Do We Know About the Rate of Recovery in Psychotherapy?

Overall Effectiveness of Psychotherapy

We begin our exploration of this topic with the blockbuster 1952 paper of Hans J. Eysenck (1916–1997). A behavioral psychologist who was born in Germany but spent most of his adult life in England, he argued against the proposal that psychologists be trained to conduct psychoanalysis, and in 1952 he published a paper comparing the effectiveness of psychoanalytically-oriented psychotherapy with no-treatment control. He concluded that approximately two thirds of the members of both groups demonstrated significant improvement. As a consequence, for many years thereafter academic psychologists and some other mental health professionals wondered if psychoanalytically-oriented psychotherapy was effective at all, notwithstanding several methodological problems in the Eysenck paper, some of which he later acknowledged.

Approximately a quarter century after Eysenck's paper there began to appear a series of meta-analyses comparing various kinds of psychotherapy to no-treatment control. In a large meta-analysis published in 1980, Smith, Glass, and Miller concluded that psychotherapy was indeed effective. The data shown in Table 3.1 are extracted from their study but include only those therapy classifications for which at least 50 effects were available. The "all psychotherapy" estimate in the table summarizes the tabled data and suggests that on average psychotherapy produces an outcome that is 0.87 standard deviations better than no-treatment control. This is equivalent to saying that the average treated patient is better off than 81% of controls.

Table 3.1 Mean effect sizes of various types of psychotherapy well represented in Smith, Glass, and Miller (1980).

Psychotherapy	No. of effects	Mean *d*
Other cognitive therapies	57	2.38
Cognitive-behavior therapy	127	1.13
Systematic desensitization	373	1.05
Psychodynamic-eclectic	103	.89
Behavior modification	201	.73
Psychodynamic	108	.69
Implosion	60	.68
Rational-emotive	50	.68
Vocational-personal development	59	.65
Gestalt	68	.64
Client-centered	150	.62
Undifferentiated counseling	97	.28
All psychotherapy	1,453	.87

Most commentators have accepted this and similar meta-analytic findings, and Eysenck's 1952 paper no longer carries any weight.

Efficacy vs. Effectiveness

Do the results of the Smith et al. (1980) meta-analysis and other studies actually shed light on the effectiveness of psychotherapy as it is practiced in everyday settings? In recent years most studies demonstrating the benefit of psychotherapy have made use of randomized controlled trials (RCTs). This is a design that psychotherapy researchers believe optimizes reliability and validity. The results of an RCT are considered to have high *internal validity* because the study is designed to emphasize differences in outcome between study arms and to minimize differences due to ancillary variables, such as variations in participants' demographic identifiers, amount of contact with a therapist, and the like. Note, however, that in contrast to drug trials, both participants and researchers are rarely "blind" to the study conditions. For psychotherapy studies, participants and study personnel are aware of what treatment is received. In the case of psychotherapy RCTs the concept of "placebo" is not as clear as it is in drug trials. What exactly do we mean by "sham psychotherapy," if we know that all psychotherapies are helpful to some extent? Nevertheless, these RCTs, known as *efficacy studies*, are considered to be the gold standard of evidence when one wishes to demonstrate that a certain psychotherapy is more or less efficacious than some other treatment.

A larger question arises with respect to the *external validity* of these efficacy studies. To what extent can we draw conclusions that relate to real-life practice of psychotherapy? In other words, is psychotherapy's *efficacy* less than, greater than, or about the same as its *effectiveness* (i.e., the outcome of routine psychotherapy offered in routine conditions to routine patients)? If efficacy differs from effectiveness, it might mean that everyday practitioners are delivering substandard treatment or that psychotherapists are "hamstrung" in research environments and cannot produce their best work. A difference between efficacy and effectiveness would call into question the generalizability of RCT findings to routine practice. Several studies have investigated the nature of differences between efficacy and effectiveness studies, and the general finding is that psychotherapy's effectiveness is roughly equivalent to its efficacy.

Perhaps the best known early effectiveness study was published in *Consumer Reports* (Seligman, 1995). Subscribers to this magazine were asked to comment on their recent experiences with psychotherapy—and with various brands of automobiles, dishwashers, vacuum cleaners, and so on. The results were very positive. Of the 426 respondents who reported they felt "very poor" prior to treatment, 87% indicated that afterwards they felt "very good," "good," or "so-so." Among the 786 respondents who felt "fairly poor," 92% reported that they felt at least "so-so," if not better, when treatment ended. The *Consumer Reports* study also demonstrated greater effectiveness for long-term than short-term therapy, but treatment model didn't affect outcome in a meaningful way.

However, subsequent reports (e.g., Nielsen, Smart, Isakson, Worthen, Gregersen, & Lambert, 2004) have raised significant concerns about the retrospective methodology utilized in the study, and at present the *Consumer Reports* study is viewed more as a satisfaction survey than as a legitimate outcome study (Nathan, Stuart, & Dolan, 2000).

There have been other, more successful attempts to measure psychotherapy effectiveness. For example, in 1997 Shadish and colleagues showed in a large meta-analysis that the degree to which RCTs were "clinically representative" did not affect overall level of patient benefit from treatment. Some years later, Minami and colleagues (2008) evaluated the effectiveness of psychotherapy provided to nearly 6,000 depressed patients in managed care by benchmarking it against psychotherapy efficacy findings for depressed participants in RCTs. In general, the patients in managed care achieved results very similar to those in RCTs, with the minor differences for patients with comorbidities. In 2013 Blais and colleagues used these same efficacy benchmarks to assess the effectiveness of routine psychotherapy offered at an academic medical center. More than 1,300 depressed outpatients were treated with psychotherapy, pharmacotherapy, or combined treatment. The three treatment modalities did not differ in effectiveness, and there were no overall differences between the effectiveness of routine treatment and the benchmark efficacy findings from the RCTs. However, the outcomes of privately insured patients were better than those of patients whose treatment was paid for by Medicare or Medicaid;

the publicly insured group did not reach the benchmarks established by research participants in the RCTs.

Dose-Response Issues

Another kind of information that helps in understanding the outcome of psychotherapy comes from a series of treatment response rate studies. In 2002 Hansen, Lambert, and Forman concluded that among a large number of RCTs, some 58% of participants showed statistically significant movement from the pathological into the normal range over the course of 13 weeks. To the extent that this finding can be generalized, it means that on average, two individuals need to be treated using the protocol to ensure that at least one will derive meaningful benefit. This statistic (often referred to as "number needed to treat" or NNT) compares quite favorably with other procedures in healthcare.

A more detailed analysis of the psychotherapy dose-response curve yields some interesting findings. It turns out that groups of psychotherapy patients demonstrate a log-linear relationship between number of sessions and improvement. In other words, within a group of patients there are rapid early gains, but change drops off at a rate that is inversely proportional to time. Generally, the curve looks something like Figure 3.1. What is not clear is whether this behavior of a *group* of patients is replicated by *individuals* within the group. One would imagine that within any sample of psychotherapy patients, some patients improve quickly while others improve more slowly. Because patients generally terminate treatment when they feel "better," one would predict that those remaining in the sample are improving less and less quickly. If one assumes that patients improve, for example, linearly, but some improve more quickly than others, and every patient drops out of treatment after achieving a certain level of improvement, this frequently yields the log-linear curve that has been observed in many population studies. In fact, several large studies have shown that mean patient improvement in psychotherapy is primarily linear in nature, with a

Typical psychotherapy response of a sample of patients

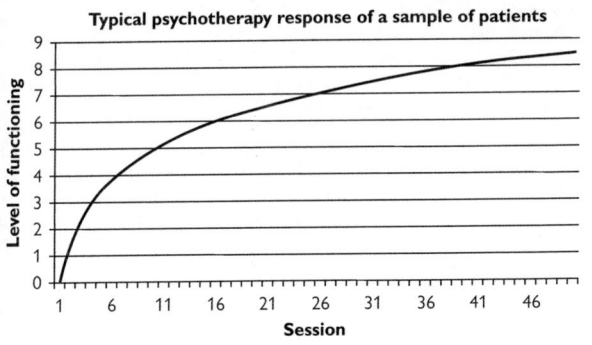

Figure 3.1. Log-linear relationship between symptomatic relief and time in treatment for a hypothetical sample of psychotherapy patients.

very limited curvilinear component (Baldwin, Berkeljon, Atkins, Olsen, & Nielsen, 2009; Reese, Toland, & Hopkins, 2011; Stiles, Barkham, Connell, & Mellor-Clark, 2008).

However, little is known regarding the session-by-session trajectory of psychotherapy patients. Some data suggest that the only way to predict the current distress level of a given patient is to know his or her status at the last session. This would mean that patients don't actually establish any trajectory of recovery, and the status at *this* session is best modeled as *last* session's status plus a random variable. If such a pattern, sometimes referred to as "random walk," does in fact apply to psychotherapy patients, it means that while groups of patients may show diminishing rates of improvement over time, a given patient within the group may or may not.

As is evident in Figure 3.1, improvement occurs rapidly in early psychotherapy, at least for some patients. Indeed, the phenomenon of sudden early gains in psychotherapy has long been of interest. Early psychoanalysts worried that such patients were engaging in a "flight into health." The idea was that patients' defense structures were threatened by the nature of treatment, and they "gave up symptoms" in order to justify leaving treatment. Psychoanalysts predicted that such patients would soon relapse. However, this has not been borne out in research data. Recent studies have demonstrated that there does appear to be a subgroup of patients who improve quickly and whose gains persist for at least a year, which is usually as long as researchers follow them.

The phenomenon of sudden early gains also occurs in other approaches to the treatment of mental disorders, including pharmacotherapy and case management. Interestingly, there are data to suggest that sudden early gains in psychotherapy may be more persistent than sudden early gains experienced by patients in other treatment modalities. This is consistent with findings suggesting that maintenance of gains following cessation of psychotherapy is often sturdier than maintenance of gains following cessation of pharmacotherapy. Some researchers have attempted to identify the treatment events in psychotherapy that may be correlated with sudden early gains. However, no consistent pattern has emerged that explains why certain patients show sudden early gains and others do not (e.g., Tang, DeRubeis, Beberman, & Pham, 2005, vs. Andrusyna, Luborsky, Pham, & Tang, 2006). Indeed, it may well be that sudden early gains result from the inculcation of hope and/or are characteristic of the natural history of some mental disorders, and the precise details of treatment are not particularly informative.

A final comment regarding dose-response issues has to do with the fact that a very large number of patients drop out of psychotherapy early on. Indeed, in large surveys fully 30% to 50% of patients fail to return after just one psychotherapy session. While it is conceivable that some of these patients may have experienced sudden early gains, it's unlikely that such rapid remission accounts for a significant proportion of individuals who do not continue treatment. We know that the median course of psychotherapy in the United States has ranged from 4 to 10 sessions. However, the mean effective dose of psychotherapy in RCTs has variously been estimated at 12 to 18 sessions, suggesting many patients are not receiving adequate doses of psychotherapy. Indeed, in a sample of more than 6,000 American outpatients receiving psychotherapy services (and possibly psychotropic medications), Hansen and colleagues (2002) found that only 14.1% of patients demonstrated meaningful clinical improvement over the course of treatment. When the authors confined their analysis to meaningful clinical improvement within the median number of sessions at each site (which ranged from 3 to 8), a mere 6.5% of patients demonstrated meaningful clinical improvement. Research suggests that patients with limited education or low socioeconomic status are more likely to leave treatment early. By contrast, patients who like their therapists, who feel that they have significant input into the nature of treatment, and who do not have significant personality disturbance are more likely to remain in treatment.

Differential Effectiveness of Psychotherapy

Psychotherapy may be generally effective, but meta-analytic results like the 1980 study by Smith and colleagues discussed previously suggest that some models of psychotherapy are more effective than others. Of course, one would expect differences in efficacy between therapy models, but the more important question is whether these differences are meaningful. It turns out that the answer may be: not so much.

Beginning in the early 1990s a series of meta-analyses examined how to understand the apparent variability in psychotherapy efficacy. Generally, these meta-analyses did show significant differences between schools of psychotherapy, but such differences usually dropped into the range of nonsignificance when the researchers' preexisting allegiances were taken into account. Researcher allegiance can be estimated by evaluating previous publication history, examining the study hypotheses, looking at the amount of detail in the paper regarding instantiation of each treatment, and so forth. Typical of the findings in this area is a meta-analysis published in 1999 by Luborsky and others. They used the data from 24 RCTs of psychotherapy delivered to outpatients with common diagnoses. The relationship between the direction of outcome and researcher allegiance was reflected in a remarkably high $r = .85$.

Some have argued that researchers establish their allegiances based on their observations of what actually works, so that perhaps the allegiance–outcome relationship doesn't mitigate the finding that one therapy is better than another. However, this argument falters in the face of a meta-analysis conducted in 2012 by Munder and colleagues, who compared the effectiveness of very similar exposure-based approaches to the treatment of PTSD. According to the literature in this area, these treatment approaches should be more or less equally effective. However, among the twenty-nine comparisons in the meta-analysis by Munder and colleagues, the allegiance–outcome relationship was significant, at $r = .35$, which supports the view that the researcher's allegiance plays a meaningful role in determining outcome.

In 1997 a research group led by American psychologist Bruce E. Wampold (1948–) took a different tack in examining the question of whether one kind of psychotherapy is more effective than another. They wondered whether studies showing that Therapy A was better than Therapy B might have been drawn from a normally distributed, homogeneous population of outcome differences, with mean difference $d = 0$. To test this hypothesis they located 114 studies published in major journals between 1970 and 1995.

Each study involved the delivery of at least two bona fide psychotherapeutic treatments to individuals with mental health problems like depression and anxiety. Because many had multiple measures, the 114 studies yielded 277 comparisons between pairs of psychotherapy. The research group concluded that the best-fitting model for the data was that the comparisons were drawn from a *highly homogeneous* population, in which the mean difference was, not surprisingly, very nearly zero ($d = .0021$). Moreover, when the authors looked at the absolute values of differences between therapy outcomes, utilizing the most liberal possible statistical treatment they found a mean difference of $d = .21$. This presumably represents an upper limit of differences, because in this portion of the analysis the authors coded as positive any difference between therapies, regardless of its direction. If in Study 1 Therapy A was more effective than Therapy B, it was counted as positive, even when Therapy B was found to be more effective than Therapy A in Study 2—that, too, was counted as positive. It is instructive to compare this upper limit of $d = .21$ with the mean effect of being in psychotherapy at all, which is about $d = .87$.

So it would appear that if there are differences in efficacy between kinds of psychotherapy, such differences are rather smaller than the overall effect of psychotherapy. This conclusion regarding psychotherapy efficacy is sometimes referred to as the *Dodo bird hypothesis*, a reference to the creature in Lewis Carroll's *Alice in Wonderland*, who judges an impromptu and completely chaotic race among strange beasts and ultimately declares, "Everybody has won, and all must have prizes." It is important to note, however, that insofar as the Dodo bird's conclusion regarding equivalent outcomes is correct, it applies only to adult treatment. There are data to suggest that in the treatment of children behaviorally oriented psychotherapies are more effective than insight-oriented and/or supportive treatments. Moreover, there has recently been a spate of smaller meta-analyses suggesting that for tightly defined adult patient populations, such as individuals with panic disorder, people with obsessive-compulsive disorder, or those with certain other conditions, some psychotherapies are more effective than others.

Empirically Supported Treatments

At the same time that evidence was accumulating to support the Dodo bird's conclusion that one psychotherapy was about as effective as another, other researchers set out to evaluate the available research literature to identify particular psychotherapies that have been clearly shown to be effective with specific groups of patients. Minor differences have arisen regarding the precise criteria that must be met to establish empirical support, but most commentators agree that if at least two RCTs from different labs demonstrate that a model of psychotherapy is significantly more effective than no-treatment control in addressing a particular diagnosis, then empirical support has been established for that treatment–diagnosis combination. Lists of such empirically supported treatments are available in various locations, including at a website sponsored by the National Institute of Mental Health (http://www.therapyadvisor.com).

Of course, it is important to underscore the fact that there are many therapy models that have not been studied, and the fact that a certain treatment–diagnosis combination has not yet been determined to have empirical support does not mean that the treatment is ineffective with the diagnosis. Absence of evidence is not evidence of absence. Indeed, it is only within the past several years that consistent empirical support has begun to accumulate for psychoanalytically-informed treatments, at least in part because studies of such treatments require much longer to complete than studies of 16-week behavioral treatments.

Just as some treatment–diagnosis combinations have empirical support, there are other models of psychotherapy about which concern has been expressed. It is known that 5% to 10% of patients experience more distress, rather than less, as a consequence of participating in psychotherapy. Obviously, one cannot conclude that all such deterioration in treatment is due to harmful treatments themselves, but a portion of it might be. Because of this, there has been increased interest in identifying potentially harmful psychotherapeutic treatments. One such list of therapies was compiled in 2007 by Lilienfeld. He identified the following interventions as "probably harmful for some individuals": critical incident stress debriefing, Scared Straight interventions, facilitated communication, the use of verbal abuse or physical restraint with attachment-disordered children, recovered memory techniques, suggestive techniques used in the treatment of dissociative identity disorder, grief counseling for individuals with normal bereavement reactions, techniques that encourage emotional catharsis without subsequent cognitive restructuring, boot camp interventions for conduct disorder, and Drug Abuse and Resistance Education programs. Lilienfeld described the following treatment models as "possibly harmful for some individuals": peer-group interventions for conduct disorder and relaxation treatments for panic-prone individuals. Some of these conclusions are more strongly supported by research than others.

In recent years there has been an interest in decreasing the frequency of poor outcomes in psychotherapy by targeting patients who fail to improve as treatment progresses. There are now consistent data (e.g., Lambert & Shimokawa, 2011) to the effect that when therapists are alerted to pay special attention to patients who are not progressing as expected, they usually take some action that has the effect of reversing the patient's deteriorating trajectory. These studies typically administer brief measures of emotional distress at the beginning of every session, and if the patient fails to make expected progress from session to session, the therapist is alerted to this fact. Some studies (e.g., Slade, Lambert, Harmon, Smart, & Bailey, 2008) show improved outcomes when therapists address, in order, these aspects of floundering treatment: therapeutic alliance, the patient's motivation, social supports available to the patient, the patient's level of perfectionism, and need for psychotropic medications.

Summary

There is no longer any real dispute that psychotherapy is effective in the treatment of behavioral disturbances. In many cases it is as effective—and sometimes more effective—than somatic treatments for mental health problems. There is no credible evidence to suggest that research efficacy studies either overestimate or underestimate the actual effectiveness of psychotherapy as it is practiced in the field. However, a significant percentage of patients may not receive an adequate dose of psychotherapy, which limits the benefit. In heterogeneous populations of adult patients one kind of psychotherapy is probably about as effective as another. However, this does not appear to be true for children, with whom behaviorally oriented therapy is likely to be more effective than other kinds of psychotherapy. As well, in more narrowly defined groups of adults with certain diagnoses, some treatments may be more effective than others. The list of empirically supported treatments continues to expand as more research is done, and it is often possible to identify several psychotherapeutic approaches from which to choose in the treatment of an individual with a particular diagnosis. It seems likely that one can rely on the Dodo bird hypothesis when choosing among empirically supported treatments for a given diagnosis: each is likely to be about as effective as the others. On the other hand, it may be that a few psychotherapeutic models carry some risk that patients will be harmed. In any event, certain patients respond more quickly to treatment than others, and a sudden early gain is not cause for alarm. Formally tracking patient distress on a routine basis helps to identify individuals who may be at risk for poor outcomes; the provision of feedback to therapists about such patients has been shown to improve outcome.

In General, How Does Psychotherapy Work?

Introduction

Studies that illuminate the internal mechanisms of psychotherapy are valuable in that they provide guidance to practitioners who wish to identify therapy skills that might have an effect on outcome. As well, such "process" studies help to clarify how apparently different psychotherapeutic models might have similar success rates.

In 2011 Norcross and Lambert reviewed the large corpus of research that attempts to predict outcome from psychotherapeutic treatment. They were unable to identify factors responsible for about 40% of psychotherapy outcome. Within the 60% of psychotherapy outcome for which they were able to identify correlates, they concluded that half (i.e., 30% of total outcome) was controlled by patient factors, such as diagnosis, willingness to change, available social supports, and the like. The quality of the relationship between the patient and therapist accounted for 12% of total outcome, the specific treatment method accounted for 8%, and the therapist variable accounted for 7% of total outcome. The remaining 3% of outcome was controlled by an assortment of other small variables. Having addressed the issue of differing treatments in the previous section, we now turn to relationship factors, patient factors, and therapist factors.

Relationship Factors

How do relationship factors affect outcome in psychotherapy? As early as 1912 Freud began to explicate the nature of the therapeutic relationship, but he had much more to say about transference issues than about the real relationship between the therapist and the patient. Over the course of the last century many theorists have pointed to the importance of the actual relationship between therapist and patient. We know from the estimates of Norcross and Lambert (2011) that relationship quality controls more outcome variance (12%) than any other known group of variables, apart from patient factors.

The quality of the therapeutic relationship is now generally referred to as the *therapeutic alliance*, and there are a number of questionnaires that appear to be good measures of it. The best known of these is the Working Alliance Inventory, which dates to a 1986 publication by Horvath and Greenberg. This measure, which can be completed by the patient, the therapist, or an observer, consists of 36 items that assess the respondent's belief about patient–therapist agreement on the *goals* of therapy, the *tasks* undertaken to reach those goals, and the affiliative *bonds* between the patient and therapist. Shorter versions of the measure with strong psychometric characteristics are also available (e.g., Hatcher & Gillaspy, 2006).

Measures of therapeutic alliance have demonstrated a consistent relationship to outcome in psychotherapy. In a 2011 meta-analysis by Horvath, Del Re, Flückiger, and Symonds, the mean correlation between various measures of alliance and outcome was $r = .275$, which corresponds to $d = .57$. Since the overall effect of participating in psychotherapy is estimated at $d = .87$, it is clear that alliance represents an important variable in this area. Most commentators believe that alliance drives outcome, although occasionally the argument is made that perhaps symptomatic improvement benefits the alliance—and not the other way around. However, there is a steady accumulation of evidence to suggest that small differences in alliance early in therapy lead to large changes in treatment outcome, while early symptomatic changes usually don't have much effect on subsequent alliance. Alliance demonstrates a somewhat weaker, but still significant, relationship to outcome in the treatment of children. It may be that alliance relates to outcome somewhat differently in the treatment of substance use disorders than in psychotherapy applied to other conditions, but the data are not yet clear on this point.

Psychotherapists are well advised to pay careful attention to the therapeutic alliance, because therapists cannot help patients who refuse to collaborate or attend regular sessions. It is important to intervene quickly when an *alliance rupture* occurs. Ruptures exist along a continuum from minor tensions between therapist and patient regarding goals, tasks, or bonds to a frank breakdown in the collaborative relationship. Minor ruptures occur often in psychotherapy, and not infrequently the therapist is unaware of them. Because of this, it is useful to track the quality of the relationship in some consistent manner, either by routinely administering a measure of therapeutic alliance or by asking the patient from time to time how things are going in treatment. Interestingly, research data suggest that when ruptures are identified and addressed directly, the outcome from treatment may actually be *better* than if no rupture at all occurs over the course of treatment (e.g., Stiles et al., 2004; Strauss et al., 2006). Of course, if ruptures are not addressed in an open and supportive environment, the risk of poor outcome increases significantly.

How might one address an alliance rupture? There is evidence that when therapists retreat to theory and address ruptures in terms of the patient's psychopathology, outcome is likely to suffer (e.g., Castonguay, Goldfried, Wiser, Raue, & Hayes, 1996; Henry, Schacht, Strupp, Butler, & Binder, 1993). Muran (2002) presents evidence that when therapists follow a certain sequence in responding to ruptures, better outcome results. The sequence begins with attention to and exploration of the rupture marker. If the patient responds with avoidance, the avoidance is explored. Finally, the patient is helped to express a basic wish or need in the therapeutic relationship. There are data to suggest that when therapists "switch gears" in response to a rupture, better outcome results. This may (but doesn't always) include changing relevant characteristics of the treatment offered.

What are the patient characteristics that predict to the quality of therapeutic alliance? Happily, level of pathology does not predict to alliance. Very ill patients are capable of forming strong alliances. One is hardly surprised to learn that patients with good interpersonal skills generally form strong alliances. More specifically, patients who wish to establish secure relationships and who expect that others will not reject them are able to form strong therapeutic alliances. Such patients are said to be *securely attached*, a concept we have mentioned before and to which we will return shortly. There are data to suggest that depressed patients with strong perfectionistic characteristics have difficulty maintaining a positive alliance late in time-limited psychotherapy, while depressed patients with fewer perfectionistic qualities demonstrate improved alliance over the course of treatment. Patients who prior to treatment expect that they will benefit from psychotherapy generally form stronger alliances, while those who are more dubious about treatment ahead of time show poorer alliances.

One study suggests that one can predict outcome much more accurately by looking at a therapist's mean alliance score across many patients than by examining a patient's alliance score after factoring out the therapist's mean score (Baldwin, Wampold, & Imel, 2007). This may mean that the therapist's contribution to alliance carries more weight than the patient's contribution, insofar as the prediction of outcome is concerned. What are the therapist characteristics that predict to the quality of alliance? Obviously, the ability and willingness to address alliance ruptures will affect mean alliance over the course of treatment. Further, in a 2001 review Ackerman and Hilsenroth concluded that the following therapist characteristics predict to poor alliance: excessive rigidity or a tendency to structure the session too much; uncertainty, tension, and distractibility; a tendency to criticize the patient or to make excessive use of transference interpretations; too much self-disclosure; and excessive interpersonal distance or use of silence.

Patient Factors Predicting to Outcome

We have noted that patient factors account for about 30% of outcome in psychotherapy; this does not include the patient's contribution to the therapeutic relationship. Which patient factors influence outcome? Research has demonstrated that a patient's ability to benefit from this treatment may depend importantly on initial level of symptoms, ethnicity, interpersonal skills, perfectionism, attachment, and expectancy.

Not surprisingly, the more symptomatic a patient is at the beginning of treatment, the less likely the patient is to experience full recovery. This is particularly true in the treatment of depression. On the other hand, Freud's belief notwithstanding, patient age generally doesn't predict to outcome from psychotherapy, with the possible exception that older depressed individuals may have poorer outcomes than younger depressed people. While women may be very slightly more likely to benefit from psychotherapy than men, this difference is not clinically meaningful.

Ethnicity does appear to play a significant role in predicting benefit from psychotherapy. In the United States, individuals of European, Asian, and Hispanic descent have roughly equivalent outcomes from psychotherapy. Asian Americans and Hispanic Americans may be more likely to benefit from psychotherapy if the therapist is of the same ethnic background. African Americans generally do less well than these other groups, and ethnic matching does not seem to improve outcome. Some have suggested that the quality of services available to African Americans is poorer than that available to other ethnicities. Data regarding the benefit of psychotherapy for other ethnic minorities in the United States, including particularly Native Americans, are too sparse to yield a clear pattern. Members of ethnic minorities in the United States report increased satisfaction with therapists who demonstrate multicultural competence. However, data are not yet available that clearly demonstrate improved outcome as a consequence of multicultural competence on the part of therapists in the United States (e.g., Owen, Leach, Wampold, & Rodolfa, 2011). One study conducted in the United Kingdom contained data to suggest that ethnic matching may lead to better outcomes (Farsimadan, Draghi-Lorenz, & Ellis, 2007).

Patients with personality disorders are less likely to benefit from psychotherapy than others, particularly those who are young and angry. More generally, patients with poor social supports benefit less from psychotherapy (and many other health interventions) than do those with better social supports. Not surprisingly, patients who prefer to talk about their problems benefit more from psychotherapy than those who don't.

We have already made reference to the fact that depressed perfectionistic patients have difficulty maintaining alliance late in treatment, which presumably affects outcome adversely. There are also data to suggest that depressed perfectionistic patients have poor outcomes through some other means (i.e., not mediated by alliance). Some have speculated that depressed perfectionists hold negative views about themselves and others, and this may interfere with their ability to profit from treatment.

We return to the issue of *attachment*. As we have noted previously, human beings are programmed to seek safety in social interactions, particularly during childhood. Based on childhood experiences and perhaps inborn predispositions, humans develop attachment styles that tend to be fairly consistent over the course of life. It is useful to think of attachment along two orthogonal axes, as in Figure 3.2.

The x-axis describes the degree to which the individual wishes to become involved in relationships. This dimension differentiates avoidance of others from attraction toward others. The y-axis describes the individual's expectation regarding others' acceptance. This dimension distinguishes the belief that one will be accepted by others from the expectation that one will be rejected. These two dimensions define an attachment plane in which a given individual can be located, and each quadrant in the plane describes a different attachment style, as shown in Figure 3.2. It is known that individuals who want intimacy and expect acceptance, a combination referred to as "secure attachment" and located in the upper right-hand corner of the

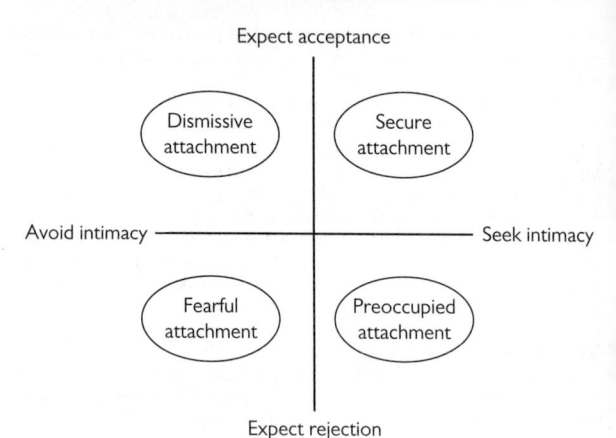

Figure 3.2. Two-dimensional depiction of adult attachment.

Axes: Expect acceptance (top) / Expect rejection (bottom); Avoid intimacy (left) / Seek intimacy (right). Quadrants: Dismissive attachment (upper left), Secure attachment (upper right), Fearful attachment (lower left), Preoccupied attachment (lower right).

plane, tend to have good outcomes from psychotherapy. Individuals who are preoccupied about attachment issues (e.g., want intimacy, expect rejection—in the lower right-hand corner) have a harder time in treatment. In a 2011 meta-analysis relating attachment to outcome from psychotherapy, Levy, Ellison, Scott, and Bernecker concluded that the attraction/avoidance dimension (on the x-axis) did not predict to outcome, but the acceptance/rejection dimension (on the y-axis) did, at $r = .22$, which is nearly as strong as the relationship between alliance and outcome. This means that patients who expect rejection in relationships have rather worse outcomes from psychotherapy than those who expect acceptance.

A final patient variable that predicts to outcome is the patient's *expectancy* prior to treatment that psychotherapy will help. In a 2011 meta-analysis Constantino, Glass, Arnkoff, Ametrano, and Smith found that patient expectancy of improvement correlated somewhat weakly, at $r = .12$, with actual outcome. There are data to suggest that the relationship between expectancy and outcome is mediated largely by patient attrition (Kwan, Dimidjian, & Rizvi, 2010) and alliance (Joyce, Ogrodniczuk, Piper, & McCallum, 2003; Meyer, Pilkonis, Krupnick, Egan, Simmens, & Sotsky, 2002).

Therapist Factors Predicting Outcome

We indicated that therapist factors, as distinct from the therapist's contribution to the relationship factor, account for about 7% of the outcome in psychotherapy. While this is not the largest variable affecting outcome, it is the variable over which therapists have the most control. A number of therapist factors play significant roles in outcome, including technical skills, therapist mental health and attitudes, management of countertransference, and the motivation to improve one's performance.

Obviously, therapist technical skills, such as the ability to demonstrate empathy and to offer interpretations in a timely, accurate manner, predict to outcome. The therapist's mental health also predicts to outcome. The effect of the *therapist's* attachment style is not well understood. A few studies suggest that when therapists and patients have complementary attachment styles, it improves outcome; however, the findings are mixed in this area. One study of mental health trainees, including psychiatric residents, showed that trainees whose primary motivators are income and excitement have more difficulty helping patients in psychotherapy than those whose primary motivators are intellectual (Lafferty, Beutler, & Crago, 1989).

A very important therapist variable that predicts to outcome is the way in which the therapist manages those reactions to patients that primarily reflect earlier experiences in the therapist's life, rather than the patient's actual behavior. Freud wrote extensively on this topic, which he called *countertransference* and conceptualized as an unconscious process (see Chapter 2). More recent definitions of countertransference include also those situations in which the therapist is consciously aware of his or her distorted perception. It is generally agreed that psychotherapy outcome suffers when therapists fail to become aware of countertransference, fail to use countertransference distortions as a source of information about the patient and the therapeutic relationship, or behave in a manner that is consistent with their countertransferential impulses.

There is probably no end to the ways in which countertransference might show itself in psychotherapy. A therapist might become unreasonably angry about a patient's behavior in the therapy session or in life outside the session. Alternatively, a therapist might begin to have unusually positive feelings about a patient, leading to sexual desire, the fantasy of developing a friendship outside of treatment, or the wish to protect the patient from all distress in life. Or a therapist might be perplexed by his or her feelings of anxiety when a particular patient brings up a certain topic. When therapists become aware of countertransference, they need to think about why it might be occurring with this particular patient and whether there is anything in the therapist's life that might be giving rise such distortions. It is also very useful to think about what the patient might be doing to trigger countertransference in the therapist, on the grounds that the patient may be doing something similar in other relationships and triggering the same feelings in others. For example, if the therapist wishes very much to help a certain patient but feels helpless to intervene effectively, is it possible that this patient is causing others to feel the same way? If so, how does the patient do this, and what purpose does it serve the patient? While countertransference can't ever be entirely avoided, and it can be informative if recognized, it can also adversely affect outcome if it is not actively managed.

It is known that when therapists are particularly anxious, they are less likely to manage countertransference successfully. As well, therapists with relatively less ability to conceptualize patients' problems in a complex and sophisticated manner are more likely to experience unmanaged countertransference. Unresolved conflicts on the part of the therapist are likely to lead to unmanaged countertransference with patients. In particular, therapists who respond to difficulty in life by failing to nurture themselves and instead pushing themselves relentlessly are likely to behave in a subtly hostile manner toward patients, and this is known to have an adverse effect on outcome.

A final therapist factor that is important to mention has to do with the concept of *therapist regrets*. At least two studies (Najavits & Strupp, 1994; Nissen-Lie, Monsen, & Rønnestad, 2010) have suggested that therapists who worry about the quality of their work and think through previous sessions with the intent of improving their performance in future sessions may have *better* outcomes than therapists who are completely satisfied with their performance. In other words, therapists who constantly strive to improve and who care a great deal about the quality of their work may be more successful than therapists who believe that their performance is fully adequate and doesn't really need to be improved.

Summary

Researchers are unable to identify the correlates for approximately 40% of the variance in psychotherapy outcome. The unique characteristics of a given model of psychotherapy account for about 8% of the variance in outcome. Patient factors account for about 30% of outcome variance, and particularly important variables in this category include the patient's initial level of pathology, ethnicity (African Americans benefit somewhat less from psychotherapy than members of other large ethnic groups in the United States), level of social supports, perfectionism in time-limited psychotherapy, predilection to talk about problems, and the expectation that one will be accepted by others. Relationship factors account for about 12% of the outcome variance, and a crucial consideration in this regard is the therapeutic alliance. It is therefore very important to address alliance ruptures as they arise in treatment. Securely attached patients are likely to form strong therapeutic alliances, while depressed, perfectionistic patients have more difficulty doing so. Therapists who are anxious, hostile, or rigid have more difficulty forming good alliances. About 7% of the outcome of psychotherapy is accounted for by therapist factors, including the therapist's technical skills and general mental health. A very important variable contributing to outcome is the therapist's ability to manage countertransference. Finally, therapists who worry a little about recent therapy sessions may have better outcomes than those who pat themselves on the back and move on.

Near the end of his career as a psychotherapy researcher, the German-born American psychologist Hans H. Strupp (1921–2006) offered ten desiderata for psychotherapists (Strupp, 1996). In abbreviated form, here they are:

1. To the extent possible, leave the initiative with patients to explore and to make their own discoveries.
2. Encourage patients' curiosity about self and the wish to collaborate with the therapist.
3. Listen for the themes of the hour.
4. Speak briefly but avoid long silences. Use a little humor, avoid jargon, and stress the tentativeness of your comments.
5. Be patient, especially when your patience is tried.
6. Identify and make use of countertransference.
7. Acknowledge your limitations, but don't apologize for them.

8. Ensure that your comments serve the patient's interests and not yours.
9. Carefully avoid criticism and pejorative communication.
10. Maintain a genuine commitment to helping.

Key Facts Box 3.1

1. Psychotherapy is effective. The difference in effectiveness between various models of psychotherapy is much less than the overall effectiveness of the treatment modality. There are increasing numbers of psychotherapeutic treatments that have shown empirical efficacy for specific conditions.

2. Groups of psychotherapy patients demonstrate log-linear recovery trajectories, but the trajectory of an individual psychotherapy patient is difficult to predict.

3. Sudden early gains in psychotherapy often predict to long-term improvement.

4. Patient–therapist relationship issues predict more strongly to psychotherapy outcome than either treatment factors or therapist factors alone.

5. Patient factors predicting outcome include level of initial severity, ethnicity, the presence of social supports, certain characterological features (including perfectionism), and attachment.

6. Therapist factors contributing to outcome include the therapist's mental health, level of skill, and, particularly, the management of countertransference.

7. Therapists are most likely to manage countertransference effectively when their anxiety level is not too high, when their conceptualization skills are strong, when they are cognizant of their own emotional "weak spots," and when they nurture themselves in the face of frustration.

8. Additional research is needed to inform individual treatment choices and response rates, particularly in understudied populations.

Research Findings from Treatment Studies

We have reviewed evidence in support of the proposition that psychotherapy is generally effective in the treatment of various mental disorders. We now address four related issues. First, we briefly recapitulate the issue of psychotherapy efficacy versus effectiveness. Next, we discuss what is known about the relative benefits of psychotherapy alone, pharmacotherapy alone, and combined treatment. Third, we ask if the provision of psychotherapy prevents relapse. Finally, we comment on how an understanding of psychotherapeutic principles might improve the outcome of pharmacotherapy.

Efficacy vs. Effectiveness

In an earlier section we reviewed studies that address the question of whether psychotherapy efficacy studies provide useful information about the outcome of psychotherapy under routine circumstances, and we concluded that in fact psychotherapy's efficacy and effectiveness are approximately equivalent. There is no body of data that points to important differences between the outcome of psychotherapy in research studies and its outcome when practiced in the field.

Monotherapy vs. Combined Treatment

Although there are other approaches to treatment, the vast majority of psychiatric patients are treated with psychotropic medications, with psychotherapy, or with a combination of pharmacotherapy and psychotherapy. What do we know about the relative benefits of psychotherapy, pharmacotherapy, and combined treatment? The answer appears to depend in part on the patient's diagnosis.

We begin with data from a meta-analysis comparing psychotherapy and pharmacotherapy in the treatment of depression (Casacalenda, Perry, & Looper, 2002). Among 883 depressed patients in six constituent studies, 46% of patients treated pharmacologically achieved remission, and this was exactly the same rate of remission among patients treated psychotherapeutically, while only 24% of control patients achieved remission. More recently, Spielmans, Berman, and Usitalo (2011) compared the effectiveness of second-generation antidepressants against clearly defined and competently delivered ("bona-fide") psychotherapies, and there was again no difference at the end of treatment, while at follow-up there was a non-significant trend ($d = .26$, based on 6 studies) for psychotherapy to outperform pharmacotherapy. In general, it appears that among unselected patients with depressive conditions, psychotherapy and pharmacotherapy yield equivalent results, particularly when one takes into account the fact that patients in research studies are more likely to drop out from pharmacotherapy than from psychotherapy (Cuijpers, van Straten, van Oppen, & Andersson, 2010).

It is true that in the National Institute of Mental Health (NIMH) Treatment of Depression Collaborative Research Program there were data to suggest that CBT was not as effective as imipramine in treating severely depressed outpatients, while interpersonal psychotherapy *was* as effective as imipramine in this population. However, there has been debate over whether the relatively poor showing of CBT may have reflected a study design problem (Elkin, Gibbons, Shea, & Shaw, 1996; Jacobson & Hollon, 1996). In any event, subsequent studies have suggested that CBT is as effective as pharmacotherapy in the treatment of severely depressed patients (DeRubeis, Gelfand, Tang, & Simons, 1999).

While psychotherapy and pharmacotherapy appear to be roughly equivalent in treating patients with depressive conditions in general, this finding may not hold true for patients who are specifically diagnosed with DSM-IV dysthymia (DSM-IV categories of dysthymia and chronic major depression have been combined into one category in DSM-5, persistent depressive disorder). In a 2012 meta-analysis of six studies comparing psychotherapy and pharmacotherapy in the treatment of DSM-IV dysthymia, Cuijpers and colleagues found that pharmacotherapy was a little more effective ($g = .28$) than psychotherapy in this population. The g statistic is very similar to the d statistic we have previously cited in discussing the effectiveness of psychotherapy as a whole ($d = .87$) and the relationship between therapeutic alliance and outcome ($d = .57$).

In the treatment of major depressive disorder, adding psychotherapy to pharmacotherapy consistently improves outcomes. In a 2004 meta-analysis of 18 studies, Friedman and colleagues found that combined treatment was slightly more effective ($d = .26$) than pharmacotherapy alone, while another meta-analysis of 20 studies (Cuijpers, Dekker, Hollon, & Andersson, 2009) yielded an effect size in the small to moderate range ($d = .40$).

However, the data are not as clear when combined treatment is compared with psychotherapy alone. In their 2004 report Friedman and colleagues analyzed data from 12 studies and found no significant difference between combined treatment and psychotherapy alone ($d = .04$) in the treatment of depressed patients. By contrast, more recently Cuijpers, Reynolds, and colleagues (2012) considered data from nine studies of depressed adult outpatients and found a significant advantage ($d = .40$) for combined treatment over psychotherapy alone. Still another meta-analysis (Cuijpers, van Straten, et al., 2009) offered a result intermediate between the two results just mentioned, having discovered a small difference ($d = .23$, based on 4 studies) favoring combined treatment over psychotherapy alone in the treatment of depressed patients. In this last meta-analysis, the authors suggested that the psychotherapy-alone condition may have been adversely affected by a relatively high number of patients with DSM-IV dysthymia.

As part of the controlled design, very few RCTs take patient preference into account, and this fact presumably limits the applicability of their results to routine clinical work. In normal treatment settings the patients' preferences are always important, and they consistently predict to outcome. Therefore, we may not be able to draw universal conclusions from these findings.

Results for specific populations, particular kinds of psychotherapy, and different phases of treatment yield ambiguous findings. For example, in the case of interpersonal psychotherapy (IPT), Cuijpers and colleagues (2011) utilized data from ten studies in which IPT was delivered in combination with pharmacotherapy and compared with pharmacotherapy alone in the acute phase of treatment. They found that the benefit of combined treatment did not reach significance ($d = .16$). By contrast, four studies compared combined treatment to pharmacotherapy alone in the maintenance phase, and the meta-analysis concluded that combined therapy was significantly more effective than pharmacotherapy alone ($OR = 0.37$). This particular finding might not extend to the treatment of patients over the age of 69, however. In one study of that population, pharmacotherapy with paroxetine alone was just as effective as combined treatment with paroxetine and monthly IPT, with two-year recurrence rates of 37% and 35%, respectively (Reynolds et al., 2006).

There is a clearer pattern of findings with regard to the treatment of chronic depression utilizing Cognitive-Behavioral Analysis System of Psychotherapy (CBASP), a CBT specifically designed to treat chronic depression. In a large therapy trial published in 2000, Keller and colleagues treated 681 adults with CBASP alone, nefazodone alone, or the combination of CBASP and nefazodone. Each monotherapy in this study yielded a remission rate of 48% in the intent-to-treat sample, while the remission rate was 73% in the combined-treatment group. A similar pattern was apparent among study completers, with response rates of 55% for pharmacotherapy, 52% for psychotherapy, and 85% for combined treatment. Manber and colleagues (2008) subsequently determined that although time to remission did not differ between the two monotherapy groups, participants in the combined-treatment group remitted more quickly than did either monotherapy group.

With regard to bipolar disorder, there have been consistent findings that psychotherapy added to pharmacotherapy decreases relapse rates. In particular, CBT, family interventions, and interpersonal and social rhythm therapy decrease relapse rates in bipolar disorder when utilized as adjuncts to pharmacotherapy (Frank et al., 2005; Otto, Smits, & Reese, 2005). Perhaps the provision of psychotherapy increases medication compliance, but it is also likely to have the effect of regularizing patients' sleep cycle and socialization patterns, as well as to help patients learn to monitor and respond more effectively to mood swings.

While there is extensive (if at times inconsistent) information regarding the relative effectiveness of various treatments for mood disorders, rather less information is available regarding other conditions. With regard to the treatment of anxiety, in 2009 Hofmann, Sawyer, Korte, and Smits combined the results of 11 studies comparing CBT plus placebo with CBT plus active pharmacotherapy. They found that combined treatment yielded better results than monotherapy immediately after treatment ($OR = 1.95$). However, this difference did not endure, and by six months after treatment, the six studies providing data showed no evidence of a significant difference between combined treatment and monotherapy ($OR = 0.66$). Interestingly, there is developing evidence to suggest that combined treatment becomes *less* effective than CBT alone when the medication is discontinued, perhaps because fear extinction is so context-dependent, and for anxiety patients the act of taking medication may serve as an important contextual cue (Otto et al., 2005). In other words, patients may assume that they were able to tolerate their anxiety because they took medication, not because they managed the anxiety differently. Thus, when they stop taking medication, that very act increases their fear of phobic cues, and their anxiety becomes worse.

With regard to obsessive-compulsive disorder the data provide little evidence that behavioral treatment (exposure and ritual prevention) is enhanced by adding clomipramine. In a 2005 study of 122 outpatients with OCD, Foa and colleagues derived response rates in the intent-to-treat sample of 62% for behavioral treatment, 42% for clomipramine, 70% for combined treatment, and 8% for placebo. A similar pattern obtained in the completer sample, where the response rates were 86% for behavioral treatment, 48% for clomipramine, 79% for combined treatment, and 10% for placebo.

In summary, it appears that among unselected depressed patients pharmacotherapy and psychotherapy are equally effective, but for patients diagnosed with DSM-IV dysthymia, pharmacotherapy may be more effective than psychotherapy. Among patients with major depressive disorder pharmacotherapy is enhanced by the addition of psychotherapy. Indeed, it is possible that combined treatment is always somewhat superior to monotherapy in this population. In the case of bipolar disorder, it is clear that combined therapy is superior to pharmacotherapy alone. Regarding anxiety disorders, it may be that the initial advantage of combined therapy over psychotherapy alone wanes over time and is actually reversed when the medication is discontinued. As for obsessive-compulsive disorder, it seems clear that behavioral treatment is superior to pharmacotherapy, and adding pharmacotherapy to behavioral treatment does not generally improve outcomes. Of course, the applicability of all of these conclusions may depend to some extent on patient preferences and individual differences.

Continuation and Maintenance Psychotherapy

We now turn from the question of remission to the issue of relapse and recurrence. Many mental illnesses are considered to be chronic conditions, with periods of relapse and remission. For example, in 2001 Keller estimated that, absent maintenance treatment, about 87% of patients who achieve remission following an acute depressive episode will become depressed again within 15 years. Clinicians have long wondered how to minimize the risk of relapse and recurrence, particularly in the case of pharmacological interventions. If one accepts the premise that drugs help patients by effecting changes in brain physiology that persist only as long as the drug and/or metabolites are present, then there is little reason to imagine that one would be protected against relapse for more than a week or two after one stops taking a psychotropic agent, given that most psychotropes have half-lives measured in hours or days. It is for this reason that many psychiatric patients, particularly those who have relapsed in the past, are encouraged to remain on psychotropic medications more or less indefinitely. By contrast, one might expect less relapse following the end of psychotherapy if one accepts the premise that psychotherapy's method of action is to effect conscious changes in cognition and coping skills over the long term, regardless of whether patient and psychotherapist have continuing regular contact with one another.

Are the data consistent with these suppositions? De Maat, Dekker, Schoevers, and De Jonghe (2006) summarized findings from six studies, evaluating the risk of relapse among 609 chronically depressed patients who were treated with either pharmacotherapy (involving various tricyclic antidepressants or paroxetine) or psychotherapy (cognitive therapy, CBT, or IPT). In the active phase of treatment, which lasted between 8 and 20 weeks, medication and psychotherapy were equally effective in bringing about remission of symptoms, each condition achieving a pooled remission rate of 39%, as one might expect based on our earlier discussion. Thirty-one percent of patients treated with medication dropped out of active treatment, but this rate was only slightly higher than the dropout rate for psychotherapy patients, at 26%. Patients were monitored for one to two years after the planned discontinuation of active treatment. Among patients treated pharmacologically, 57% relapsed after discontinuing medications, but among patients treated psychotherapeutically, only 27% relapsed after treatment ended.

One might reasonably predict that psychotherapy in the continuation and maintenance phases of treatment would reduce the risk of relapse or recurrence. There are in fact several specific psychotherapeutic treatments, such as mindfulness-based cognitive therapy for chronic depression, maintenance IPT for depression, and Twelve-Step facilitation for addiction, that have been shown to decrease relapse, and we review these in the corresponding sections of Chapter 5. At present we confine our discussion to a different question: Is relapse/recurrence reduced when pharmacotherapy is followed by a course of psychotherapy?

The literature in this area is somewhat limited, and we review here only two meta-analyses summarizing studies of patients with depressive disorders, bearing in mind that these findings may or may not generalize to other conditions. In 2011 Oestergaard and Møldrup demonstrated that the addition of psychotherapy to pharmacotherapy at any point in the acute or continuation phase of treatment decreases the risk for relapse ($OR = 3.28$–4.56, depending on the time of assessment). In the same year, Guidi, Fava, Fava, and Papakostas also investigated the effect of adding psychotherapy in the continuation phase of treatment, either concomitantly with antidepressant medication or after medication was discontinued. Five clinical trials provided data about the effect of adding psychotherapy while continuing antidepressant medication. In this case, it appears that the addition of psychotherapy decreases the risk of relapse, but the difference is not significant ($OR = 0.84$). Three studies provided data about the effect of starting psychotherapy while antidepressant medication is being tapered. Here there was a significant advantage of sequential treatment over simple tapering ($OR = 0.65$) in terms of decreased risk for relapse. Of note, the demonstrated efficacy of sequential treatment—that is, of using psychotherapy as a continuation treatment for depression after remission has been achieved with pharmacotherapy in the acute phase—underscores psychotherapy's potential as an important continuation or maintenance treatment option, one that may allow the safe discontinuation of antidepressant medication following remission, even in patients at significant risk of relapse or recurrence.

In summary, it does appear that psychotherapy, either alone or in combination with pharmacotherapy, confers resistance to relapse or recurrence in the continuation and maintenance phases of the treatment of depressed patients. Moreover, psychotherapy decreases relapse rates when delivered either during the acute phase or in the continuation phase of treatment. This appears to be the case even when psychotherapy is delivered concomitantly with pharmacotherapy during the continuation phase, although in that case the advantage conferred does not reach significance. Again, one must be cautious in applying these findings to the treatment of a particular patient, as the patient's preference is always significant, and research findings typically represent group outcomes that may or may not apply to an individual

Bringing a Psychotherapeutic Understanding to Pharmacotherapy

We now briefly address the topic of how a psychotherapeutic approach to the patient can improve outcomes from pharmacotherapy. It is probably self-evident that patients are likely to benefit when clinicians conceptualize the act of prescribing medication in both psychobiological and psychotherapeutic terms. It is clear that the effect of medication depends on more than its biological properties, and it is never possible to disentangle the influence of the human relationship between clinician and patient from the biological effect of the treatment offered. The patient's attitude about the clinician and about other people in general certainly affects the degree to which the patient will comply with treatment and will actually respond to it. Not only is the patient's attitude about the clinician important, but the patient's attitude about the particular treatment is significant. As we have said, there are consistent data to suggest that patients are more likely to respond to treatments that they believe will help them. In other words, when patients are given a treatment that doesn't make sense to them, the result is generally less than desirable. It seems likely that the placebo effect (for better or worse) is best understood in terms of the patient's beliefs and expectations, not only about the treatment but also about the ability of the clinician to be helpful.

The patient's views and attitudes are important predictors of outcome, and the same can be said of the views and attitudes of the clinician. There are data to suggest that providers who frequently refer patients for psychotherapy are more realistic regarding the benefits of psychotherapy and are themselves better psychotherapists than those who refer infrequently for such treatment. Just as one's own beliefs regarding psychotherapy correlate with one's competence as a psychotherapist, so too one imagines that one's attitude regarding medications would correlate to one's success as a pharmacotherapist. Indeed, some have suggested that, in the same way that the psychotherapy alliance predicts to outcome, the "pharmacotherapy alliance" can make or break the patient's response to a particular medication or to all medications. At the simplest level, if the patient doesn't take the prescribed medication, it will not help. Of course, even if the patient does faithfully follow the pharmacological treatment regimen, there are endless psychological considerations that may affect the outcome.

The act of prescribing always involves the elucidation of a diagnosis and development of a treatment plan, as well as the development of an optimal relationship between doctor and patient. It is sometimes difficult to balance these tasks, but it becomes even harder when psychotherapy and pharmacotherapy must share the stage. In addition to the clinician's need to attend to diagnosis, treatment, and the relationship, substantial effort and time must be devoted to the task of exploring and coming to understand the patient's psyche. It is not so easy to juggle these tasks simultaneously. When psychotherapy goes well, there is a tendency to give short shrift to pharmacotherapy, and vice versa. Moreover, since many clinicians harbor preconceptions to the effect that either psychotherapy or pharmacotherapy is the better route to help with the "real" problems of the patient, there is a risk that the emphasis on one and lack of focus on the other may deprive the patient of optimal benefit from both treatment modalities. Patient and doctor sometimes find themselves on opposite sides of an implicit debate about whether the primarily somatic targets of medication are more or less important than the primarily social and psychological targets of psychotherapy. Such a disagreement may imperil the alliance, particularly if neither side raises it as a topic of discussion.

The clinician's countertransference can always interfere with optimal pharmacotherapy, but this is particularly likely to occur when the clinician is also conducting psychotherapy with the patient. There is a risk that the clinician may unknowingly respond to feelings of anger, fear, or frustration about the patient's problems by over- or under-prescribing. Such increased emotional arousal may prevent clinicians from conceptualizing their patients in a sophisticated manner and may cause them to fall back on treatment strategies that are less likely to be effective, such as exhortation, emotional withdrawal, or inappropriate closeness. Clinicians' beliefs about and tolerance for human suffering may lead them either to seek to assuage distress to such an extent that the patient becomes "numb," on one hand, or to withhold needed comfort, on the other. Of course, these issues can and do arise when the tasks of pharmacotherapy and psychotherapy are split between two providers, but such conflicts become all the more difficult to sort through when there is only one provider, and clinician and patient are working in the context of the increased intimacy that naturally arises in psychotherapy.

Psychotherapy Within Psychiatry: Narrowing Indications and Broadening Options

We end our review of useful perspectives with some comments designed to increase psychotherapeutic flexibility within the range of mental health problems commonly seen in psychiatry. We have indicated that our focus in this text is on models of psychotherapy that are designed for use in the treatment of significant mental disorders. Of course, there are other kinds of psychotherapy that have particular application to the problems of individuals who seek insight for its own sake, who seek "growth" experiences, or who are functioning within the normal range but view themselves as having some minor difficulties ("the worried well"). Examples of psychotherapy appropriate for such reasonably well-functioning individuals might include certain variants of Gestalt psychotherapy, "hobby analysis," encounter groups, and the like. Psychiatrists are likely to have less call for the use of such treatment modalities than are other mental health professionals, who may have some relatively well-functioning patients in their caseloads. In this text we have intentionally limited our investigation of psychotherapy to only those kinds of psychotherapy that apply to individuals who have clinically significant impairment or distress. The psychotherapy research we have cited may not apply to patients without significant mental disorders. Importantly, many psychotherapeutic modalities are designed to target specific symptom profiles. As such, these techniques do not necessarily extend to all psychiatric diagnoses and often require modification for efficacy in certain populations.

Within this more limited scope of patients and psychological models we have suggested that learning about two overarching psychological theories (psychoanalytic and behavioral) and then integrating these theories with useful knowledge from several research perspectives (neurobiological, psychological, and treatment studies) allows providers to develop the ability to conceptualize each patient broadly and flexibly, and it permits one to create a treatment plan that has the best chance of success.

We would suggest that it is *always* appropriate to think about the patient from the perspective of the information presented in this text. It is always helpful to try to understand the patient from a psychodynamic and also from a behavioral perspective, although in the case of any particular patient one of these theoretical perspectives may turn out to be more useful than the other. Similarly, it is always appropriate to think about how the research findings that we have presented might apply to a particular patient and what the research leads one to predict about how well a particular patient will respond to the various treatment options available. The application of theories and research to a patient's problems will permit a more sophisticated conceptualization of the patient, and enhanced individualized treatment plans are based on broad understanding and experience. Moreover, it is well established that when clinicians are able to think about patients in a complex manner, they are less likely to make countertransferential errors in treatment.

However, it is not necessarily the best thing to offer psychotherapy to every patient. We have already made the point that certain kinds of psychotherapy may be more likely to cause deterioration in treatment, and one would wish to have a strong rationale before encouraging a patient to accept any of those riskier treatments. Moreover, we know that patient preferences are important in predicting treatment outcome, a relationship that is presumably mediated by patient expectancy—or, perhaps equivalently, by the effect of placebo. If a patient specifically requests psychotherapy, it is probably a good idea to provide it or to make an appropriate referral. By contrast, if a patient indicates a disinclination to participate in psychotherapy, it will probably not be helpful to insist upon it, especially if the patient continues not to be interested in psychotherapy after having been told about the research findings that support its value in the patient's case. In either scenario, the ideal situation is to discuss the patient's feeling openly, provide education, and explore resistance or other intense feelings regarding treatment using the most appropriate methods for the individual.

If clinician and patient do agree that psychotherapy might be helpful in treatment, what kind of psychotherapy should be offered? Of course, many psychotherapeutic modalities are available, and there are varying levels of empirical support for different conditions and populations. Such information can provide useful guidance regarding the choice of a psychotherapy model. Treatment manuals are now available for more and more psychotherapy–disorder pairs, and such manuals can be very useful. However, it is possible that over-adherence to manuals may have adverse outcomes in some settings (e.g., Castonguay et al., 1996). Care should be taken to use manuals in the appropriate setting and to receive proper training before embarking on manualized therapies. Happily, most manuals nowadays are written in such a way that the clinician has reasonable flexibility and can exercise judgment in how to apply the manual to a particular patient, while continuing to maintain a supportive and responsive relationship with the patient.

Should clinicians stick to one treatment method in a given case, or should they pick and choose among treatment methods? There are two related considerations in this regard. First, it is often difficult to identify an empirically supported treatment model for which the research data exactly conform to the patient's personal characteristics and symptom constellation. In other words, the therapist is often in the position of trying to apply an empirically supported treatment model, based on the patient's general similarity to a group of research participants. Extrapolation to one individual must be based on clinical judgment as well as sum of the science. Second, many patients have multiple problems, for which a sequence of empirically supported approaches is indicated and seems most practical. However, it is almost impossible to find research evidence to support the sequential application of multiple psychotherapy models to a given set of symptoms. At some point in the future there may be data in support of more flexible protocols, and some promising early work has begun to appear on the development of "unified protocols," such as one proposed in 2010 by Barlow and colleagues, utilizing behavioral principles to address a range of anxiety and depression symptoms.

Most experts recommend against picking and choosing treatment techniques on a session-by-session basis to meet the momentary needs of patients, an approach to treatment often referred to as "eclecticism." The only research evidence that demonstrates the effectiveness of the eclectic approach is the general finding that much of psychotherapy has similar effectiveness. (Note here that we are not using the term "eclecticism" to refer to therapists' diverse training or the ability to provide a tailored protocol based on a variety of therapeutic principles and philosophies.) Many experts recommend that one pick a given treatment protocol and stick with it until either the patient recovers or there is clear evidence that the treatment has failed. Such an approach to treatment is intellectually consistent and conforms to the design of many research studies. It permits one to establish a clear relationship between technique and effect in a given case. It may also be somewhat dogmatic, and it risks wasting time and effort on a method that has diminishing returns for the patient but has not yet entirely ceased to be effective. A possible middle ground between undisciplined eclecticism and rigid consistency might be referred to as "pluralism," in which the clinician applies models of psychotherapy sequentially and intentionally, addressing one symptom or condition first, and then another, based on research showing a link between the psychotherapy model and the particular symptom or condition. Thus, to treat an individual with panic disorder who misuses alcohol or drugs and also has an underlying personality disorder, one might begin by addressing the panic symptoms by utilizing an empirically supported behavioral approach, such as Brief Therapy for Panic Disorder, after which one might interpose a few sessions of Motivational Interviewing to address ambivalence about accepting treatment for substance abuse. If this is successful, one could utilize Twelve-Step facilitation or CBT to treat the substance abuse itself, after which one might apply psychodynamic techniques to treat the underlying personality disorder.

It is, of course, always useful to track the patient's progress in some formal way, if only to increase the likelihood that one will have early warning that therapy is not succeeding. However, it is particularly important to track progress when one makes use of one or more procedures in a manner that has not been specifically validated, so that one has objective evidence regarding the trajectory of treatment and can intervene quickly when problems develop. The routine use of formal symptom checklists provides a measure of safety when one ventures beyond what is known from research findings.

In sum, we suggest that psychiatrists may benefit from focusing primarily on those kinds of psychotherapy that are known to address symptoms of clinically significant mental disorders. We further suggest that while it is always helpful to think psychotherapeutically about patients, clinicians and patients must work together to determine the best choices and understand resistance to treatment. We suggest that clinicians apply empirically supported models of psychotherapy to patients, perhaps with the flexible use of a manual, and we suggest avoiding the extremes of rigid consistency and undisciplined eclecticism by adopting a more pluralist approach, applying research-based interventions on a sequential basis, even as one carefully tracks the patient's progress in treatment.

Summary

1. In the treatment of many mental disorders, psychotherapy and pharmacotherapy are often equally efficacious. The addition of psychotherapy may improve pharmacotherapeutic treatment, while it is less clear that the addition of pharmacotherapy to psychotherapy improves outcome.

2. Psychotherapy is a useful strategy to decrease the likelihood of relapse or recurrence of depression. Psychotherapy has the potential to confer longer-term benefits than pharmacotherapy following the discontinuation of the acute phase of treatment. Also, if continuation or maintenance treatment is provided, psychotherapy is an efficacious option, either alone or in combination with medication, regardless of the type of treatment employed in the acute phase.

3. The application of psychotherapeutic principles to pharmacotherapeutic treatment is likely to improve outcome, but the provision of both modalities by the same clinician requires special attention to the art of balancing both treatments and to transference and countertransference issues.

4. The sequential application of several empirically supported treatment models may be justified in a case in which the patient presents with several problems, not all of which can be treated using a single model of psychotherapy.

Recommended Reading

Norcross, J.C. (Ed.) (2011). *Psychotherapy relationships that work: Evidence-based responsiveness* (2nd ed.). New York: Oxford University Press, USA.

Chapter 4

Learning Psychotherapy

Introduction *114*
Basic Skills *116*
    Attending and Listening skills *116*
    Restatements *117*
    Questions *119*
    Showing Empathy *120*
    Challenges *122*
Common Psychotherapeutic Techniques *124*
Proposed Learning Sequence *130*

Introduction

While it is certainly useful to begin learning psychotherapy by reading about it and then discussing the topic with others, the development of reasonable proficiency as a psychotherapist requires considerable practice, some of which includes expert feedback and advice on how to improve one's performance, which is referred to as *supervision*. Indeed, many therapists continue to receive supervision throughout their careers. In this text we present didactic information relevant to psychotherapy. We would encourage the reader to discuss this material with peers who are still early in the learning sequence and with individuals who have had more experience doing psychotherapy. Ultimately, however, becoming a competent psychotherapist is a process that takes years, and there is no substitute for extensive practice under supervision.

We begin our survey of this topic by discussing the basic skills that cut across all kinds of psychotherapy: attending and listening skills, restatements, questions, showing empathy, and challenges. Earlier in the text we introduced the *Dodo bird hypothesis*, which asserts that in large groups of adult patients one version of psychotherapy is probably about as effective as another. To the extent that this is true, it raises the probability that outcome is heavily influenced by therapist behaviors that are common across many kinds of psychotherapy. More specifically, one might reasonably conclude that fundamental relationship skills play a central role in affecting outcome, given the fact that the therapeutic alliance has about two-thirds as strong an effect on outcome as being in psychotherapy at all (i.e., $d = .57$ vs. $d = .87$).

The basic skills—attending and listening, restatements, questions, showing empathy, and challenges—describe most of what psychotherapists do on a moment-by-moment basis in session, and if these skills are expertly executed, they have the effect of improving the therapeutic alliance, and outcome improves. If they are not well executed, the therapeutic alliance suffers, and outcome suffers. Most people are moderately competent in executing these basic skills on an everyday basis. However, to maximize outcome, psychotherapists need to become experts in the basic skills, and for this reason we focus on them first. Moreover, it is perhaps strange but true that one can help many psychotherapy patients simply by executing these skills very well. Patients feel understood and respected when therapists demonstrate these skills consistently, and we know from the therapeutic alliance literature that such feelings predict good outcomes.

As an example of "feeling understood," we make reference to a major school of psychotherapy that bases its techniques on the proposition that patients will lose their symptoms if and only if a certain kind of relationship is established with the therapist. *Client-centered psychotherapy* was developed in the 1940s and 1950s by an American psychologist called Carl R. Rogers (1902–1987), one of the first researchers to adopt a rigorous approach to the study of psychotherapy. For example, in many client-centered studies, psychotherapy sessions were transcribed and subjected to somewhat reliable methods of content analysis. Rogers took the position that symptoms of psychopathology arise when one no longer relies on one's *organismic valuing system*, an internal "felt sense" that helps one decide the best course of action in a given situation. The organismic valuing system helps one make decisions based on one's particular needs and goals. Rogers believed that people stop paying attention to their organismic valuing system because they value the love and support of parents and important others who may contingently reinforce behavior that meets others' needs but not one's own. In other words, some people have early family experiences that cause them to make decisions to please others without taking their own needs into account.

Rogers suggested that the task of psychotherapy is to help patients to begin relying once again on their organismic valuing system, and he believed that therapists could bring this about by demonstrating "genuineness" in the therapeutic relationship, by communicating unconditional positive regard for patients and their internal experiences and ideas, and by communicating empathic understanding to patients. At a concrete level, this involved reflecting patients' thoughts and feelings and encouraging patients to explore topics about which they had mixed feelings, in the expectation that the process of exploration would lead them to sort through their conflicts. Client-centered therapists rely very heavily on the basic skills we are about to describe, and these, together with a therapeutic attitude informed by the above treatment goals, constitute much of the technique of client-centered psychotherapy.

After we discuss the basic skills, we introduce a list of specific psychotherapeutic techniques that appear in a variety of types of psychotherapy. Not only is this list helpful in giving the reader a sense of the strategies used in psychotherapy, but it will simplify the task of describing important models of psychotherapy, as we do in Chapter 5. Finally, we propose a sequence of learning experiences that will help lay the groundwork for readers to produce good outcomes in psychotherapy.

Basic Skills

Few research studies link the execution of basic skills to outcome in psychotherapy, but such research as does exist suggests that the skills are helpful. The literature also suggests that skills are likely to be most effective when they are executed in a manner that is consistent with the session's verbal content. For example, it is known that when therapists lean slightly forward, it helps the therapy process, but trunk lean is much more helpful when it is flexible and is consistent with the content of discussion. Similarly, it is known that when therapists paraphrase patients' statements about feelings, patients respond by introspecting further, and at the end of the session they report decreased anxiety. However, outcome is much more directly benefited when therapists speak in a way that complements the patient's style.

Attending and Listening Skills

Psychotherapy patients lack information about their problems, or they don't know how to use the information they do have to generate workable solutions, or both. Thus, one very important goal of psychotherapy is to help patients make sense of their thoughts and feelings. Ultimately, patients need to learn to think, feel, and act differently, but the process begins with careful attention to the content of their mind. Every school of psychotherapy requires patients to learn to attend to thoughts and feelings in a new way, and therapists model this by listening and attending very carefully. If patients are exposed to this behavior on the part of therapists, they are more likely to engage in the behavior themselves. When therapists attend and listen, it communicates respect for patients and encourages them to continue to explore their thoughts and feelings. Patients then discover perspectives on and details about mental phenomena that may expand or even contradict their habitual understanding of them. A classic definition of psychotherapy is that we keep patients talking until they finally hear themselves.

When therapists engage in attending and listening behavior, they sit up, present themselves as kind and interested, and work to ensure that their verbalizations don't get in the patient's way. This is not to suggest that therapists should withhold support from their patients by maintaining stony silence. Silences should always communicate warmth, support, and respect. Ideally, therapists will establish an environment in which patients feel comfortable with thoughtful silence and can use the time to introspect. Obviously, one of the big rewards for therapists in mastering the skill of tactical silence is that they gain time to plan carefully what to say and don't feel pressured to respond before they are ready to do so.

It is important that therapists avoid little motor habits that may signal their internal state. Professional poker players rely on "tells" to read other players, and some patients may be skilled at reading such nonverbal behavior. Therapist motor habits may include stereotyped finger movements, repeatedly glancing around the room or at the clock, jiggling one's leg, playing with one's hair, and the like. This is not to suggest that therapists should sit stock still. Rather, therapists should sit comfortably, if alertly, and should move easily in their chairs, but they should avoid any motor habits that may "tell" the patient that the therapist is feeling uneasy, anxious, or otherwise distressed.

Cultural issues loom large with regard to attending and listening. Of course, diversity issues are always important in psychotherapy, but it's particularly useful to mention them in regard to nonverbal behavior. Behaviors such as silence, interpersonal distance, eye contact, and the like are interpreted differently by different cultures, and one isn't always aware that one is making a culturally dependent interpretation.

For example, in most European American subcultures, speakers make fleeting eye contact, but listeners fix their gaze on speakers. By contrast, in many African and East Asian cultures the respectful listener looks down. With regard to interpersonal distance, certain Mediterranean cultures are comfortable with close distances when talking to someone else. When therapists and patients have different expectations regarding interpersonal distance, it can lead to discomfort and misunderstandings on both sides. Even silences have different meanings in different cultures. For the most part in European American culture, it is considered rude for a conversation participant of lower status not to offer a response to the participant of higher status. Offering a response is viewed as evidence that the lower-status individual is listening carefully to his or her superior. In some other cultures, it is seen as evidence of respect when the lower-status individual *doesn't* respond.

How should therapists negotiate these cultural differences? One strategy is to find out as much as possible about a new patient's cultural background and then, during the first few minutes of interaction, to rely on expectations based on what one may have learned about this culture in general. As quickly as possible, however, therapists should gather specific information about how *this particular patient* interprets nonverbal behavior and should then replace expectations based on stereotypes with expectations based on actual experience. More generally, it is helpful to approach *every* patient as if he or she comes from a different cultural background, and learn from that patient what he or she prefers and expects.

Restatements

In one way, this basic skill is just a logical extension of attending and listening. Restatements focus on what the patient just said, either in the form of a *paraphrase* or a *summary statement*. Paraphrases are seldom longer than one sentence, and they summarize a sentence or two of what the patient has just said. An example might be, "You didn't know what to think when your boss came into the office." Summary statements may be several sentences long, and they usually pull together the last few paragraphs of the patient's verbalizations. An example might be, "We've been talking about the confusing relationship with your boss. Sometimes it feels like she ambushes you at the office, but at other times she seems to be quite supportive. It is frustrating that this hot-and-cold relationship causes anxiety and distracts you so much from your work."

Restatements serve the purpose of communicating that the therapist is following the patient's verbalizations. In particular, summary statements are a way to pull together several ideas so that the patient grasps the import of what has been said up to that moment and can then continue to explore the topic. Restatements also permit the therapist very gently to lead the patient in a direction that is likely to be helpful. At any given point in a therapy session, there are usually several directions in which the conversation might go, and therapists can use restatements as a way to contingently reinforce patients for addressing some topics and not others. Questions can serve a similar purpose but are experienced by patients as more intrusive. Patients are often unaware that therapists manage the therapeutic discussion through the strategic use of restatements; they usually respond better to this management technique than to other attempts to keep the session "on task."

If therapists can use restatements gently to lead the session, in which direction should the therapist lead? This is, of course, a question that is not easy to answer in every instance. However, it is usually true that the best direction in which to lead the patient is the one that is consistent with one's case conceptualization. If the therapist has a theory about the patient's problems and about how to ameliorate them, then it's best to direct the conversation in a way that is consistent with that conceptualization. Unfortunately, one doesn't always have such a conceptualization, or one's theory of the case may not cover the particular topic that the patient has raised at the moment. In such a situation, one can rely on the *psychotherapy fallback rule*, which is that it's best to direct the conversation toward the patient's thoughts and feelings, rather than to focus on the patient's observable behavior or on the actions of other people.

Not infrequently, the therapist may be unsure about exactly what the patient is thinking or feeling, and for this reason paraphrases and summary statements can be slightly off the mark. This is actually not a problem, because when patients believe that therapists are working hard to understand their point of view, they will almost always offer clarification so that they are better understood. This actually has the benefit of forcing patients to think more clearly about what they are trying to say. However, given that the therapist often fails to deliver a perfect restatement, it's best to offer restatements in a manner that invites the patient to clarify or correct. Some therapists do this by asking questions like, "Am I getting that right?" or "Does that sound correct to you?" Therapists can transform the restatement into a question by raising the pitch of their voice at the end (as if asking a question) or by giving a slightly questioning look. Particularly when starting with a patient, it is important to facilitate a more open discussion and not to over-interpret, because patients have varying levels of comfort in "correcting" the therapist. Not infrequently, patients allow an incorrect line of discussion to proceed if the therapist over-emphasizes his or her interpretation. Later in therapy it isn't necessary to invite a response so directly, because by then the patient will have learned that any correction of a restatement will be always welcomed by the therapist.

Finally, it is important that therapists strive to offer *succinct* restatements in which the therapist *does not* parrot the patient's exact words. One exception to the virtue of using different words occurs when patients are struggling with ambivalence; at such times a technique called Motivational Interviewing, which we review in the Chapter 5 section on other individual psychotherapies, prescribes that the therapist use the patient's exact words so as to prevent the patient from quibbling with the therapist over wording as a way to direct attention away from the ambivalence itself. In almost all other circumstances, however, patients respond best when the therapist slightly rephrases what was just said.

Questions

There are two kinds of questions that therapists use in psychotherapy. *Closed questions* can be answered in a few words—yes, no, or a discrete fact. They are useful to gain specific and generally simple kinds of information. Closed questions are sometimes also effective in slowing down the patient. *Open questions* cannot be answered in a few words. They are useful to encourage the patient to explore further in a certain direction. While closed questions do have a place in psychotherapy, most of the time therapists use open questions. Many therapists find this skill hard to learn, because the majority of day-to-day conversation involves closed questions. It is important to realize that good therapy rarely models regular conversation; instead, it utilizes the therapist's skills to help patients understand their own thoughts and motivations.

Here are some important guidelines regarding questions. First and foremost, it is important to remember that patients experience questions as more intrusive than restatements or attending and listening behavior. *It is therefore a good idea to precede the first question in a series with a restatement.* Thus, "You were taken aback when your boss accused you of failing to ring up that sale the right way. Can you tell me more about what you were thinking right after she said that?" Or, "So your mood has been down since yesterday, and you've had trouble making yourself do anything at home. What was going on when your mood dropped yesterday?" Each time the therapist asks a question that moves the conversation in a slightly new direction, the question should be preceded by a restatement. This may seem artificial and takes considerable practice under supervision to do well.

Another important guideline states that *psychotherapy sessions should never fall into a pattern of questions and answers*. When the patient realizes that the therapist has established a Q&A routine, the patient will stop thinking and will simply wait for the next question. When that happens, the therapist ends up doing the active work, and the patient is permitted or even encouraged to take a passive role in the session. Obviously, it's fine to pose a series of questions to complete a formal evaluation, but once the actual psychotherapy begins, the Q&A needs to end. Within any list of questions the therapist should interpose restatements and other kinds of verbalizations so as to keep the patient as active as possible in the session. In particular, one way to break up the Q&A routine is to ask questions in the form of statements. Many therapists ask questions in this form: "I'm wondering about . . .," "I'm curious about . . .," "I wonder if you could say more about . . .," or "Tell me about . . ."

Another guideline for questions is that it is usually best to *avoid asking patients any question that begins with "why."* There are many ways to understand an individual's reasons without asking why, which for many people reminds them of accusatory parents who are about to punish them for having misbehaved. Instead of asking "why," therapists can say, "Help me understand what you were thinking there." One might also say, "I'm curious about what some of the alternatives were that you considered in that situation." Therapists can also ask, "What was the thought you had about that situation that led you to feel (or act) that way?" It's also fine to ask, "Do you have a theory about what's going on with this?" As with many of these skills, it takes considerable practice to avoid using conversational language such as asking "why." Most therapists need training to avoid this word.

Just as therapists are encouraged to utilize the *psychotherapy fallback rule* to decide how to direct the conversation through restatements, this rule is also useful when the therapist must decide which questions would be helpful to pursue. Thus, therapists are encouraged to ask questions that are consistent with their conceptualizations; failing that, questions should direct the patient to focus on his or her own thoughts and feelings, rather than to focus on observable behaviors or the actions of others.

As was the case with restatements, therapists are encouraged to ask questions succinctly. Therapists may be tempted to make additional comments instead of waiting for a response. This can pose a real problem, since it over-directs the patient. Here is an example of the kind of question string to avoid: "Can you tell me more about what happened? I mean, what exactly were you thinking when your wife said that she would be home late? Were you upset? Is this typical of how things are in the marriage? I mean, what thoughts did you have right after the phone call?" In response to such a question the patient can only feel perplexed and may feel the need to answer in a way that pleases the therapist. With practice and supervision, therapists can learn to deliver elegant and precise questions, after which they must **stop** and **wait**.

One advantage of asking questions is that by gathering details, therapists are able to move beyond patients' conceptualizations of their problems. Patients may come to therapy with a theory about their problems in life, and the theory may or may not be helpful in solving those problems. It is important for therapists to communicate that they understand the patient's point of view, that they are able to see the world as the patient sees it. It is, however, crucial that therapists also develop an alternate view of the patient's problems and that this alternate view readily lead the patient to consider recommendations about how to make helpful changes in his or her life. Therapists gather details by asking questions: "Can you tell me exactly what happened in that conversation with your boss? Lead me through it." When the patient begins to generalize or otherwise wanders off track, the therapist says, "Wait a moment. We were talking about what happened right after your boss started to raise her voice about entering the sales data. What exactly did she say, and then what did you say?" This may be a situation in which closed questions are more useful than open questions, particularly if the patient has difficulty remaining on task or the patient has prematurely decided what the core problems are in his or her life. In general, open questions and restatements encourage patient exploration. Closed questions may be useful in gathering information, clarifying, and helping to keep the patient on-task.

Showing Empathy

In our discussion of client-centered therapy, we noted that Carl Rogers was interested in the construct of empathy. Indeed, many systems of psychotherapy make explicit reference to empathy, and virtually all encourage the therapist to behave in a way that leads the patient to believe that the therapist is empathic. There is evidence that empathy and outcome are correlated nearly as strongly as are alliance and outcome. However, there is much better agreement on how to measure alliance than on how to measure empathy, because in psychotherapy empathy has to do with the patient's perception that the therapist understands and resonates to the patient's feelings—not such an easy thing to measure.

At a concrete level, therapists are encouraged to demonstrate empathy through reflection of the patient's feelings. Such reflection can be in the form of a restatement, "You're feeling pretty sad about that," or through nonverbal behavior that mirrors the patient's feeling state. Not only do patients interpret the therapist's reflection of feelings as evidence of empathy, but such reflection of affect helps to orient patients' attention more directly to their emotions, about which some patients have only limited information. A focus on feelings also has the effect of short-circuiting intellectualization and other avoidance strategies patients may employ. Patients usually attend more acutely when they are aware of their emotions, and they introspect more deeply.

Here are some suggestions about reflecting feelings. First, every therapist should routinely track the patient's feeling state. At any point in a session, the therapist should be able to answer the following question after a delay of no more than two seconds: "What is the patient's emotional state right now?" Obviously, therapists can track affect by paying attention to the content of the patient's verbalizations. However, it's also useful to notice the patient's nonverbal behavior and to pay attention to verbal dysfluencies. Is the patient's conversation speed or vocal quality different than it was a moment ago? Might this reflect a shift in affect?

One template for reflecting feelings is as follows: "You feel . . ." + feeling label (state the observed emotion) + context (in named situation). Therapists should try to match the *intensity level* of the patient's feeling and should be as specific as possible about the *context*, exactly what it was that triggered the affect. It is fine for the therapist to be slightly off the mark, but then the patient must feel that he or she is free to correct the therapist. As was the case for restatement more generally, patients benefit from thinking through the way in which the therapist didn't precisely grasp their experience, since it sharpens patients' understanding of the experience in question and increases the collaborative bond between patient and therapist. After offering a feeling reflection early in treatment, it's good to ask the patient something like, "Does that sound right to you?"

Most patients respond very well to the therapist's reflection of affect. However, this may not be an appropriate technique for every patient. Indeed, there are some patients who for cultural or other reasons may become uncomfortable when discussion turns to their feelings. Sometimes therapists have to proceed gently when it comes to feelings. It is important constantly to monitor for changes in affect and to respond accordingly. If the patient gives evidence of distress in response to the therapist's reflection of affect, the therapist might comment on this, might reflect affect again, or might move away from affect for a little while. Again, practice and supervision improve mastery of these skills and allow therapists to diversify their responses during uncomfortable situations.

Challenges

The last of the basic skills is the delivery of challenges, a therapeutic maneuver in which the therapist points out a discrepancy between how the patient thinks, feels, or acts and something else. This is clearly the riskiest of the five skills; there is research evidence to suggest that all too often challenges go awry in psychotherapy. Certain models of psychotherapy, like Motivational interviewing, which we discuss in detail in Chapter 5, offer very precise guidelines for delivering challenges, whereas other modalities avoid challenges altogether. We discuss here a general approach to challenges that is useful in most other kinds of psychotherapy.

Most often therapists offer challenges that point to the discrepancy between two of the patient's statements: "If I'm understanding you correctly, on one hand you want to keep seeing your girlfriend, and on the other hand, you'd like to date someone else. Can you say more about that?" Another common purpose of challenges is to help the patient understand the irrationality of a belief: "So you felt guilty about reacting against your mother's attempts to control you. Can you talk a little more about that?" Less frequently, therapists offer challenges to point out the disparity between what patients say and how they act: "On one hand, it seems to you that the most important thing is for parents to exert a healthy influence on their children. On the other hand, you find yourself spending very little time at home because of work. How do you put these two together?" On rare occasions therapists challenge patients by pointing out the difference between patients' desires and the needs of others in their lives: "So part of you thinks that it's your paycheck, and you should be able to spend it in a way that makes sense to you. But another part of you recognizes that your family needs to have some input into spending decisions. Is that right?"

When patients are clearly working toward change in their lives, challenges should be delivered in a very gentle, supportive manner, and they should occur infrequently—in most treatment models no more than 5% of therapist verbalizations should be challenges, and in many instances challenges should occur *much less frequently* than that. With patients who are not interested in changing behavior, the frequency of challenges may climb toward the 5% limit, but if this continues for very long, the alliance is likely to become so damaged that the outcome of treatment will be in doubt. Moreover, certain populations may appreciate challenges more than others, and it is important to monitor for comfort and outcome if challenges are used in session.

Before offering challenges, therapists should make sure an *inconsistency really exists* by carefully listening to and observing the patient. Therapists then need to think through their intention in pointing out the patient's inconsistency. Is it possible that the therapist's primary motivation in challenging the patient is to discharge frustration? Challenges like this can be cathartic for the therapist, but they *rarely help the patient*. It is also very important to consider whether an intervention less direct than a challenge might be more effective. As well, the cultural implications of a challenge should be considered. If after all this the therapist decides that a challenge is the least direct intervention possible in the situation, the therapist should formulate the challenge using one of the following templates. (Remember first to make sure the inconsistency really exists within the patient!)

1. "On the one hand, X, and on the other hand, Y. How do you put these two together?"
2. "I'm confused. I think you're saying X, but it sounds like you're also saying Y. Can you help me understand that a bit more?"
3. "Can we back up a bit? You said you felt X, because you thought Y. Can we talk some more about that?"
4. "So part of you feels X, and part of you feels Y. Is that right?"
5. Or even more simply: "It sounds like *part* of you is feeling X. Am I getting that right?"

After delivering the challenge, it is important to encourage the patient to provide feedback. The therapist should pay careful attention to the result of the challenge.

There was once a television series called *Columbo*. In it, actor Peter Falk played a detective who solved cases by presenting himself to the suspect in a friendly but slightly confused manner. Lt. Columbo's approach to the interview was so disarming that the miscreant usually stumbled into confessing by the end of the episode. Many successful psychotherapists take such a tack in treatment: "I think I'm getting confused . . ." or "I'm sorry that I'm not with you here. Can you slow down and say that again?" These are implicit challenges, but they are so indirect that patients are unlikely to become defensive. As a result, patients often verbalize the discrepancy themselves, which is certainly much more fruitful than when the therapist has to do so.

Summary

1. Basic psychotherapy skills include attending and listening, restatements, questions, showing empathy, and challenges.
2. Through practice and supervision with a highly experienced provider, therapists must develop a very high level of performance in these skills.

Common Psychotherapeutic Techniques

We have suggested that when psychotherapists develop expert competence in the execution of certain basic, pan-theoretical skills, the likelihood of good outcome increases. We now offer a list of more specific psychotherapeutic techniques that are utilized in a number of different models of psychotherapy. This alphabetical list will give the reader a sense of the strategies that psychotherapists use. We will refer to this list later on, when we discuss the major models of psychotherapy. These techniques are used to varying degrees, depending on the treatment modality.

Activity scheduling: In one variant of activity scheduling, patient and therapist agree on certain activities in which the patient will engage during the coming week. These can be new activities or activities in which the patient wishes to engage more frequently. Activities typically tracked include physical exercise, working on household tasks, sleep, socializing with others, and the like. The patient tracks the target activities using a suitable form, typically a log or calendar that breaks each day into one-hour segments. Sometimes patients are also asked to rate the target activities along certain dimensions, such as the associated pleasure or sense of mastery. The other variant of activity scheduling involves having patients simply log their main activities during each one-hour period over the course of several days. Both variants of activity scheduling rely on the fact that charting is usually *reactive*: people increase desired activities and decrease undesired activities when they keep careful track of them.

Analyzing defenses: Some might argue that this technique is specific to psychoanalytically-informed psychotherapies, but something like defense analysis actually occurs in many kinds of psychotherapy. Analyzing defenses involves the therapist's exploration with the patient of hypothesized mental phenomena that interfere with the patient's ability to accept and act directly on his or her impulses, wishes, and predictions. This technique involves uncovering beliefs about the world that shed light on why the patient doesn't act in a manner that would be more directly gratifying or effective, even though the patient possesses the skills to do so.

Assertiveness training: Patients are directly taught skills to enable them to assert themselves in a variety of social situations. There are any number of assertiveness training manuals (e.g., Alberti & Emmons, 2008) that provide information about the differences among passivity, self-assertion, and aggression. Such manuals also provide sequenced instructions and specific homework assignments to help patients learn how to make "I" statements, how to express direct requests, how to respond appropriately to the other person, and so forth. Frequently in assertiveness training the therapist demonstrates assertive behavior for the patient and encourages the patient to copy the demonstration as closely as possible. Therapist and patient may also practice scenarios in which the patient plans to behave assertively in the coming week.

Assigning homework: While some psychotherapy models take the position that the patient can find relief simply by working hard in therapy sessions, many models of treatment explicitly require the patient to try out new behaviors or to conduct "experiments" during the week, reporting back to the therapist at the beginning of the next session. Patient and therapist use data collected from the assignment to understand the patient's problems better and to evaluate the patient's current status. In most psychotherapy models that utilize homework, assignments are developed collaboratively by patient and therapist, and it is important to anticipate and resolve ahead of time any obstacles to their completion prior to the next session. When therapists assign homework, it is very important to ask the patient about the homework at the next session. If the patient comes to expect that the therapist will *not* inquire about homework, the patient will be much less likely to complete future assignments.

Behavior monitoring: If the patient is attempting to change the frequency of a certain behavior, it is often helpful to monitor the behavior's frequency between sessions using an appropriate form. Behavior monitors may consist of simple counts, or they may provide more specific information, such as when the behavior occurred or other circumstantial information. As previously noted, monitoring is almost always reactive; the simple act of monitoring can be helpful all by itself. Behavior monitoring is also helpful to gather data regarding the frequency of behaviors that might become problematic, such as disturbed sleep patterns, aggressive outbursts, consumption of alcohol or drugs, and so forth.

Catharsis: Sometimes patients benefit from having a strongly emotional experience with the therapist, in which they understand themselves or some aspect of their lives in a new way. Catharsis occurs when the patient has a sudden insight that is accompanied by a great deal of affect, usually sadness or relief.

Constructing hierarchies: When a patient is fearful of a certain situation or behavior, the therapist can increase the patient's cooperation with and eventual outcome from exposure treatment by developing a hierarchy that starts with a stimulus that evokes minimal fear and ends with one that evokes a great deal of fear. For example, the hierarchy of a patient with snake phobia might involve a dozen steps that differ from one another along dimensions of the actual distance from the snake and the size or color of the snake. The hierarchy of a person with social phobia might involve steps that differ from one another in terms of the number of people in the interaction, the status of people, the degree to which the patient calls attention to himself or herself, whether the interaction is structured or informal, and so on. Most patients are willing to confront items that are low on their fear hierarchy, and as they become comfortable with the easier items, they are willing to move on to more frightening items.

Contingent reinforcement: This technique, essentially equivalent to operant conditioning and sometimes referred to as *contingency management*, involves organizing the environment in such a way that the performance of a target behavior is consistently followed by a pleasurable consequence. Contingent reinforcement may also involve the consistent nonreinforcement of behaviors that compete with the target behavior. An example of contingent reinforcement is a child's behavioral chart (sometimes called a star chart), in which parents affix special stickers to a chart when the child engages in certain target behaviors, such as performing chores, coping with frustration, and so forth. As well, adults can contingently reinforce themselves by "earning" desirable consequences for performing target behaviors or by depriving themselves of certain pleasurable activities if they fail to do so.

Downward arrow: This is a technique that helps patients discover the underlying meaning of a distressing thought. The therapist begins by helping the patient to verbalize a belief; for example, the patient may say, "My wife was upset with me when my paycheck was short." The therapist then asks, "If that's true, what would it mean?" The patient may then reply, "If I don't give my wife what she wants, she won't love me." Each time the patient offers a response, the therapist again asks, "*If that's true, what would it mean?*" Finally, the patient arrives at a fundamental belief, such as, "I'll be all alone, and no one will care for me."

Exposure: Patients who fear certain stimuli are exposed to those stimuli in a controlled manner, as a consequence of which they learn that the feared stimuli are not actually dangerous. Exposures can be constructed to overcome a variety of anxiety conditions, including phobias, panic, and obsessions and compulsions, among others. There are data to suggest that the behavioral treatment of almost all anxiety disorders depends to a greater or lesser extent on exposure. Exposure treatment frequently requires the use of anxiety hierarchies (cf. "constructing hierarchies," above).

Extinction: This is a technique that can be used to decrease the frequency of undesirable behaviors. Patient and therapist first identify the reinforcers that maintain an undesirable behavior, and they then organize the patient's environment such that the expected reinforcers are not delivered in response to the undesirable behavior. As a consequence the behavior frequency and strength drop off, and the behavior is ultimately said to be *extinguished*.

Feedback: When a patient is told directly by a therapist or psychotherapy group member how the patient affects the other, this is referred to as feedback. Feedback may take the form of a comment on the relationship between the speaker and the patient, on the speaker's feelings toward the patient, on the patient's behavior, or on the speaker's belief about the patient's psychological makeup.

Free association: Referred to as the "fundamental rule" of psychoanalysis, free association requires that patients say whatever comes into their minds during the therapy session, without exercising any control or censorship at all. The resulting stream of verbalizations provides the therapist with raw data from which to develop hypotheses about the patient's mental activity, including the structure of the patient's defenses.

Interpretation: This technique involves the therapist making the patient aware of the relationship among current thoughts, feelings, and behaviors. Alternatively, the therapist may draw parallels between current issues in the patient's life and the patient's important experiences in the past.

Journaling: This is a form of homework in which the therapist encourages a patient to write about emotionally meaningful experiences that occur during the week. Alternatively, the patient may be asked to write down thoughts and feelings on a particular topic.

Mindfulness: This is a state that Kabat-Zinn described in 1994 as "paying attention in a particular way: on purpose, in the present moment, and nonjudgmentally." Many people develop a state of mindfulness through meditation practice. In psychotherapy therapists encourage patients to develop mindfulness skills as a way to remain aware of their feelings and impulses. If one remains mindful, one is less likely to react ineffectively to certain thoughts and feelings; instead, one simply observes or is aware of previously troubling thoughts and feelings, without reacting.

Modeling: When therapists demonstrate target behaviors to patients, they are said to be using modeling to assist the patient in behavior change. Modeling may be explicit, as when the therapist demonstrates the difference between passive and assertive responses in a given situation, or it may be implicit, as when the therapist works through a specific problem with the patient in a manner that the patient has never before experienced.

Planning experiments: Patients can challenge beliefs about themselves or their lives by planning experiments to conduct between sessions. For example, a patient with social phobia who expects to be viewed by others as boring or unworthy can evaluate this prediction by planning to participate in a mildly feared social interaction after agreeing with the therapist on the precise criteria by which the patient will assess others' reactions. Alternatively, an individual with alcohol addiction may believe that controlled drinking is possible; patient and therapist can plan experiments to determine if this is so.

Problem solving: Some patients don't have a consistent and reliable strategy to make important decisions or solve problems. Therapists can teach a step-by-step approach to solving problems, including activities like defining the problem clearly, brainstorming possible solutions, listing the advantages and disadvantages of each alternative, and so forth.

Psychoeducation: In this technique the therapist provides technical information to the patient about the patient's illness. Such information may include diagnosis, treatment alternatives, and prognosis, or it may include more specific information about symptom patterns and the like.

Reframing: When patients harbor inappropriately negative views of themselves or their experiences, therapists can help them by offering a different view. For example, a mother may chastise herself for failing to spend every minute with her children. The therapist may help her to see that she spends as much time with her children as anyone reasonably could, particularly in view of the fact that she works hard to improve their environment by maintaining a job outside the home. Similarly, a person who has recently achieved abstinence from addiction may feel worthless for having had such a problem, but the therapist can point out that overcoming addiction is evidence of real strength that not everyone has.

Rehearsal: When patients are learning new behaviors, it is worthwhile to rehearse them repeatedly with the therapist and outside of the session before implementing them in target situations. Sometimes therapists encourage patients to rehearse behaviors covertly by imagining them in sequence before actually executing them.

Relapse prevention: Originally designed to decrease the likelihood of relapsing into addiction, relapse prevention is now viewed as a good way to help patients avoid relapse in any chronic disease. The technique involves identifying cognitive, emotional, and situational triggers and warning signs of relapse so that the patient can take steps in a timely manner to forestall a relapse. Such steps might involve reviewing therapy notes, increasing physical or social activity, contacting treatment personnel, talking with significant others, and so forth.

Relaxation training: This technique involves teaching the patient techniques (including progressive muscle relaxation, visualization strategies, and special breathing techniques) to achieve a deep state of relaxation, with the intention that the patient will then use this technique to decrease autonomic arousal as needed in daily life. Relaxation training is used for its own sake to manage anxiety and can also be used in service of treatments for phobia and the like.

Role plays: Patients can practice new behavior with the therapist by acting out short scenes in which the new behavior is demonstrated, either by the therapist or by the patient. Role plays are also used to provide the therapist with more detailed information about important interactions that the patient wishes to discuss in the therapy session. It is often helpful for role plays to be executed twice. First, the therapist plays the role of the patient, and the patient plays the interlocutor. This permits the therapist to get a better sense of the patient's interlocutor while modeling the desired behavior for the patient. Then the roles are reversed, and the therapist can assess how well the patient has learned the approach previously modeled by the therapist.

Setting goals: Many models of psychotherapy require that patient and therapist set clear behavioral goals for treatment. These goals should be fairly concrete and amenable to achievement through treatment, and it is important to review them from time to time as treatment progresses. The therapist uses the patient's agreement with goals as a way to motivate an individual who may feel disinclined to do certain kinds of hard work in therapy.

Setting time limits for treatment: Therapy models that use manuals are sometimes time-limited, with a course of treatment often lasting from 12 to 20 sessions. The patient is told about the time limit at the beginning of treatment, and the therapist may occasionally remind the patient about it as treatment progresses, with the expectation that this will help the patient remain focused in sessions and will lead the patient to redouble his or her efforts to work through problems. Time limits also allow patients to anticipate and prepare for closure.

Skill building: Many patients lack the skills necessary to resolve certain problems in their lives. They may not know how to behave assertively, how to make small talk in social situations, how to make decisions, how to decrease autonomic arousal, how to focus attention, or how to distract themselves. Therapists may teach these skills directly, using a combination of psychoeducation, role plays, and homework.

Socratic questioning: It is usually best for patients to arrive at their own conclusions rather than to wait for the therapist to tell them what to think. One method to help patients view their problems in a new way involves the use of Socratic questioning, in which therapists pose a series of questions designed to lead patients to understand their problems differently. The key here is that therapists must remind themselves beforehand to remain genuinely curious about which conclusion the patient will ultimately reach. Such an attitude of openness and acceptance on the part of the therapist decreases the likelihood that the patient will feel manipulated by the Socratic approach.

Stimulus control: When patient and therapist have discovered a relationship between a target behavior and the presence of specific environmental stimuli, it can be helpful to manipulate those stimuli. For example, people with alcohol dependence should limit the amount of time they spend in bars, while depressed people should spend more time socializing with others. At a more sophisticated level couples might use certain cues to remind themselves to interact in a calmer, more supportive manner.

Transference work: One of the basic tenets of psychoanalysis is that when a patient comes to understand the ways in which he or she *misperceives* the therapist and the historical reasons for such misperception, the patient learns to relate to other people in a more veridical and effective manner. As well, examination of the transference offers clues regarding the patient's defense structure. Transference work, the portion of therapy conversation that focuses on such transference distortions, also occurs in many other models of psychotherapy, if only because the patient's difficulties are reflected in interpersonal problems that become manifest in the therapy relationship.

Proposed Learning Sequence

In this section we present a sequence of activities for you to undertake in order to work toward becoming a competent psychotherapist. Not surprisingly, the development of professional competence in psychotherapy takes a number of years. Mastery increases with education, practice, and supervision. Similar to many other complex skillsets, there is always more to learn, and one's performance can always improve.

At the outset, we encourage you to consider whether you would be prepared to undertake a course of psychotherapy with yourself as the patient. There is no better way to learn a complex skill than to observe it at close range, and your experience as a patient will give you information about how psychotherapy works at a level of detail that no book, class, or video can ever match. It is immensely helpful to acquire a clear understanding of the patient's experience in psychotherapy; once you have been a patient yourself, you will experience less frustration when your own patients fail to progress quickly or don't seem to understand what you are telling them. Perhaps most importantly, when therapists understand themselves better and can recognize their own biases and triggers, they will have a better understanding of their own countertransference when treating patients.

Regardless of what you decide about seeking psychotherapy for yourself, there are a number of other activities that will help you to develop skills as a psychotherapist. First of all, most psychiatry residents in training talk with other trainees about their thoughts and ideas in response to what they read in this and other texts and, in a similar way, discuss and digest what they hear in classes on the topic. It is hard to resolve subtle points or to answer complicated questions without discussion of this kind. However, it is important to check with your institution about the limits of discussing actual cases with peers or supervisors. A certain level of anonymity of the patient may be required, depending on the educational setting.

The next step is to practice short sequences of therapy sessions through role play. Locate a partner who can play a generally cooperative, mildly depressed or anxious patient. Your partner should play a real patient or should act out a more anxious/depressed version of himself or herself. The "patient" should not be fabricated, because it's unlikely that the resulting role play will be realistic. If it makes sense, you and your partner can switch back and forth between the roles of therapist and patient. It's also extremely helpful to have a third person to provide feedback after each role play, because you won't be able to observe yourself very well, and the "patient" will be focused on acting his or her role. Use a timer, and set it for just three minutes to begin. Focus your attention on one basic skill at a time, progressing through the skills in the order we presented them in the earlier section: attending and listening, restatements, questions, showing empathy, and challenges. You should do at least three or four role plays per skill (and perhaps rather more than that). When you recognize clear improvement in one skill, move on to the next, but remember in each role play also to incorporate the skills you have practiced in previous role plays. This is one of the most common mechanisms for learning therapy skills—practice with each other first, ideally under the supervision of highly experienced therapists.

4 LEARNING PSYCHOTHERAPY

Tips for Role Playing to Learn Psychotherapy Skills

1. For attending and listening, do your best as "therapist" not to say anything of significance during the role play. If you feel comfortable doing so, aim to mirror the mood or content of the "patient" with your facial expression or body language. Whenever you feel the impulse to speak, **count silently to yourself for five seconds before you say anything**. Work on increasing the length of time that you feel comfortable with silence. After the session is over, talk to each other about what increased or decreased comfort, anxiety, and other emotions. Ask observers what they noticed about your nonverbal behavior, and ask for specific feedback regarding any distracting motor habits. Were there approaches that seemed more sincere? Did anything appear to be condescending? Discuss how slightly different approaches may have yielded more desirable results. You should discuss each role play for at least 10 to 15 minutes afterwards. Feel free to let the discussion lead to the consideration of larger issues in psychotherapy. This is a good time to think through questions or worries you may have about it.

2. For restatements, focus on speaking briefly. Make sure to encourage the "patient" to clarify or correct any misunderstanding on your part. Try gently changing the direction of the conversation solely through the use of restatements. Experiment with what happens when you rely on the "psychotherapy fallback rule" described above. Consider also making a restatement that is very slightly off the mark in order to see how the "patient" actually responds. Ask the "patient" about his or her experience of this. If you record the interaction, watch it later and stop the tape each time you have completed speaking. Now try to say what you just said in half as many words.

3. When you begin working on questions, you may want to lengthen role plays to four minutes or so. Pay very careful attention the use of open questions, as well as to whether you offer a restatement prior to each question. Avoid closed questions if at all possible. Try to ask two to four questions over the course of a four-minute role play. Afterwards, ask the "patient" how he or she experienced your questions. Were they relatively on the mark, unobtrusive, and helpful? If not, can you identify what may have gone wrong?

4. When working on empathy, strive to offer about two feeling reflections over the course of four minutes. Practice responding empathically by saying the emotion the "patient" seems to be experiencing and also mirroring the affect in your face. As well, practice using the template described above: "You feel . . ." + feeling label + context. Be careful to specify the context unambiguously (but briefly), and make sure that you use a feeling label that correctly gauges the *level* of affect. Don't say "nettled" when the patient is enraged, and don't say "suicidal" when the patient is mildly dysphoric. However, if you believe it would be helpful to modulate the patient's level of affect, you can do so by intentionally "overshooting" or "undershooting." Whether you wish to help the patient regain some control or to experience affect more deeply, you can *slightly* overstate or understate the level of affect, and the patient will probably move in the direction

that you would like. Obviously, the result of misstating level of affect is very much dependent on context.
5. Challenge role plays need to be longer still, perhaps five minutes in length. Take your time to gather information, and adopt a neutral-to-curious tone in stating the challenge. Try to utilize the on-the-one-hand/on-the-other-hand template described above, and strive to deliver no more than two challenges in five minutes. Carefully observe how the "patient" responds. Afterwards, ask whether the "patient" felt supported or threatened and whether you as therapist seemed to be curious or more insistent. Try to identify which challenges were particularly effective or ineffective—and why.

Having done multiple practice role plays for each of the basic skills, try some longer role plays in which you integrate all the basic skills. These role plays might be 10 to 15 minutes long to begin, and if you can videotape them, you'll find it's very helpful to review the videotapes with another student or with a more experienced psychotherapist. In preparation for reviewing the videotape, select a portion in which you weren't sure how to handle the situation, and play that portion of the tape for the other viewer. Following discussion of the problem portion, watch the entire tape together, stopping as needed to review any sections that you might have executed differently. At this level in your training, you should still focus primarily on basic skills. Speak with your supervisors to determine which skills need additional work before seeing patients for the purpose of therapy. When you begin seeing actual psychotherapy patients, you will feel more comfortable having done several longer practice sessions, including at least one session that lasts 45 to 60 minutes.

It may now be appropriate to consider learning one method of psychotherapy. You may have a particular preference, you may be required to use a modality due to your training, or one method of psychotherapy may be much more accessible than another in your particular setting. All things being equal, it's best to begin with a manualized, short-term treatment model, assuming that a supervisor is available to meet with you on a regular basis regarding your work with the patient. After you've read a text on the model you wish to learn, locate your supervisor and a relatively uncomplicated patient. It is best to work with a patient who has not been in psychotherapy before, so that you don't have to "re-educate" the patient regarding the model of treatment you are employing. You should *not* begin doing psychotherapy without arranging for **weekly** supervision sessions. The supervisor should be an expert in the modality you are learning. Consider recording your sessions, assuming that the patient gives all necessary written permissions for this to occur. Recording sessions is strongly encouraged for certain methods. It is far more helpful to have the supervisor hear or watch your sessions directly than to rely only on your summary of what occurred. If you find that you spend too little time in supervision playing the tape, consider playing "Russian roulette" on occasion. This involves picking—entirely at random—a five- or ten-minute segment to play during the supervision session. You are also encouraged to team up with another student (ideally, one with a little more experience than you, but it's all right to work with a student at your skill level) with whom you can play your tape in its entirety. In your discussion with the other student, focus primarily on basic skills.

Leave discussion of conceptualization and overall strategy to meetings with your supervisor. While reviewing videotapes with a colleague, reserve some time to talk about your feelings in sessions with this particular patient and your general feelings about conducting psychotherapy. Ask your colleague whether he or she sometimes feels the way you do.

Another commonly used method for weekly supervision with psychodynamic therapy is review of the *process note*. A process note is created by the therapist immediately or very soon after the patient session. Although there may be different approaches, typically the therapist attempts to recreate the entire session from start to finish by literally writing down his or her entire memory of the session. This note is read out loud by the therapist during supervision. Together, the supervisor and trainee consider the content of the session and how the therapist filtered the session during the creation of the process note. The supervisor helps the therapist to see themes (in the patient and in the therapist) and provides valuable pointers for skill building and handling the session content. Considerable insight can be gained during this exercise, particularly with regard to transference and countertransference, which is otherwise typically challenging to recognize. Many therapists continue to create process notes and to maintain supervision as a regular part of their work. It is important to be aware that process notes are not considered part of the chart or medical record. They must not contain identifying information of any kind and are handled according to institutional rules and laws.

Some manualized treatments come with therapist compliance checklists, usually consisting of five to ten specific therapist behaviors that should be evident in each session. In other cases such checklists can be found in the research literature. The use of therapist checklists will help you to identify areas of your performance that might be improved. If you identify several such areas, make a concrete plan for how you might increase or decrease the behaviors in question. You should discuss this with your supervisor. To improve your performance on these target behaviors, make use of the reactivity of monitoring by formally tracking your performance in each session.

Focus on learning one therapy model at a time. Treat at least three or four patients in one model of supervised psychotherapy before moving on to a second model of psychotherapy. The second model of therapy might be more complicated, less well structured, or longer than the first, and it will almost certainly involve a different mindset and skillset. With the second therapy model you can simply repeat the learning sequence just described. You should again arrange to have weekly supervision meetings with a psychotherapist skilled in the new model. Once you have learned two models of psychotherapy, it is easier to learn a third or fourth. As well, having learned more than one model of psychotherapy, you will begin to develop a "style" of psychotherapy that particularly suits you. You may elect to focus on just one model of treatment, or you may find that you prefer practicing psychotherapy within a pluralistic model, applying different psychotherapies in sequence in order to treat a range of presenting problems with patients. Many therapists rely primarily on one model of treatment but utilize techniques from other approaches in a modular fashion.

Summary

Steps to the development of competence as a psychotherapist:

1. Learn about the theory that underlies various psychotherapeutic techniques.
2. Practice specific skills in brief role plays with another student.
3. Videotape longer role plays with a partner who plays a specific patient.
4. Learn in detail about the techniques of a specific (preferably manualized) psychotherapy.
5. Locate a skilled supervisor and a patient, and consider videotaping therapy sessions (after you have obtained all necessary written permissions), to be reviewed weekly with the supervisor. Use a therapist compliance checklist, if possible.
6. After treating three or four patients using one treatment model, learn a second model and treat several patients, again reviewing videotapes on a weekly basis with a supervisor.

Recommended Reading

Ivey, A.E., Ivey, M.B., & Zalequett, C.P. (2010). *Intentional interviewing and counseling: Facilitating client development in a multicultural society* (7th ed.). Belmont, CA: Brooks/Cole, Cengage Learning.

Chapter 5

Current Psychotherapies

Psychotherapy Training 140
Individual Psychodynamic Psychotherapies 142
    Psychoanalysis 142
    Psychodynamic Psychotherapy 150
    Transference-Focused Psychotherapy (TFP) 156
    Mentalization-Based Treatment (MBT) 161
    Supportive Psychotherapy (Including Psychoeducation) 165
    Play Therapy 168
Individual Behavior Therapies 174
    Cognitive-Behavior Therapy (CBT) 174
    Exposure and Response Prevention (ERP) 192
    Brief Cognitive Therapy for Panic Disorder 196
    Prolonged Exposure for Posttraumatic Stress Disorder
       (PE-PTSD) 200
    Dialectical Behavior Therapy (DBT) 205
    Applied Behavior Analysis (ABA) 211
Other Individual Psychotherapies 214
    Interpersonal Psychotherapy (IPT) 214
    Motivational Interviewing (MI) 219
    Twelve-Step Facilitation 223
    Eye Movement Desensitization and Reprocessing
       (EMDR) 227
    Biofeedback for Mental Disorders 231
    Therapies from Complementary and Alternative
       Medicine 233
Psychotherapy for Multiple Patients 236
    Group Psychotherapy 236
    Mindfulness-Based Cognitive Therapy (MBCT) 240
    Family Therapy 242

In this chapter we describe the psychotherapeutic techniques currently used by most psychiatrists. We begin by describing individual psychotherapies that are based on psychodynamic principles. We then review individual psychotherapies based on behavioral principles, after which we cover a number of individual treatment models that are more evenly influenced by both theories. We end by touching briefly on group therapy and family therapy. Throughout the chapter we will refer in bold font to specific techniques, such as **free association** and **assertiveness training**, that are used by several models of psychotherapy that we describe. The reader is encouraged to refer to the definitions of these techniques in the section entitled "Common Psychotherapeutic Techniques" in Chapter 4.

Within the description of each psychotherapy we offer information regarding the model of psychopathology, specific treatment strategies, and a brief summary of supporting research. We then offer a case example. The case example is meant to be an illustration of the most important concepts relevant to each treatment approach. The examples are necessarily brief and simplistic, and they generally ignore many of the complexities, uncertainties, and contradictions that occur in the treatment of actual psychotherapy patients.

Psychotherapy Training

It is important to understand that training varies widely within a given psychotherapeutic modality. The most intensive clinical education in psychotherapy is related to psychoanalytic training, which requires at least four additional years after completion of a psychiatric residency, a clinical Ph.D., or the equivalent (see http://www.apsa.org for more information). Cognitive-behavior therapy (CBT) certification is offered by the Academy of Cognitive Therapy (see http://www.academyofct.org/); however, few therapists claiming skills in CBT are certified. In the United States, psychiatry residents are required to demonstrate proficiency in several treatment modalities; however, each program offers a different structure, and skillsets (and interest in therapy) vary widely among psychiatrists.

Titles such as therapist, psychoanalyst, psychodynamic psychotherapist, or CBT specialist are not regulated, and anyone can claim to have any of these skills. Moreover, training or even certification in a specific modality does not always imply competence in special populations requiring additional training (e.g., for children or for individuals with schizophrenia or trauma). Patients and providers are advised to familiarize themselves with the optimal level of training for treatment models so that a good fit can occur between patient needs/expectations and provider skillsets.

Individual Psychodynamic Psychotherapies

Psychoanalysis

Model of Psychopathology

Formal psychoanalysis is based on the principles of mental functioning and psychotherapeutic techniques originally developed by Sigmund Freud and is conducted as long-term analytic work—with the analysand lying on a couch. The model of psychopathology involves the full gamut of psychodynamic theory described in detail in Chapter 2 and therefore will not be repeated here.

Treatment Strategies

Formal psychoanalysis, often simply referred to as analysis, is an intensive treatment model that consists of usually hour-long sessions held three to five times per week over a long-term period, often extending multiple years. As noted above, psychoanalysis is conducted with the analysand (the patient) lying on a couch. The initial goal of analysis is to investigate and uncover the unconscious material that gives rise to the defenses, resistance, and transference distortions that are the subject of study in the analytic setting. The ultimate goal of analysis is to achieve insight. In the Freudian model (indeed, in all psychodynamic therapy) insight equals health.

The focus on insight should not be misinterpreted as evidence that the goal of psychoanalytic treatment is simply increased self-knowledge. Insight can bring symptomatic relief. When employed within psychiatry, all psychotherapy is intended for the mitigation of symptoms, and that is the case here as well.

Symptomatic relief through psychoanalysis and other forms of psychodynamic therapy comes in many forms. One important means to relief is the development of an observing ego that allows the patient to establish a different psychological relationship with the intrapsychic material. This new relationship affords the opportunity to learn and implement more effective, less symptom-inducing strategies, both internally and in relationships with others. Another mechanism is the important shift that comes from acquiring the ability to verbalize and to think differently about material that previously existed only as a nameless feeling tone. Still another route to significant symptomatic improvement may come from making meaning and sense out of experiences that were previously distressing to the point of being disabling.

One of the conceptual conundrums inherent in psychoanalysis is the need to bring unconscious material into conscious awareness. The problem is that conscious awareness of instinctual material is the very thing that the ego resists most strongly, leading ultimately to the development of symptoms. Understanding permits change, but understanding occurs only by accretion, and, as a consequence, uncomfortable material has to be addressed again and again in the slow process of *working through*.

One means by which to bring unconscious material into awareness is through the use of **free association**, a technique designed to provide therapist and patient with a large sample of verbal material, over which less ego control is exerted than is typically the case. The analyst pays careful attention to the content, sequence, and affect attached to material arising in free association in the hope of identifying patterns that might permit the development of hypotheses about unconscious material and defenses against it. Analysts also make use of the analysis of dreams. While the recognized range of primary process thinking that can be revealed through dreams has expanded since Freud, contemporary analysts continue to believe that during sleep the ego is less efficient in its censorship of unconscious material than when one is awake. Therefore, dream analysis continues to be a good method of accessing information about the functioning of the unconscious and any defenses against awareness of instinctual material.

A very important means by which psychoanalysis helps to bring unconscious material into awareness consists of **transference work**, in which the analyst pays careful attention to the patient's incorrect beliefs about the analyst. As a strategy for promoting the development of the transference, the patient is generally not permitted to have much personal information about the therapist, and the therapist avoids playing a direct role in the patient's conflicts. Analysts' strict adherence to the role of therapist and their refusal to offer advice or to respond with other than genuine curiosity about the patient's problems is often referred to as therapist *neutrality*. In formal psychoanalysis, having the patient lie on a couch assists in this promotion of transference distortions by limiting the patient's awareness of the actual analyst, who typically follows Freud's model and sits behind the patient. By making the transference the object of study in analytic treatment, patients have the opportunity to become aware of their habitual interpersonal distortions. For many patients this focus on the transference may represent the first time they have consciously and successfully worked through such complicated interpersonal conflicts with another person.

Analyzing defenses and analysis of resistance constitute another important activity in psychoanalysis. The analyst helps the patient to understand the structure and history of his or her preferred but problematic defensive strategies, in the hope that by making this information conscious, the patient will develop new and more effective strategies by which to cope with uncomfortable material.

At strategic points, the analyst may offer **interpretations** intended to shift the patient's attention toward material that may promote insight. The idea here is that this shift is gentle, only one slight step ahead of the patient's own awareness, rather than presenting a radical revelation.

Psychoanalysis is a lengthy process that is typically thought to unfold across three phases. Early on, therapist and patient develop a working relationship, and the transference gradually develops. The middle part of treatment involves analyzing the transference, exploring defenses, and encouraging the patient to make connections among thoughts and feelings, as well as earlier experiences that the patient previously viewed as unrelated. As the defense structure begins to shift and symptoms remit, the termination phase of treatment begins, in which therapist and patient address the patient's anxiety about ending treatment. This is a particularly fruitful period of treatment, in that it emphasizes issues of dependency and loss, which are at the root of many patients' difficulties.

Research Findings

For many years the complaint offered about psychoanalysis was that there was little convincing evidence of its efficacy. For the most part, the evidence offered in its support consisted of case reports and idiosyncratic, uncontrolled studies. Practitioners of psychoanalysis pointed out that research was hard to conduct on such a lengthy treatment, and they suggested that it was extremely difficult to design valid measures of intrapsychic functioning, given that changes in defense structure represent the goal of treatment. Moreover, such research as there was tended to conflate formal psychoanalysis with "psychodynamic treatment." There is no bright line that separates these two models of treatment.

More recently there have been a few "modern" studies of psychoanalytic treatment, although definitional problems continue. In 2001 Blomberg, Lazar, and Sandell followed a large number of Swedish patients receiving state-sponsored psychoanalysis. Patients met with therapists three to five times per week for an average of 51 months. Symptomatic change was measured in a variety of ways, and at the end of treatment these patients showed improvement in the range from $0.4 < d < 1.5$, depending on the measure. Recall that the average change in all psychotherapy is estimated at $d = .87$. In the study by Blomberg and colleagues the only control group consisted of patients receiving less intensive "psychodynamic" treatment (in which sessions occurred once or twice a week for an average of 40 months), and those patients showed improvement in the range of $0.4 < d < 0.6$.

In a 2008 Finnish randomized controlled trial (RCT) Knekt and colleagues showed that although long-term psychodynamic treatment (mean = 232 sessions) was less effective than short-term psychodynamic treatment (mean = 18.5 sessions) at twelve-month follow-up, it was decidedly more effective than short-term treatment at three years after the end of treatment.

Finally, in a 2008 meta-analysis Leichsenring and Rabung combined seven RCTs and one effectiveness study that compared long-term psychodynamic therapy (mean = 103 sessions) with various short-term treatments (mean = 33 sessions), including cognitive interventions, family therapy, and "psychiatric treatment as usual." Between long-term psychodynamic psychotherapy and various short-term treatments there were significantly different effect sizes with regard to overall effectiveness ($ES = 0.96$ vs. 0.47), target problems ($ES = 1.16$ vs. 0.61), and personality functioning ($ES = 0.90$ vs. 0.19). Differences were even larger for patients with personality disorders, chronic mental disorders, or multiple mental disorders.

In summary, there is now evidence to suggest that psychoanalysis—or, perhaps, long-term psychodynamic treatment—is an effective treatment modality, although it works slowly. This treatment model may be particularly effective in treating patients with personality disorders and other complex symptomatic presentations, as one might well expect in view of the theory and structure of treatment.

Case Example

Alan is a 44-year-old, married father of one child. He works as a tax attorney. He has long been dissatisfied with his job, and he feels distant from his wife and their 12-year-old daughter. Alan reports that his energy and motivation have been impaired for as long as he can remember, and for at least ten years he has felt sad three or four days each week. However, his mood usually rises somewhat on the weekends, which he often spends holed up in his basement practicing guitar. Alan states that he has difficulty sleeping, and he believes that he will always feel just as bored and dissatisfied as he does now. He indicates that he has been in and out of psychotherapy for years and has taken a variety of antidepressant drugs, but nothing has ever seemed to help for very long. He now presents for treatment with Dr. Reilly.

Alan is the fourth of five children of a law school faculty member and a homemaker. His next older sibling, a brother 18 months his senior, was impulsive and often got into trouble when Alan was growing up; Alan learned to avoid trouble by staying mostly to himself. His father was often away from home and seemed more interested in his career than in spending time with the children, although on occasion the father did attend the athletic events of Alan's eldest brother. As a child Alan felt closer to his mother than to his father, and he was also close to the sister two years his junior.

In school Alan earned respectable but not outstanding grades. In high school he tried out for football, at least in part with the hope that this might afford a means to spend more time with his father. However, Alan was athletically not nearly as talented as his brothers, and he soon quit the junior varsity team. After that he participated on the school golf and tennis teams. His mother and younger sister attended some of Alan's matches, but whenever he played, his father seemed to have to work. Alan also took up the guitar in high school. His mother arranged for him to obtain lessons, and Alan enjoyed playing.

Upon graduation from high school Alan attended the state university. He majored in political science, although this never really interested him. He began dating in college, and in his senior year he met his future wife. After graduating from college he immediately enrolled in law school, where he maintained a B+ average. His father urged him to establish a specialty practice in the law and pulled some strings to permit Alan to obtain postgraduate training in tax law. After completing the additional training Alan married his wife, and they moved to a city about 200 miles from Alan's home town. Here, he has worked for the same firm for the past 18 years. Alan reports that he and his wife seldom argue, but their sex life is limited. He is proud of his daughter but doesn't share any real interests with her. Alan sees his parents once or twice a year in Florida, where they moved after the father's retirement. He also maintains regular contact with his younger sister but has less contact with his brothers.

Upon interview Alan presents as a socially competent but distant man who gives little evidence of anxiety, other than that his palms are sweaty when he and Dr. Reilly shake hands. Over the course of several sessions Dr. Reilly determines that Alan is a suitable candidate for analysis. He concludes that Alan is in a stable situation, is able to commit to and can pay for long-term treatment, is able to observe his own psychological processes, and in his life has been able to establish affectively charged relationships, including with his mother and his sister. Dr. Reilly recommends that he and Alan schedule sessions three times a week.

In the first formal treatment session Dr. Reilly asks that Alan lie on the couch, while Dr. Reilly sits in a chair behind Alan's head. Dr. Reilly instructs Alan regarding the technique of free association and encourages him to talk about fantasies, dreams, or anything else that comes to him. Although Alan is not surprised about these instructions, he finds himself feeling mildly annoyed at the apparent pointlessness of such activity. After a few sessions, however, he notices that he has begun looking forward to his meetings with Dr. Reilly, to whom he can talk about whatever comes to his mind. He appreciates Dr. Reilly's evident interest in him and believes that Dr. Reilly is listening carefully. He looks forward to the interpretations or recommendations that he believes Dr. Reilly will eventually offer.

One day, after about four months of treatment, Alan tells Dr. Reilly about a dream he had the night before. In the dream Alan was running late for work, and this worried him because he knew he needed time to prepare for a meeting with a client. There were people in his kitchen that Alan didn't recognize, as a consequence of which he had to wait before he could prepare his breakfast. Finally, Alan was able to get to his car and started to drive to work, but the trip was slow and difficult because traffic was heavy. Once at work, Alan quickly tried to review his notes, but he couldn't entirely understand what he had earlier written down. As the meeting started, Alan began his presentation, but the client often looked away and said nothing. Alan tried to engage the client by asking him a question, changing the subject, and even telling a joke, but he received no response. At that point Alan awakened to his alarm.

Alan falls silent after recounting the dream to Dr. Reilly. The latter asks Alan to say more about his thoughts and feelings in the dream. Alan replies that he was especially focused on engaging this client, because the latter came from a wealthy family, and Alan hoped that the client might refer his relatives and acquaintances. Alan comments that in the dream he was very much puzzled by the client's reaction. Was the client dissatisfied with Alan, was he feeling irritated, or was he not really listening at all? Alan says that he was most upset about the fact that he had no idea what the client was thinking.

Dr. Reilly wonders with Alan if the client might be a stand-in for Alan's father. Alan can easily see this connection, and they discuss Alan's feeling of distance and alienation from his father. Alan comments that he often feared his father's wrath, even though his father seldom expressed any emotion toward Alan. Dr. Reilly asks Alan if he might have worried that his father was angry because Alan was close to his mother. Alan is nonplussed and simply suggests that it might have been easier to imagine that his father had angry feelings than no feelings at all.

Dr. Reilly then wonders aloud if Alan's dream might also reflect his feelings about their work together in treatment. Alan initially rejects this idea until Dr. Reilly explains that dreams can usually be interpreted in several ways. Even so, Alan comments that he doesn't feel disconnected from Dr. Reilly. Dr. Reilly doesn't reply directly but suggests that in future sessions they watch for feelings of alienation on Alan's part, either in his daily life or in their relationship with one another.

Over the course of the next several months Alan continues to speak about whatever comes into his mind, although in some sessions he has more difficulty than in others. He realizes that he is becoming a little bored. Alan sometimes comments on his uncertainty about what to say, to which Dr. Reilly usually replies by asking Alan how he felt just before his thoughts seemed to stop. Alan tries gamely to respond but finds that going forward his thoughts are still unclear. By the eighth month of treatment this is happening quite often, and Alan is aware of becoming frustrated. He now frequently tells Dr. Reilly that he doesn't know what to do and would like some guidance. Dr. Reilly consistently responds with mild encouragement to keep trying and then asks Alan what he was thinking and feeling a few minutes previously.

One day in the ninth month Alan begins the session by saying to Dr. Reilly, "We need to talk." Alan says he appreciates Dr. Reilly's concern and support, but he needs some direction in order to know how to proceed. Alan comments that previous therapists have been more directive than Dr. Reilly, and in this regard he makes particular reference to his last therapist, Dr. Smith. Dr. Reilly remarks on the fact that Dr. Smith is a woman, and he adds that perhaps there's a part of Alan that feels as if he's being left to flounder on his own. Alan replies that he does sometimes feel like that, and he says he has to remind himself that Dr. Reilly really does want to help him. "Sometimes," Alan adds, "I think that even if you've helped other patients, you might not know how to help in a case like me."

Alan then asks if Dr. Reilly is annoyed that he mentioned his previous therapist. In response, Dr. Reilly wonders aloud whether Alan might be worried about whether a male might become jealous over his feelings for certain women. Alan replies that he's not sure what to think about this. Finally, Alan acknowledges that he is becoming bored with treatment, and he wonders if Dr. Reilly is turn bored with him. With the hour nearly at an end, Dr. Reilly suggests that they pick up their discussion at the next session.

However, Alan misses the next session because of a sudden increase in work at the office, and when he returns to see Dr. Reilly, he spends most of the session talking about his frustration dealing with a particular administrative law judge on behalf of a client. Dr. Reilly expresses interest and encourages Alan to say more about this but then asks Alan what he makes of the fact that they were going to talk about whether their time together was useful, but Alan then missed the next session and, upon returning, talked about work instead. With slight annoyance, Alan replies that he intended to get to the issue of their relationship, but the work problem seemed more important at the moment. He then states that he is committed to treatment, even though he can't always see how it will help. Asked to elaborate, Alan replies, "Basically, that's where it stands. Isn't our time up for today?"

Over the next few weeks Alan notices that he is thinking more and more of leaving treatment. He discusses these thoughts with Dr. Reilly, who comments that Alan might feel a sense of relief or even a kind of victory when he thinks of stopping their work together. He wonders aloud if Alan may sometimes have had similar thoughts vis-à-vis his father. Alan replies that he has long thought of writing off his father, but he hoped that at some point his father might soften and show some interest. Besides, he says, cutting off his father would make the relationship with his mother more complicated. Dr. Reilly replies, "There must have been a lot of times growing up when you wanted just one parent, your mother, and not the complete set."

Now in the second year of treatment, Alan continues to struggle with frustration and lately sadness in his sessions with Dr. Reilly. He expresses these feelings directly to Dr. Reilly and is becoming more affectively engaged in the sessions. He notices that although he is more aware of painful feelings, he is also less bored in the sessions, and he no longer worries that Dr. Reilly might be daydreaming or asleep. Instead, he now worries that Dr. Reilly might be angry with him. He has the thought that eventually Dr. Reilly will find him too demanding and will want to transfer him to another therapist. He is afraid to say this to Dr. Reilly, however, imagining that if he does, Dr. Reilly will confirm his worst fears.

Alan reports another dream. He says in the dream he was helping his daughter program her smart phone. Although he felt confident in his ability to help her, the phone continued not to function properly, and Alan became increasingly anxious as more and more functions on the phone ceased to work. His daughter was unhappy, and she commented repeatedly that one of her classmates was good with phones and could help her. However, Alan kept trying. At last, the phone went dead altogether, his daughter was crying, and his wife appeared in the room asking what was wrong, glaring at Alan as she did so.

In discussing the dream, Dr. Reilly asks Alan what he makes of the fact that he was trying to fix a telephone, in particular, and together they wonder about whether communication might have been a theme of the dream. Alan also talks about his recent attempts to do more with his daughter, particularly in response to his sense that she is pulling away from him and his wife. More than anything, Alan comments that he wishes he hadn't touched the phone, because then he wouldn't have made the problem worse than it already was.

Dr. Reilly asks Alan whether the dream might reflect something about the therapy relationship. Alan replies that he hadn't thought about it, but perhaps there's a part of him that is afraid to communicate to Dr. Reilly what's at the deepest level inside him. He says he sometimes thinks he'll just end up pushing Dr. Reilly away. In response, Dr. Reilly asks, "So who's rejecting whom?"

Alan is struck by this question. He begins to wonder if his father rejected and ignored him, or was it the other way around? Did he expect his father to reject him for some reason? For example, was he worried about his father's reaction to his close relationship with his mother? Alan also wonders whether it's really the case that when he expresses his feelings, others are likely to pull away. As he discusses this with Dr. Reilly, the latter encourages Alan to think about how he believes Dr. Reilly has responded to Alan's increased expression of emotion over the course of their work together. Upon reflection, Alan replies that they have worked together more productively since he has expressed a wider range of affect.

This session marks a turning point in Alan's treatment. He begins to notice outside sessions that he is experimenting with letting people know his feelings. He and Dr. Reilly discuss this, and they also work through the anger that Alan experiences when important people in his life are less than fully responsive to his newly developing interpersonal style. Alan says he sometimes believes that Dr. Reilly has misled him by promising that if he engages more with those around him, his problems will disappear. Alan and Dr. Reilly discuss whether this might reflect his idea as a child about how life would be if his father had been more interested in him. At first Alan denies any connection between this childish belief and his frustration about making changes in his life now, but in time he comes to accept that in both instances his expectations may have been unrealistic. He also acknowledges that he can't remember when Dr. Reilly actually told him to open up to others, after which everything would be fine. Alan feels a little sad as he considers the idea that there are no magic answers.

After three years of psychoanalysis, Alan and Dr. Reilly review his progress. Alan reports that he no longer feels so isolated and uninvolved with other people, and his mood is definitely improved. He has a more comfortable (but at times still frustrating) relationship with his father. He is closer with his wife, and their sex life has improved. He has become involved in several musical groups in his free time and is developing friendships with other men. In view of this progress, Alan and Dr. Reilly decide to terminate treatment in three months.

During the last three months of therapy, Alan and Dr. Reilly discuss Alan's fears about being on his own, without the support of treatment. They also spend time working through feelings of sadness about Alan's painful awareness that no one person can give him the supplies of love and understanding he once craved from his father. Alan says this is somewhat balanced by his recognition that he feels a degree of satisfaction when he engages a range of people by confiding in them about his thoughts and feelings.

> At the end of treatment Alan looks back with wonder at how he used to act, and he is pleased with his progress, even though he continues to experience days on which he feels depressed and lonely, and his sleep is still less than optimal.

Psychodynamic Psychotherapy

Model of Psychopathology

By way of introduction, we note that psychodynamic psychotherapy is often viewed as a less intensive and more personable version of psychoanalysis. Psychiatry residents are generally required to demonstrate basic competency in this treatment model and may pursue additional training if desired, typically in association with a psychoanalytic institute. The skillset of individual providers varies widely, from no formal training to full psychoanalytic training. As with any modality, patients should inquire about training and work history to understand the skillset of the therapist.

Practitioners of psychodynamic psychotherapy believe, as did Freud, that at bottom psychopathology results from ego defense gone awry. While many psychodynamic psychotherapists view the vicissitudes of human instincts as the prime movers in human development, others suggest that humans grow in response to different challenges, such as striving for superiority, the need to self-realize, or the tension between union and separation, to cite a few examples. Some psychodynamic theorists have attempted to graft Existentialist philosophy onto psychoanalytic thinking; they believe that the need to establish meaning is a fundamental human drive, and the failure to do so leads to emotional distress, resulting in the development of symptoms.

In the previous section, we presented the essential features of formal psychoanalysis and its application within psychiatry as the prototype of psychodynamic psychotherapy. In this section, we expand our scope and review the remainder of the diverse category of psychotherapy treatments based on psychodynamic theory. As with psychoanalysis, the model of psychopathology encompasses the full body of psychodynamic theory described in detail earlier in this book and therefore will not be repeated here.

Treatment Strategies

As one might imagine in view of the broad range of psychodynamic theory, psychodynamic psychotherapists utilize an extremely wide range of formats and techniques. Beginning with Sándor Ferenczi and Otto Rank, psychotherapists who identify with psychodynamic thinking have advocated less intensive treatment than is offered in formal psychoanalysis. A typical pattern consists of weekly 50-minute sessions, in which therapist and patient are seated face to face. This may be structured as either short-term or long-term treatment.

All the mechanisms we have reviewed in the psychoanalysis section to mitigate symptoms of mental disorders also apply within psychodynamic psychotherapy. In general, however, with regard to technique there may be less reliance on certain psychoanalytic techniques such as **free association** and formal dream interpretation. However, in face-to-face therapy spontaneity of discourse performs much the same role as **free association**, and dream material remains important. The treatment focus depends on the model of psychodynamic theory that the therapist is using.

In addition to psychodynamic psychotherapy broadly based within a particular model of theory, there are also some more carefully defined psychodynamic treatment formats now available. These include treatments that focus primarily on specific targets, such as the Oedipus complex (e.g., Sifneos, 1992) and self-image and separation issues (e.g., Mann, 1980). In 1985 Strupp and Binder published the first treatment manual for short-term psychodynamic treatment. Their particular approach grew out of a major research program conducted over many years at Vanderbilt University. Transference-focused psychotherapy and mentalization-based treatment are other examples, and these two therapies will be discussed separately.

While psychodynamic psychotherapists may not agree on all of the details of the treatment they offer, they generally agree on the importance of the value of **analyzing defenses** and resistance and offering **interpretations**, and they emphasize the significance of some variety of **transference work** as a means to promote useful insight. Psychodynamic psychotherapists are usually less obviously neutral vis-à-vis the patient than are formal psychoanalysts, and there is an increased focus in psychodynamic treatment on providing an overtly supportive environment and addressing alliance ruptures more directly.

Research Findings

In the section on formal psychoanalysis we cited some research findings of relevance to psychodynamic psychotherapy. One implication of the research already cited is that shorter psychodynamic treatment may be less effective than longer treatment. Indeed, in a 1991 meta-analysis Svartberg and Stiles showed that psychodynamic treatment lasting fewer than 12 sessions may be less effective than lengthier treatment. Even so, in 2004 Leichsenring, Rabung, and Leibing conducted a meta-analysis using 18 high-quality RCTs that compared short-term psychodynamic psychotherapy with other treatments (mostly CBT) or wait-list control. These authors found that short-term psychodynamic psychotherapy was effective and did not differ in effectiveness from other approaches to treatment. As well, in 2009 de Maat, de Jonghe, Schoevers, and Dekker investigated psychodynamic psychotherapy of moderate length (at least 50 sessions over at least a year) and found significant change at post-treatment ($d = 0.87$) and even greater change at follow-up between one and three years later ($d = 1.18$).

In the face of such findings, there is increasing acceptance in the field that psychodynamic psychotherapy probably qualifies as an empirically supported treatment.

Case Example

Barbara is a 33-year-old, never-married, childless woman who works as an administrative assistant in an engineering firm. She reports that she has always been a worrier. She worries about losing her job (and about whether she could pay her bills if she did), she worries about whether her friends are upset with her, and she worries about her mother's physical and emotional health. She also worries about the direction of the national economy, what will happen when she grows old, and whether her boyfriend of three years will ever pop the question. When, on rare occasions, Barbara discusses her fears with a friend, she is usually able to see that her anxiety is unrealistic. Nonetheless, she has been troubled by multiple worries virtually every day at least since late adolescence, and the worries are accompanied by poor concentration, muscle tension, shakiness, and difficulty sleeping. Barbara otherwise denies symptoms of a mental disorder. She is in good physical health.

Barbara is the eldest of three children of working-class parents. Her father was alcoholic and often unemployed, as a consequence of which Barbara's mother was the primary breadwinner and had to depend on Barbara to look after Barbara's younger brothers. The mother confided extensively in Barbara about her unhappy marriage. Then, when Barbara was 14 years old, her father died in a car accident, presumably while intoxicated. After that, Barbara's mother seemed to worry even more and spent long hours recounting her concerns to Barbara. Barbara did her best to shoulder the responsibility that her mother placed on her, and she rather liked the fact that her mother seldom disciplined her—although Barbara was in fact exceptionally well behaved.

Barbara performed well in school and was popular. After graduating from high school she could have gone to college but instead felt obliged to find a job. She continued to live at home and contributed to her brothers' upkeep until the boys left home and Barbara's mother remarried eight years ago. After that, Barbara sensed that her mother wanted privacy, and as her stepfather was earning adequately, the next year Barbara decided to move into a place of her own about a mile from her mother's house.

Barbara reports that she enjoys her job, and she says her love life is pretty good. She began dating more actively after she moved out of her mother's house seven years ago, and during the past three years she has had a steady boyfriend. She would like to marry her boyfriend, but he never mentions the topic, and she doesn't feel comfortable asking about their future. Sometimes Barbara worries a little about the fact that her boyfriend likes to drink on the weekend.

When Barbara meets Dr. Thompson, she presents as a socially engaging and very pleasant woman who makes an effort to respond directly and succinctly to Dr. Thompson's questions. Dr. Thompson has the thought that Barbara is likely to be an easy patient, because she appears to have the capacity for insight and is highly motivated to change. He also admits to himself that he finds Barbara to be a rather attractive woman. He and Barbara agree to meet on a weekly basis.

In the first formal treatment session Dr. Thompson asks Barbara what she would like to discuss. Barbara hesitates for a moment, glances quickly at Dr. Thompson, and begins talking about worries regarding her performance at work. When Dr. Thompson asks about Barbara's performance evaluations, she responds that they are consistently very good. Dr. Thompson admits to confusion about this, after which Barbara giggles with embarrassment and comments that this is typical of her worries—so many of them are unrealistic. Even so, the worries keep returning, and she can't ever seem to resolve them fully.

Over the course of the next few sessions Barbara continues to discuss her various worries. She feels relieved when Dr. Thompson asks a question or makes a comment that helps her see that a worry is unrealistic, but the pattern is always the same: the worry comes back later on. After this happens a few times, Dr. Thompson comments that reassurance doesn't seem to be helpful. Barbara responds that she finds Dr. Thompson's comments to be very helpful, and she has the private thought that she doesn't want Dr. Thompson to feel he isn't helping her. She's sure he must be helping, and he seems like such a nice man.

One day Barbara tells Dr. Thompson about a dream she's had. She goes on to report that a few nights ago she dreamt that her mother had been diagnosed with cancer and was refusing chemotherapy. Somehow, her stepfather was not in the picture, and Barbara was responsible for taking care of her mother. Barbara recalls being very frightened that her mother might die. In the dream she tells her mother how devastated she would be and begs her to accept treatment. Her mother reluctantly agrees. In the final scene of the dream, Barbara's mother dies in spite of having had the chemotherapy she didn't want. Barbara woke up in a panic and then burst into tears over the loss of her mother.

After Barbara recounts the dream, Dr. Thompson asks what she makes of it. Barbara replies that it was just too horrible, and she doesn't know what to think. She adds that maybe she should ask her mother whether she is having regular medical checkups. Dr. Thompson asks Barbara to say more about the emotion associated with the dream. Barbara replies that in the dream she alternately felt frightened, burdened, and also pleased about her ability to convince her mother to accept treatment. When her mother died in the dream, she felt as if the floor had dropped out from under her.

Dr. Thompson then asks Barbara what it's like to be responsible for a parent. Barbara replies that family members have to look out for each other, and she begins to recount how hard her mother's life has been. Dr. Thompson agrees that life has treated her mother harshly, but he states, "Still, it must bother you just a little that you have to pick up the slack." Barbara replies that she loves her mother and would do anything for her. However, a few moments later she adds, "But maybe I do resent it in a way, and I just don't know it."

As treatment continues Barbara talks more and more about her relationship with her mother. She is able to acknowledge that while she liked helping her mother and brothers when she was younger, she did miss out on certain activities in high school. For example, she couldn't attend a number of dances because she had to look after her younger brothers while her mother worked the afternoon shift. She says that sometimes she thinks about what her life would have been like had her mother remarried ten years earlier. Perhaps she could have gone to college and eventually gotten a better job.

By this time Dr. Thompson has arrived at the conclusion that Barbara represses awareness of her own needs in order to care for her mother, her adult brothers, her boyfriend, her coworkers, her boss, and everyone else with whom she comes in contact in her life. Dr. Thompson suspects that every time Barbara experiences the impulse to do something for herself, she defends against it, as she somehow senses that meeting her own needs might decrease her ability to meet the needs of others. She has long since fallen into the pattern of failing to notice these impulses, as they are diverted before they even become conscious. Instead, Barbara experiences a kind of free-floating anxiety that attaches itself to whatever she happens to be thinking about at the moment.

In Session 16 Barbara mentions that the previous Saturday night her boyfriend again drank too much, and the bartender called her to come and pick him up. She brought him to her apartment and put him to bed. During the night he threw up, and the next morning he was irritable with her. When Dr. Thompson asks Barbara how she feels about taking care of her boyfriend in this way, she initially responds it doesn't bother her when he blows off a little steam on the weekend, especially given that he works so hard during the week. Dr. Thompson then expresses interest in the fact that the boyfriend was out drinking while she stayed home on a Saturday night. Barbara laughs this off but acknowledges that she worries about his drinking. She then glances at Dr. Thompson and says, "But, of course, you're right. I know I should set better limits with him. I'm probably being silly, right?"

Dr. Thompson suggests to Barbara that part of her seems to want to accommodate to her boyfriend's point of view, while another part seems to want to agree with Dr. Thompson's point of view. He wonders aloud, how can she reconcile these two impulses?

Barbara struggles with this question. She begins by saying that her boyfriend is a great guy—he's not perfect, but who is? She says it's her responsibility to love him as he is. At the same time, she recognizes that Dr. Thompson has her best interests at heart, and although he hasn't said it directly, she believes that he doesn't approve of how she deals with her boyfriend. In fact, none of her friends approve. Starting to tear up, Barbara says, "It's like I'm stuck. My boyfriend needs me to be one way, but everyone else needs me to be another way. I don't know what's the right thing to do. Are you disappointed with me, Dr. Thompson?"

After this session Dr. Thompson feels unsettled. He has the thought that Barbara is very responsive to the idea that she must meet his needs. He wonders if he has somehow communicated how warmly he feels toward her. He acknowledges to himself that part of him wants Barbara to stay his patient forever. He actually doesn't want her to lose the accommodating quality that makes her such pleasant company. He feels a little embarrassed to have these thoughts about his patient but decides, on balance, that his countertransferential impulses are unlikely to have interfered too greatly with treatment so far. Besides, he reminds himself that if part of him is invested in preventing Barbara from changing, something similar is probably happening in virtually every one of her other relationships. Dr. Thompson resolves to remain aware of his impulses during sessions with Barbara and to look for opportunities to explore with her how other people might press her not to change.

In the next three sessions Barbara and Dr. Thompson discuss her habit of doing whatever she thinks others want her to do. However, they have some difficulty determining what the fear is behind this habit. Barbara says she just knows that she's always been like this.

In Session 20 Dr. Thompson asks Barbara if she sometimes worries about what he wants from her. She pauses, begins to reply in the negative, but then admits that she tries to do as she thinks he wants her to do. She explains, "I'm coming for help, and if I don't do what you think I should, why am I wasting your time?"

Dr. Thompson presses further. He points out that most patients have difficulty doing exactly what the therapist would like them to do. Barbara professes surprise about this. She thinks for a moment and then says, "I guess I'm afraid that if I don't do what you think I should, you'll see me as an uncooperative patient and won't want me to come back. If you didn't want to work with me anymore, I'd be so upset."

Dr. Thompson asks Barbara if this abandonment idea sounds familiar. She says she's never thought much about it. Dr. Thompson reminds her of the dream about her mother's cancer, in response to which Barbara says, "Hmm. That's a good point."

Barbara then asks, "So if I just ignored your advice, wouldn't you be mad?"

Dr. Thompson replies, "If you ignore my advice, it's because I'm not giving good advice." He adds, with genuine warmth, "I think you're a great person, Barbara, and I like you just as you are. But I think you'd feel more comfortable if you began taking better care of yourself, rather than to direct so much of your attention to meeting everyone else's needs."

Over the course of the next eight sessions Barbara and Dr. Thompson focus on a particular recurrent sequence: Barbara has the impulse to act in a certain way, she then fears that someone else will be injured or will reject her, after which she is frightened about the prospect of abandonment, forgets what it was she wanted to do in the first place, and instead feels unsettled and worried. In time Barbara can recognize this sequence both historically and in real time. She struggles to weigh the costs and benefits of meeting others' needs versus meeting her own needs, and over time she experiences a gradual shift toward caring for herself. As this shift occurs, she reports fewer irrational worries, but she notes that she is now troubled by a new, more rational worry. She says she is concerned about how much people will like her when she stops taking care of them. Will other people tolerate this shift in her behavior?

Dr. Thompson consistently directs Barbara's attention to this dilemma, and he highlights those instances in which she chooses to ignore her own impulses, even when Dr. Thompson implies she might do otherwise. After they disagree, he points out that they're still working well together, and he says directly to Barbara that he can't fault her for making her own decisions, because ultimately she knows what's best for her.

At the end of Session 29 Barbara reports that her anxiety is moderately decreased, and she's feeling more comfortable asserting herself. She has broken up with her boyfriend and is dating a new man. She still worries about her mother and tries hard to meet the needs of coworkers and her boss, but she is experimenting with setting more limits with friends and other family members. She and Dr. Thompson decide that it might make sense to begin scheduling appointments every two or three weeks. After six months of less frequent sessions, they decide to end treatment altogether. However, Dr. Thompson encourages Barbara to return in the future for more treatment, should she wish to do so.

Transference-Focused Psychotherapy (TFP)

Model of Psychopathology

Based on the mixed-model psychodynamic theory of psychiatrist Otto F. Kernberg (1928–), borderline personality organization is understood within TFP as a failure to integrate the "good" and "bad" aspects of objects, as well as a failure to integrate extreme perceptions of the self. In response to such splitting and the emotional arousal that follows from it, the individual with borderline personality organization becomes extremely sensitive to any threat of rejection, leading to the development of problematic relationships with others. This results at least in part from the fact that splitting prevents one from recognizing the transient nature of conflict. Individuals who engage in splitting at any given moment tend to see significant others as either all good or all bad, and they have little tolerance for normal variations in the moods and behavior of others. Instead, the individual who engages in splitting responds in an exaggerated manner to minor shifts in interactions with significant others, failing to appreciate the stability and continuity inherent in important relationships.

The goal of TFP is to help the individual with borderline personality organization to integrate objects and aspects of the self that have been split off, so that he or she can respond with equanimity to the normal ups and downs of important relationships. A direct byproduct of integrating "good" and "bad" objects is that one has less need to utilize primitive defenses, and one's reality testing improves as a consequence of decreased emotional arousal and the recognition that self and others have both positive and negative features and are neither perfect nor terrible. Successful treatment is expected naturally to result in decreased self-injury, fewer hospitalizations, and fewer suicide attempts.

Treatment Strategies

TFP is a manualized treatment that lasts at least a year and involves twice-weekly sessions. Following completion of a detailed treatment contract, therapist and patient focus primarily on **transference work**, with the intention of helping the patient to integrate split-off aspects of the self. More specifically, transference distortions are identified, and this is followed by an investigation of the therapeutic relationship in order to identify the ways in which errors in the perception of self or other are consistent with the transference distortion in question. As well, the patient is made aware of how such distortions played themselves out earlier in life, and the therapist offers the **interpretation** that the patient's emotional distress over the risk of losing important relationships works to perpetuate the split between an all-good and all-bad view of significant others. Patients are helped to develop a more realistic view of self and other in the therapeutic relationship, so that over time they develop a more balanced view of self and other in relationships outside of therapy. In particular, patients are encouraged to acknowledge both good and bad aspects of the self and are helped to see that such a mixed picture of self and others is both accurate and useful.

Research Findings

There have been encouraging findings regarding the efficacy of TFP in the treatment of borderline personality disorder. In a one-year study TFP was as effective as dialectical behavior therapy (DBT, reviewed later in this chapter) in decreasing suicidal behavior, but TFP appears to have been more effective than DBT or supportive therapy in decreasing a wide range of symptoms associated with the diagnosis of borderline personality disorder (Clarkin, Levy, Lenzenweger, & Kernberg, 2007). On the other hand, in a study lasting three years comparing TFP with schema-focused therapy (a version of CBT with particular application to personality disorders), TFP was effective in decreasing general psychopathology and borderline psychopathology, in particular, but the outcome from TFP was less strong than the effect of schema-focused therapy (Giesen-Bloo et al., 2006). In a more recent one-year study TFP was more effective than treatment by experienced community psychiatrists in retaining patients in treatment, in decreasing suicide attempts, and in a number of other domains, including particularly decreasing symptoms of borderline personality disorder (Doering et al., 2010).

Case Example

Charlene is a 35-year-old, recently married, childless woman who is referred for evaluation for TFP. She does not work outside the home. Charlene recounts her history quickly and in a tone that communicates that she is desperately in need of assistance. She states that she has had two brief psychiatric hospitalizations in her life, most recently three years ago. Both followed overdoses of non-lethal amounts of antidepressant medication. Charlene states that she has engaged in cutting since early adolescence. She overspends and sometimes drinks too much. She says she can't seem to maintain an intimate relationship (with either sex) for longer than two or three years. Indeed, Charlene states that her husband is tiring of the emotional roller coaster, and she can hardly blame him, because in just two years she's put him through the wringer. Charlene says that previous therapists have tried to help her, but something always happens, and either she leaves or they fire her. Charlene denies current symptoms consistent with major depression, persistent depressive disorder, generalized anxiety disorder, or any psychotic disorder. She does comment that she worries she's on her way to another depressive episode, particularly in response to her awareness of increasing tension in her marriage.

Upon interview Charlene appears to be anxious and physically somewhat shaky, but her presentation is otherwise unremarkable, apart from the neediness that Dr. Underwood senses.

Dr. Underwood tells Charlene that TFP is a challenging treatment method that requires her to commit to a year of twice-weekly psychodynamic psychotherapy. He explains that he will push Charlene to look at herself and her relationships in a way that may make her feel uncomfortable, but he says that if treatment is successful (which is not a foregone conclusion), she will end up feeling less anxious in relationships and will view herself as less helpless and frightened. He states that in treatment they will need to focus particularly on how she punishes herself (as contrasted with periods in which she feels angry toward those around her), and they will investigate the difficulty she has seeing both sides of herself and of others.

Charlene admits that this description of treatment frightens her, particularly the fact that it might not work. Dr. Underwood suggests that Charlene bring her husband to the next session so that they can all discuss treatment together. Charlene says she would like that, because she's not sure whether to go ahead with TFP or to have herself admitted to the hospital.

When Charlene brings in her husband at the next session, Dr. Underwood reviews the expectations of treatment, and he underscores the fact that it will be his responsibility to stick to the treatment plan, regardless of what happens, as long as Charlene attends sessions regularly. However, if she skips more than three sessions in a row or establishes a pattern of frequently missing nonsequential sessions, treatment will end.

Charlene's husband presents as a somewhat overcontrolled man who asks a number of questions about the plan and eventually indicates his concurrence. "She needs something," he says. "I can't take much more of this."

After her husband leaves the room, Charlene immediately agrees to initiate treatment under the conditions outlined. She and Dr. Underwood spend the rest of the session discussing what it's like for Charlene when her husband is upset with her.

In the first few full treatment sessions, Charlene discusses her anxiety about her marriage, and she admits that she becomes so worried about this that she sometimes cuts her thighs in order to relieve her distress. Dr. Underwood points out that Charlene consistently describes herself as the cause of all marital problems, and she denies that her husband has any responsibility for their difficulties. Charlene replies that her husband has his problems, but if it weren't for her, things would be much better in his life—and in the lives of a lot of people. She says she sometimes thinks the world would be better off without her, although she assures Dr. Underwood that she's not feeling suicidal, at least not right now.

Dr. Underwood also points out in the first few sessions that Charlene seems to view herself as entirely helpless and may be harboring the fantasy that Dr. Underwood will tell her what to do so that her life will miraculously improve. Charlene replies that even though she knows that's impossible, she does wish it were true, and it frightens her to be reminded that she has to help herself. She admits that she doesn't believe she has it in her to get better on her own.

During the ensuing couple of weeks Charlene complains less about her marriage, and she says her husband seems to be less angry with her. Then, in Session 7, Dr. Underwood notices a shift in Charlene's manner. She describes having gotten into a minor dispute with her mother-in-law. Charlene admits that this woman often manages to irritate her. She adds that she has noticed some similarities between her husband and his mother. Sometimes, she says, she wishes she hadn't married into this family. Charlene is a little more assertive in this session, and in the next session she reports that she's actually feeling angry with her husband because he won't take her side in the disagreement with his mother. In a tone that is uncharacteristically level and firm, Charlene avers that her husband is a wimp when it comes to his mother. Maybe, she says, her husband would be happier sleeping with his mother than with Charlene.

Dr. Underwood expresses surprise about this shift in Charlene's tone. Charlene admits that she's irritated, adding that she feels irritable more often than most people know. Dr. Underwood asks if Charlene sometimes feels irritable with him. Charlene replies, "Yeah, maybe, but actually I don't think so much about you between sessions. I have other problems to deal with."

Dr. Underwood states that he's feeling confused. Just a month ago, when they started treatment, Charlene seemed to be feeling helpless and desperate, and she appeared to be willing to agree to almost anything. Now, he says, she's much less anxious and implies that therapy isn't all that important to her.

Charlene replies, "Well, I guess I'm feeling better. Is that a problem? Aren't you happy that I feel better?"

At this point Dr. Underwood explains that it's not uncommon for people with problems like Charlene's to shift back and forth between aggressor and victim, and he wonders if this shift is occurring right now. Charlene snaps, "Hey! Real person over here. I'm not some specimen."

Over the next couple of weeks Dr. Underwood continues to focus on the shift in Charlene's mood and her view of other people. In a kind but clear way he reiterates that she now views him as much less significant in her life, but not so long ago she harbored the wish that he rescue her. Charlene can agree that this is so, but she admits that it's hard for her to remember how she was actually feeling when treatment began.

At the beginning of Week 6 Charlene presents as less irritable. She says she is worried that her husband might be having an affair, based on the fact that he didn't leave his phone lying out so that Charlene could quickly scan his email while he was asleep, as is her habit. She says she is afraid that her husband might leave her, and if that happened, she would have a hard time managing. She asks Dr. Underwood what he thinks she should do.

Dr. Underwood again points out the shift, and he challenges Charlene to try to think about the ways in which she loves and depends on her husband, on one hand, and she is upset with him, on the other hand. Charlene finds this task difficult, but with assistance from Dr. Underwood, she is able at least to mention pluses and minuses of her marriage within the same five minutes of discussion.

Over the course of the next few months Dr. Underwood repeatedly addresses Charlene's splitting behavior, not only in terms of her marriage, but also in terms of the way she sees herself and in the therapy relationship itself. They discuss the fact that Charlene has long viewed family members and other intimates in extreme (but temporally inconsistent) terms, and they talk about how difficult it is to manage a relationship when her view of the other keeps shifting. Charlene begins to show a glimmer of understanding in this regard, but she finds it almost impossible to recognize when she is splitting until she discusses it with Dr. Underwood after the fact. She also has difficulty in the moment preventing herself from trying to modify her husband's behavior rather than to work on modifying her own behavior. Meanwhile, her mood bounces around by the week, and she feels alternately angry and then ashamed of her earlier behavior. Dr. Underwood points out that as Charlene's variable behavior creates conflict with important people in her life, her relationships tend to be marked by extremes, which perpetuates her view of self and others as either all good or all bad.

Dr. Underwood decides to narrow the focus of therapy, insofar as he is able, to their relationship with one another. He does not discourage Charlene from discussing the current problems in her life, but when he can, he points out the ways in which she views both herself and Dr. Underwood in extreme (and usually opposing) terms. If she describes herself in negative terms, he reminds her of the positive, and vice versa. If she idolizes him, he reminds her that he's disappointed her on occasion, and when she's angry with him, he reminds her of how important their work together really is.

By the end of the first year of treatment, Charlene is having increased success viewing herself and others in a more balanced manner, particularly after Dr. Underwood points out to her that she is most likely to distort when she is aroused. He therefore suggests that she monitor her arousal level as a way to decrease the likelihood that she will overreact. Charlene begins to report less conflict with her husband, she describes a more stable marital relationship, and she reports that the frequency of cutting has dropped from two or three times a week to about once every six weeks. Charlene continues to spend excessively on occasion, but she is no longer bingeing on alcohol.

When the first year of treatment comes to an end, Charlene and Dr. Underwood decide jointly that continued treatment is in order. They do not renew their formal treatment contract, but they begin meeting weekly in order to continue their work to stabilize Charlene's behavior and mood.

Mentalization-Based Treatment (MBT)

Model of Psychopathology

MBT is another psychodynamic treatment for borderline personality disorder, in this instance falling within the intersubjective school and based on the premise that individuals with disorganized patterns of attachment, presumably due to early interaction with unresponsive or inconsistent caregivers, are not likely to relate effectively to others or to understand the connection between intentional mental states and their own or others' behavior. In other words, they lack the most rudimentary sort of psychological-mindedness, and they find it difficult to understand how subjective intent is related to why they or others do what they do. Alternatively, people with limited mentalizing skills may be able to connect intent and behavior at some times, but the capacity for mentalization becomes unavailable at moments of emotional arousal. It is proposed that by resolving attachment difficulties and by helping patients to understand and to predict the behavior of others, they will naturally feel safer in relationships, will develop a stronger sense of self, and will learn to regulate affect more effectively.

Treatment Strategies

Formal MBT involves twice-weekly sessions that alternate between individual and group psychotherapy. The therapist strives to provide a stable attachment experience and focuses on helping the patient understand the intentions and experiences of each participant in the therapy dyad or group. The therapist carefully manages the therapeutic relationship in such a way that the patient feels neither overwhelmed with affect nor excessively detached, thus providing a model for optimal interpersonal functioning and ensuring that the patient experiences the kind of mild arousal that facilitates learning. After helping the patient to modulate affect within the therapy session, the therapist repeatedly directs the patient's attention to discussion of what each person is feeling and experiencing in the current interaction.

While MBT involves a great deal of **transference work**, this differs from the nature of such work in many other psychodynamic treatment models, in that the goal is something other than the patient's increased insight about defenses and relationships or the patient's ability to understand his or her history in a new way. Rather, the MBT focus on the transference is intended to permit therapist and patient to understand the perspectives and intentions of one another. This is referred to as "mentalizing the transference," and one might think of it as practice for the patient in understanding the intentions that lead people to think, to feel, and to act as they do. In the context of the relatively secure attachment between therapist and patient, the therapist begins each investigation of a transference event by validating the patient's feeling about the relationship, after which the events immediately preceding the current moment are explored. The MBT therapist is expected to acknowledge his or her own inevitable mentalization failures due to countertransference, after which therapist and patient collaborate in arriving at an interpretation of the interaction. Finally, the therapist may offer an alternate view of what has occurred.

Research Findings
Bateman and Fonagy reported in 2008 on the long-term follow-up of 44 patients with borderline personality disorder who were treated with either routine outpatient care or MBT in a partial hospitalization program. All but three patients were followed for eight years, at which time only 14% of those treated with MBT met diagnostic criteria for borderline personality disorder, in comparison with 87% of those patients treated with routine care. In 2009 Bateman and Fonagy reported on a larger study in the form of an RCT comparing outpatient-based MBT with best clinical practice. They showed that while patients in both treatment arms experienced improvement, change happened more quickly for those treated with MBT.

Case Example

Dave is a 39 year old, divorced father of two children. He reports that since his divorce three years ago, he has dated at least 15 women but hasn't been able to establish a lasting relationship. He adds that women have always been the most important thing in his life, and if he's not in a relationship, he sometimes thinks he might as well just pack it in. He says, "It's like I'm just floating out there, and I don't belong anywhere." Dr. Vanderzee asks Dave if he has thoughts of harming himself. He replies, "Not really. Why?"

Dave explains that he still doesn't understand why his wife left him, because he felt that their marriage was okay. He comments that one of the most difficult things about being single is the lack of sex. He muses, "Sex kind of like keeps my head straight or something." Since the divorce, Dave says his mood has been down much of the time, and his inability to "get a girl" makes him feel worthless, although he denies sleep or appetite disturbance, unrealistic guilt, or crying spells. He states that he never felt depressed like this until just before the end of the marriage. About a year before his wife left him, he began drinking a case of beer every other day, and this continued until about 18 months ago. He comments that he doesn't know why he drank like that, because he doesn't actually like the taste of beer. Maybe he was just lonely and enjoyed spending time at the bar, he suggests. At present he indicates that he consumes an average of two mixed drinks on each weekend night. Dave states that when he was drinking heavily, he got into frequent physical altercations. At present he doesn't fight very much, although he admits that he feels irritable quite often, particularly while driving. He says, "You know, there are a lot of idiots in the world." However, Dave denies anger problems on his job as an insurance adjuster. He says, "I just do my job, and if a customer doesn't like it, I can't help that."

Upon interview Dave presents as a generally cooperative but mildly depressed individual. He relates his history in a very matter-of-fact way. He generally denies any other symptoms of a mental disorder.

Dr. Vanderzee recommends to Dave that they begin weekly individual therapy sessions, and she also asks that he join a weekly therapy group for people with problems like his. She offers the opinion that Dave has mood problems and is feeling confused about relationships. She suggests that the combination of individual and group psychotherapy is likely to address his problems in an efficient way. Dave replies that he was thinking he would receive individual treatment, but if the doctor wants him to join a group, he imagines that he could give it a try.

Early on in Dave's individual sessions, Dr. Vanderzee notices that he doesn't really seem to have a clear idea of what to do in therapy. While he tries to follow her instruction to talk about whatever is on his mind, he usually just describes recent events and recounts the conversations he has had with others.

Dave continues to date but remains perplexed about why his relationships don't last, and he expresses frustration about his dates' behavior. He says, "Women nowadays—I guess they want a guy with money or someone who's going to give them a child." Dave points out that he doesn't have much money because he has to pay child support, and he certainly doesn't want any more kids. "So I'm just out of luck," he says.

Dr. Vanderzee begins to encourage Dave to contemplate what his current date might actually be thinking and feeling, and she also encourages him to consider his internal reaction to the date's behavior. She finds that she actually has to suggest to Dave what might be going on inside the mind of his date. He acknowledges that he has never really understood "how women think." However, it also becomes clear that he doesn't recognize the choices he has in reacting to the world. Most of the time, he just does what he does and moves on.

When she has the opportunity, Dr. Vanderzee encourages Dave to focus on their interaction within the therapy session, and she helps Dave to understand both what she might be thinking and feeling, as they talk with one another, and what Dave himself is thinking and feeling. Further, she asks him about his experience in the psychotherapy group and helps him to analyze interactions with other members from the perspective of both his and their mental states. Dave finds this work frustrating, and he begins to express more and more distress as

Dr. Vanderzee keeps returning to the issue of people's thoughts, feelings, and intentions. In several sessions he exclaims in exasperation that he is "not a mind reader," and on one occasion he says, "You women just think differently from us guys!"

Dr. Vanderzee responds to Dave's frustration by backing off a little and then suggesting that Dave might be feeling confused and a little lost. She also suggests that she probably misjudged his level of frustration at the moment, which led her to push him harder than was desirable. This has the effect of settling Dave. Dr. Vanderzee then asks him to say more about the idea that it's hard to communicate because she's a woman and he's a man.

Dave begins talking about his childhood. He recounts that he was never especially close to his mother, who he says was "too emotional" and with whom he could "never win." By contrast, he says he was more comfortable with his father, who he says didn't talk a lot and was "just a regular guy." Dave comments that his father was more effective in stopping conflict between Dave and his siblings, while his mother's intervention usually consisted of blaming Dave for being a "bully." Dave suggests that he respected his father more than his mother, in response to which Dr. Vanderzee points out the connection between Dave's view of each parent and the quality of his relationships with each of them. She also asks if, based on Dave's knowledge of her, he believes that Dr. Vanderzee is like his mother and is "too emotional." Dave thinks for a moment and then replies, "Maybe not."

Over time Dave begins to have more success in talking about his mental state and in speculating about the mental state of others. Dr. Vanderzee suggests that Dave use this new understanding to think about how to act on dates. He admits that the prospect of thinking all the time about his and his date's mental state sounds exhausting, and he would prefer to "go on automatic pilot." Still, he agrees that it might be worth trying a different approach. Such a shift in behavior does actually lead to more satisfying dates, and in time Dave finds a woman who appears to be interested in a relationship. Dave and Dr. Vanderzee discuss the developing relationship in quite a bit of detail in their sessions together.

Dave's mood begins to lift as the new relationship develops, and he reports less general irritability. Episodes of road rage decrease to nearly zero. Dr. Vanderzee underscores the connection between Dave's mood and the sense of connection he feels with his new girlfriend. They also discuss the ways in which the girlfriend has an inner life that differs from that of Dave's mother. Dave begins to take pleasure in understanding the new girlfriend in a way that contrasts significantly with the experience of his marriage.

After 1½ years of individual and group therapy, Dave and Dr. Vanderzee decide that he is doing well, and they plan to end treatment within the next month. At the last session Dr. Vanderzee talks about her feelings regarding their work together, and Dave talks about his experience of treatment. Dr. Vanderzee encourages Dave to contact her again if he feels the need.

Supportive Psychotherapy (Including Psychoeducation)

Model of Psychopathology

The term "supportive psychotherapy" is used in a number of ways and sometimes refers to basic counseling or talk therapy. We use it here to mean the application of psychodynamic principles, but not with the goal of effecting fundamental change in an individual's defense structure. Instead, supportive psychotherapy uses psychodynamic principles with the intention to "shore up" ineffective defenses of the patient and to promote optimal functioning in general. Supportive psychotherapists agree with their psychodynamic brethren that psychopathology results from the ego's failure to cope effectively with unconscious conflict, but they do not aim to promote insight or to clear away ineffective ego defenses and substitute more effective defenses in their place. Rather, they help to suppress unconscious conflict by reinforcing whatever defenses the ego may be using at present, effectively adding the therapist's voice to the particular strategy the ego uses to cope with conflict. As is the case for psychodynamic psychotherapy, there may be disagreement among supportive psychotherapists regarding the nature of instinctual material with which the patient struggles (sexual, striving for superiority, Existential, and so forth), but there is no disagreement about the idea that the ego is failing to cope with unconscious conflict of some kind.

Treatment Strategies

In supportive psychotherapy the clinician makes less use of interpretation, observation, and confrontation than is the case in psychodynamic psychotherapy. These therapeutic interventions are more appropriate for psychodynamic psychotherapy, in that they encourage patients to reflect on their coping strategies, and they draw patients' attention to thoughts, feelings, and behaviors that they may previously have ignored. On balance, these interventions lead patients to consider changing the way they deal with problems in life. By contrast, the supportive psychotherapist gives more advice, praise, and affirmation than does the psychodynamic psychotherapist. Such interventions lead patients to "do more of the same" or perhaps to try another behavioral strategy without examining the associated assumptions and defenses.

Another strategy commonly used by supportive psychotherapists involves educating patients about their condition, about what is needed to achieve remission of symptoms (i.e., elements of the treatment plan), and about relevant aspects of normal functioning. While **psychoeducation** can be utilized in any model of psychotherapy, it is particularly suited for use in supportive psychotherapy. Psychoeducation often includes the implicit admonition to make specific behavior changes, and patients may understand the provision of such information as evidence that if they follow the therapist's instructions, they will feel better. This contrasts with the fundamental assumption of psychodynamic psychotherapy, which suggests that improved insight translates into improved mental health. In psychodynamic psychotherapy the field of operation occurs much more within the patient's mind than in supportive psychotherapy.

Research Findings

Because the term "supportive psychotherapy" is used in so many ways, it is difficult to summarize research concerning its efficacy. However, two recent studies may shed some light on the topic. In 2012 Cuipers, Driessen, and colleagues examined the effect of "non-directive supportive therapy" in the treatment of adult depression. They located eight studies that compared such treatment with a control group, yielding a mean effect size in the moderate range ($g = .54$). Recall, however, that psychotherapy in general has an effect size of $d = .87$. (The g and d statistics are roughly comparable.) Of course, it isn't clear whether "non-directive supportive therapy" is entirely equivalent to the way in which we have defined supportive psychotherapy.

By contrast, in 2008 de Maat and colleagues evaluated a version of supportive psychotherapy called "short psychodynamic supportive psychotherapy" with 313 mildly or moderately depressed adult outpatients; their treatment model does appear to accord with our definition of supportive psychotherapy. Some patients in the study were treated with supportive psychotherapy alone, some with pharmacotherapy alone, and some with both modalities. In general, supportive psychotherapy was as effective as pharmacotherapy, while combined therapy was more effective than pharmacotherapy alone, but combined therapy wasn't necessarily more effective than supportive psychotherapy alone. Patients and therapists generally preferred that supportive psychotherapy be included as an element of treatment.

> **Case Example**
>
> Ella is a 60-year-old, married mother of two adult children. She presents for psychotherapy in connection with escalating conflict in her son's marriage. Ella states that since her children have grown up, she has consistently avoided becoming involved in their problems. However, when her son lost his job four months ago, Ella and her husband offered to let the son and his wife stay in their finished basement until they could get back on their feet financially. Ella says it soon became evident that the son and daughter-in-law were arguing frequently about money. Further, Ella says her daughter-in-law confided in Ella that the son was using cocaine on a regular basis. Ella says she talked to her son, who reported that he was insufflating a couple of lines every other week, and he denied any other drug use or alcohol abuse. He complained that his wife was not reliable, and he admitted that because of this and other reasons he was unhappy in his marriage.
>
> Ella says that now she doesn't know what to believe. She states that she is very worried about both her son and daughter-in-law, and she finds herself ruminating about them day and night. Her husband seems intent on keeping his distance, and when she tries to talk to him about the young couple, he changes the subject after a few minutes. Ella says that her sleep is disturbed, and she worries that she's becoming depressed. However, she denies symptoms consistent with a major depressive episode now or at any time in her life.

Upon interview Ella presents as a pleasant and cooperative, somewhat anxious older woman. Dr. Wilson suggests that they meet in weekly sessions for a few weeks or months to see what they can work out.

In the first two therapy sessions Ella recounts in further detail the recent events in the lives of her son and daughter-in-law. She reiterates that she doesn't want to interfere in the young couple's relationship, and it becomes evident that she is worried that such interference might lead to bad feelings and/or to injury on the part of the young people. At the same time, Ella notes that her older brother, who died three years ago, was alcoholic, and she is aware of how much her brother's wife and children suffered as a consequence of the brother's drinking. She says she worries about whether her son might have inherited a tendency to become addicted.

Dr. Wilson provides Ella information regarding the diagnosis of substance use disorders. Ella states that in light of the diagnostic criteria, she doesn't really believe that her son is an addict, although she doesn't approve of his use of cocaine, particularly given the couple's current financial situation. Dr. Wilson also talks with Ella about family dynamics and comments on the attempt by the daughter-in-law to "triangulate" Ella—that is, to pull her into the marital relationship in the hope of stabilizing it. Dr. Wilson suggests that Ella can indeed stabilize the young people's relationship by becoming a part of their marriage, but this will deprive the son and daughter-in-law of the opportunity to work out their own difficulties and will cause Ella to experience their distress even more. Ella comments that she finds this information very helpful, at least in part because it offers a way of understanding the basis of her impulse to stay out of other people's affairs.

A few sessions later Ella begins to explore in greater depth her fear of responding to others in a way that might injure them. With Dr. Wilson's assistance, she traces this back to certain experiences in her childhood. She says that she learned by watching her older siblings that words can hurt. Moreover, she recalls that on several occasions in the third grade she made fun of another girl in her class, only to learn later on that the other girl was very upset about her poor peer relationships and two years later changed schools because of this.

Ella states that since about the age of ten she has therefore avoided saying anything too direct to other people for fear of hurting them. Dr. Wilson responds that lack of self-assertion might be a problem in some situations, but in this circumstance it is not. He suggests that Ella's impulse is the right one, and she should continue to avoid mixing herself up in her son's marriage.

Ella asks Dr. Wilson how she can stop ruminating about the situation that continues to unfold in her basement. Dr. Wilson suggests that they try to figure out when she has more success and when less success in stopping the ruminations. Ella thinks about this and then states that when she talks with her husband or a friend about her worries, they become larger. When she distracts herself by reading or doing volunteer work, the ruminations recede. Dr. Wilson suggests that Ella consider doing more of what works and less of what doesn't, and he also suggests that she might benefit from the behavioral technique of scheduling her worry, which would involve picking out one 15-minute period, at the same time every day, when she can worry about her son and daughter-in-law. If ruminations arise at other times, she is to remind herself that she has a designated worry time and should try to defer her worries until then.

After ten sessions Ella reports that she is feeling better. She says that somehow her son and daughter-in-law have stopped talking to her about their problems. Dr. Wilson suggests that perhaps Ella may have signaled in some way that she wasn't receptive; Ella agrees that that could well be the case. She says she has managed to limit her worry time to the designated 15 minutes daily, and she is otherwise generally able to view the young couple's problems from an emotional distance. She says she reminds herself that every marriage is different, and her son and daughter-in-law need to get through this rough patch in whatever way they can. She thanks Dr. Wilson for his assistance, and therapy comes to an end.

Play Therapy

Model of Psychopathology

It was Freud who in 1909 first applied psychoanalytic concepts to the treatment of a child. Five-year-old Little Hans was afraid of horses, and based on reports from the child's father, Freud believed this reflected the boy's fear of his father in the Oedipal triangle. In fact, Freud had minimal personal contact with Little Hans, and the direct treatment of children using psychoanalytic principles had to wait for the next generation of theorists, particularly ego psychologist Anna Freud and object relations theorist Melanie Klein. Notwithstanding their fierce rivalry with one another over many years, these two women are together credited with having established the use of play as a means to understand and ultimately modify a child's defense structure. They both believed that children who present for mental health treatment have experienced some sort of block to their development, and they established the goal in treatment of resolving or removing whatever is preventing healthy development. Melanie Klein and Anna Freud believed that if child and therapist played together, the content and quality of the child's play would perform the same functions as free association, thereby providing the data necessary for the psychoanalysis of children. Consistent with the intervention offered Little Hans, both women believed that the children would benefit from the therapist's interpretations of their play.

However, after a number of years there was a shift in understanding regarding the therapist's task in play therapy. Rather than offering interpretations regarding the meaning of children's play, in the hope of reorganizing the child's defense structure, play therapists came to believe that children benefit from learning to think and to speak about play in a rich, imaginative way, and they are particularly likely to benefit from developing both the ability to connect behavior with intent and the ability to imagine the perspectives of others. Often, the play therapist concludes that a child has not developed in a healthy way because of an attachment failure, and therapists therefore place great emphasis on the development of a stable, supportive, consistent relationship with the child. Play therapists believe that such a relationship provides an opportunity for repair of attachment insecurities.

Play therapy has been utilized in the treatment of children with a wide range of mental disorders. It has even been applied to the treatment of autism spectrum disorder utilizing a variant of play therapy called Floortime. This treatment model emphasizes the development of specific skills that are often lacking among children with this disorder, including regulation and interest in the world, engagement and relating, two-way intentional communication, continuous social problem solving, symbolic play, and bridging ideas.

Treatment Strategies

Play therapy sessions are often held once a week but may be scheduled to occur less frequently. Therapist and child meet in a room that contains a variety of toys and other objects that are specifically chosen to encourage imaginative play. Early on the therapist may simply need to help the child engage in play, but as time goes on the therapist's role shifts to one of encouraging the child to verbalize about the content of play, emphasizing imagination and, particularly, the varying perspectives of characters in the child's play. As children come to trust their therapists, they may be willing to begin discussing emotional problems or difficult circumstances in their lives, to which the therapist responds supportively and may offer suggestions about how the child might cope more effectively.

The therapist may or may not have regular contact with the child's parent, and the parent may or may not actually engage in the play therapy sessions from time to time. If there is regular contact between therapist and parent, the therapist offers suggestions to the parent that are designed to strengthen the parent–child bond (thus addressing attachment issues) and to modify ineffective parental behavior toward the child. This may include input regarding reasonable developmental expectations, as well as encouragement that parents respond to children in terms of the children's interests and current level of functioning. Play therapists often place particular emphasis on helping the parent to perceive the child more accurately, rather than to view the child through the lens of the parent's current conflicts or difficult history.

Research Findings

In general, psychotherapy with children that includes a behavioral component has been shown to be more effective than treatment without a behavioral component (Weisz, Weiss, Han, Granger, & Morton, 1995). This general finding suggests that play therapy may be less effective than psychotherapeutic approaches that involve behavioral interventions more directly. However, in a 2005 meta-analysis of 93 studies of play therapy (broadly defined), Bratton, Ray, Rhine, and Jones showed that play therapy was in fact effective ($d = .80$). Within this large group of studies the authors showed that certain non-psychodynamic kinds of play therapy were more effective than other play therapy, and they also found that play therapy was more effective when parents were involved in treatment than when they were not. Research on the use of play therapy with children diagnosed with autism spectrum disorder (e.g., Floortime) has yielded limited results.

Case Example

Federico is a four-year-old boy who resists going to preschool. The elder of two children, Federico consistently reports stomach problems and general distress on Monday mornings, and he asks that his mother not take him to school. Federico's mother usually insists that he go to school, reminding him that he goes there for only a few hours every other day. Sometimes, however, she says that Federico really does appear to be ill, and she lets him stay home. She notes that he usually attempts to stay home from school on either Wednesday or Friday as well.

Federico's mother reports that her son has many worries, and she says he has always been an anxious child, certainly more so than his younger brother. She states that he often has difficulty falling asleep at night, and he is a picky eater. She says that Federico reminds her of her younger brother when they were growing up, and she worries that, like her brother, Federico will remain a timid individual who will eventually begin abusing alcohol. Federico's mother states that her son generally achieved developmental milestones on time, and she says he is physically healthy. She states that she has a closer relationship with Federico than does the child's father, who is an active and gregarious, at times even boisterous police officer. The mother is trained as a nurse but has worked very little outside the home since Federico was born.

Upon interview Federico does indeed appear to be an anxious child. He remains near his mother and says little to Dr. Yao. When the latter asks him about what worries him, Federico replies that he's not usually scared, but he doesn't like monsters and doesn't like going to bed when it's dark.

Dr. Yao refers Federico and his mother to a behavior therapist who will address the child's school refusal, and she begins seeing Federico individually for play therapy. Federico is initially reluctant to separate from his mother, but after the mother accompanies her son and Dr. Yao to the play room, Federico seems more content to permit his mother to wait in the lobby until the end of the session. Dr. Yao shows Federico around the play room, and she asks which toys he would like to play with. Federico gravitates to a track with some small race cars, and he arranges some races. Dr. Yao comments on Federico's activity, and when he asks that she help him with the races, she joins in.

In the next session Dr. Yao asks Federico if he would like to play with puppets. He indicates his willingness to do so, and he then organizes a fight between his and Dr. Yao's puppets. Dr. Yao asks Federico to say why the puppets are fighting, and she wonders what each of them is thinking. Federico is quite competent in verbalizing each puppet's point of view. He says the little puppet (assigned to Dr. Yao) is afraid that the big puppet (assigned to Federico) will hurt him. The big puppet thinks the little puppet is stupid. After that Federico has Dr. Yao's puppet go off by himself to cry, while the big puppet exults over "winning." In the last few minutes of the play therapy session, Dr. Yao asks Federico if he sometimes feels sad or afraid like the little puppet. Federico replies that he does, and he says he also cries.

In the next few sessions Federico appears to settle in comfortably to his relationship with Dr. Yao. In one session they build a fort with cardboard bricks, and while they do so, Dr. Yao asks Federico what he does to feel safe when he's scared. In another session Federico plays school with Dr. Yao, and it becomes evident that he is frightened of some of the bigger children. Dr. Yao asks Federico what happens if he talks to the teacher about mean kids, and he replies that maybe the teacher will believe him—or maybe not. Dr. Yao asks Federico to pretend that she is a mean kid, and she encourages Federico to tell her to stop being mean. Then she asks Federico to pretend that she's the teacher, and she encourages Federico to tell her about the mean kids. Afterwards, Dr. Yao congratulates Federico on how well he spoke to the mean kid and to the teacher. Federico beams.

By this point in treatment Federico has begun attending school regularly, presumably in part because of the behavioral intervention. Dr. Yao decides to work with Federico on his more general anxiety. In the next session Dr. Yao tells Federico she's heard that he's going to school regularly, and she says she's so happy that he is feeling better about it. She asks Federico what other things make him feel sad or scared. Federico doesn't respond directly, and Dr. Yao suspects that he can't call his worries to mind at the moment. She therefore hypothesizes that he might be afraid to sleep by himself, and she also wonders if he might be afraid of his father.

Dr. Yao gets out an empty doll house and suggests that she and Federico put dolls and furniture in the house. Federico comments that dolls are for girls but soon sets out to furnish the house and to place dolls in various rooms. Federico places the three doll children in a room with the doll mother, while the doll father is working in the backyard. Dr. Yao asks why the older brother isn't with his father in the backyard. Federico responds that the mother is nice, but when the father wants to play catch with the older brother, he yells when the older brother can't catch the ball. Dr. Yao says she wonders if the older brother would like to do easier things with his father. Federico changes the subject.

Dr. Yao arranges a meeting with Federico's parents (but without Federico), and when the father comments that he and his son don't do much together, Dr. Yao suggests that they go for walks and also play with toys in the basement, gently suggesting that the father try to follow Federico's lead without "taking over" the interaction. Dr. Yao also suggests that the child's mother encourage interaction between Federico and her husband, including perhaps having the father read Federico a bedtime story on the nights that the father doesn't work.

In subsequent sessions Federico and Dr. Yao again play with puppets and build more forts. In one session they play a game about bedtime, and Federico talks about all the different people he could have read him a story before switching out the light. It develops that Federico does not have a nightlight in his room, and when Dr. Yao brings Federico to the lobby to meet his mother, she pulls the mother aside to suggest that she might want to consider buying a nightlight for the child's room.

After ten sessions Federico's mother reports that her son is attending school without difficulty, and she says he seems less anxious. She reports that Federico now spends more time with his father, and he seems to be developing a taste for roughhouse play. The addition of a nightlight has decreased Federico's anxiety about bedtime, as has perhaps the occasional involvement of Federico's father in the bedtime routine. Federico is still a picky eater, but Dr. Yao suggests that parental encouragement is the best thing to try at this time, and she predicts that over time Federico will become more adventurous about food. Dr. Yao suggests that they have accomplished their goals and can end treatment. She tells Federico goodbye and encourages the family to return in the future if there is a need.

Individual Behavior Therapies

Cognitive-Behavior Therapy (CBT)

Model of Psychopathology

It is useful to note that competency in CBT is a common requirement for psychiatry residents. However, skillsets of CBT practitioners vary widely according to level of training and personal interest. Patients and providers should be aware that many therapists state they use CBT but may not actually employ basic skills learned by those with formal training in CBT. Providers and patients should inquire about specific practices to understand how closely a therapist follows the anticipated CBT model.

CBT is the quintessential second-wave behavior therapy, relying as it does on behavioral principles that are applied in the service of changing both observable behaviors and cognitions. There are multiple variants of CBT. We discuss here the most widely practiced version of CBT, which is the cognitive therapy developed by the American psychiatrist Aaron T. Beck. Beck takes as his point of departure the proposition that cognitions mediate between situations and one's reaction to them, according to a model like the one shown in Figure 5.1.

Upon experiencing a specific situation, the individual appraises or interprets it in a way that is consistent with his or her beliefs about the world. This leads the individual to react in some way, by experiencing a feeling, by acting overtly in some manner, or by having another thought. This reaction becomes the new situation that he or she then appraises, and the sequence continues. In time other external situations may occur, leading to new sequences of appraisals and reactions. Symptoms of mental disorders are thought to correspond to the presence of thoughts that lack accuracy or utility and/or to behaviors that are ineffective. Causality is not implied, however; the theory does not assert that symptoms cause disordered thoughts and behaviors, or that the presence of such thoughts and behaviors causes symptoms. They are simply correlated.

When an individual presents with symptoms, multiple interventions are possible. One can modify the initial situation; one can modify an appraisal or two along the way; or one can modify a consequential behavior or thought. Direct modification of emotions is considered to be more difficult.

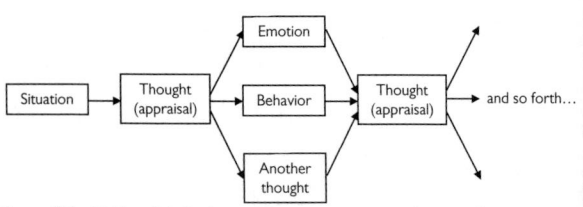

Figure 5.1. CBT model of relationships among situations, thoughts, feelings, and behaviors.

Consider one possible sequence. I come home from work, and I notice that my wife is not talkative. Depending on my core belief and on my experience in the marriage, I might appraise this situation in any number of ways. Perhaps I say to myself, "She's angry at me for something, but she probably won't tell me what it is." This thought leads to another thought, "It's unfair that I have to deal with her behavior." This might then lead to yet a third thought, "I'm tired of this," which will be followed by feelings of anger. I might then try to avoid her all evening; if we have to interact, I might behave in a passive-aggressive manner.

In this sequence, a situation (quiet wife) leads to a thought (she's mad at me), which leads to another thought (it's unfair), leading to another thought (I'm sick of this), which leads to an emotion (anger) and two behaviors (avoidance and poorly disguised irritability). If this sequence runs its course, it will probably lead to an increase in thoughts of hopelessness and other symptoms of depression. Where can the CBT therapist intervene? One might modify the situation in the first place (e.g., by having me check in with my wife by phone during the day), or one might question the sequence of my thoughts in response to the situation. Is my wife actually angry with me? How might I determine if my appraisal is correct? If she is angry, will she really not talk about it directly? If indeed I have correctly assessed my wife's mood and intentions, is there a more useful way to think about what this means? Given several options, what are the virtues of thinking about the situation as previously described or in some other way (e.g., that my wife is herself depressed or doesn't know how to solicit support from others)? What other behavioral responses might I consider, apart from my plan to "fight fire with fire"?

Treatment Strategies

The CBT therapist works to change specific situations, cognitions, and behaviors that maintain or exacerbate symptoms on a minute-by-minute basis in the patient's daily life. The therapist also encourages the patient to make more fundamental cognitive and behavioral changes that will prevent symptoms from arising in the future. The therapist helps the patient **build new skills** (e.g., through **assertiveness training**, **problem solving**, or **activity scheduling** to increase the frequency of target behaviors), helps the patient to manage distorted cognitions on a more routine basis, and teaches the patient **relapse prevention** skills.

There are three levels of cognition at which CBT therapists work: automatic thoughts, intermediate beliefs, and core beliefs, as illustrated in Figure 5.2. The most superficial level of cognition is the *automatic thought*, one's very quick appraisal of a situation. Automatic thoughts are often hardly noticed until the therapist points them out. Beck (2011) suggests that people have hundreds of automatic thoughts during the day; when these automatic thoughts lead to emotional distress, they are referred to as *automatic negative thoughts*. Much of the work of CBT involves identifying and helping the patient to challenge automatic negative thoughts. No attempt is made to change the thought if upon analysis it is clear that it is both accurate and useful. However, if an automatic thought is either *inaccurate* or *lacks utility* (i.e., doesn't help the patient), then therapist and patient work together to substitute a thought that is more accurate and/or useful. Some patients

```
"She's upset with me. I'm annoying her by asking a silly
question while she's busy with something else."
```

SITUATION:
Sales clerk mumbles response to question about an item on sale.

AUTOMATIC THOUGHT

INTERMEDIATE BELIEFS
(e.g., If I make decisions based on my own needs, other people may reject me; if I do things for others, they might tolerate or even appreciate me.)

CORE BELIEF
(e.g., I am unlovable.)

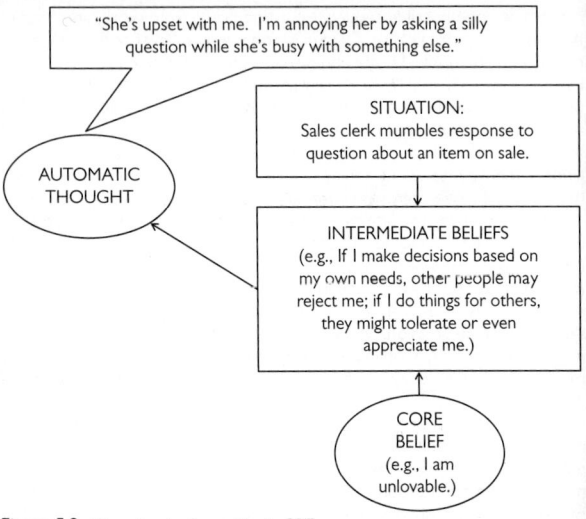

Figure 5.2. Three levels of cognition in CBT.

may find it helpful to categorize the kinds of cognitive distortions to which they most often subscribe, such as catastrophizing, black-and-white thinking, selective abstraction, emotional reasoning, overgeneralization, mind reading, and so forth.

At the most profound level of cognition, there are *core beliefs*, which summarize one's basic ideas about the world. When depressed, individuals are thought to hold one of these three main core beliefs: unlovability, helplessness, and worthlessness. Individuals with the core belief of unlovability are certain that no one will care for them as they are. At best, they may believe that if they are helpful to others in some way, they may be tolerated or even appreciated for the services that they provide. Individuals with the core belief of helplessness believe that they cannot cope with problems in the world and must rely on powerful others to survive. Those with the core belief of worthlessness view themselves as fundamentally flawed, immoral, or bad.

Patients with other kinds of psychopathology may hold different core beliefs. In the case of anxiety, one might strongly believe that the world is a dangerous and unpredictable place. Personality disorders can also be described in terms of their core beliefs. For example, individuals with strong avoidant tendencies believe that they are too fragile to cope with painful feelings, and they must protect themselves by avoiding a wide variety of thoughts, feelings, and situations. People with paranoid tendencies believe that they are weak and vulnerable. They therefore remain constantly on guard and scan the environment for threats.

When individuals are asymptomatic, they hold more forgiving core beliefs, such as that they are fundamentally likeable and can cope effectively with most of the problems they face in life. During episodes of illness, however, the negative core beliefs are likely to be activated. In CBT it is hypothesized that people accept their core beliefs in an unquestioning way; they are simply viewed as true. If therapists challenge patients about the shift in core beliefs between asymptomatic periods in the past and the current period of active illness, patients usually reply that they had never thought about this discrepancy, or that they were mistaken in the past but now see the world more clearly, or that they never *really* subscribed to the more forgiving core belief.

There are a number of ways for therapists to identify core beliefs. One commonly used technique is the **downward arrow**, in which the therapist moves from the patient's automatic negative thought to the underlying core belief by repeatedly asking something like, "If that's true, what would it mean about you?" Another way to identify core beliefs is to sample a wide array of the patient's automatic negative thoughts and then to look for themes. CBT offers a number of strategies to help patients shift their core beliefs, including the provision of **psychoeducation** regarding the nature of core beliefs, keeping a diary of events that argue either for or against the core belief, undertaking an historical review to understand how the core belief developed, and other specialized techniques. Patients find that core belief work is difficult, and this is particularly true for individuals with personality disorders, at least in part because they (unlike people with relapsing and remitting disorders) have never held more forgiving, flexible core beliefs. CBT therapists generally defer addressing core beliefs until the patient has been successful in modifying more superficial cognitions, such as automatic thoughts and intermediate beliefs, which we discuss next.

Between the automatic thoughts and core beliefs is a third level of cognition, the *intermediate beliefs*. These are the rules, attitudes, and assumptions that individuals live by, given their particular core beliefs. We have already mentioned one intermediate belief in talking about the individual with a core belief of unlovability. Such an individual might subscribe to the following pair of assumptions: "If I make decisions based on my own needs, other people will reject me; if I do things for others, they might tolerate or even appreciate me." Intermediate beliefs are generally harder to modify than automatic negative thoughts, but they are easier to modify than core beliefs. It is hypothesized that since intermediate and core beliefs underlie automatic thoughts, if the deeper-level cognitions can be modified, the automatic negative thoughts will occur much less frequently.

CBT is a highly structured model of treatment. At the beginning of treatment therapist and patient collaboratively **set goals**, as a way to ensure that therapy remains focused and the patient remains engaged. These goals should be concrete and, if possible, should refer to observable behaviors. A CBT session typically begins with a very brief check-in about the patient's primary symptom (mood, anxiety, and so forth) and major events during the week, after which therapist and patient agree on the problems they wish to address in the therapy hour. Homework from the previous session is reviewed, and then the main portion of the agenda is addressed. This involves discussion of no more than two or three current problems in the patient's life. Problems might include conflict with a significant other, difficulty motivating oneself, or anxiety about an upcoming event, among many other possibilities. While working through the agenda, therapists help patients to conceptualize problems in terms of situations, thoughts/appraisals, and reactions. Therapists also frequently point out the steps they are taking together to work on each agenda item, in the expectation that this will *teach patients to become their own therapists*.

CBT therapists try not to tell patients to think or act differently, preferring instead to lead patients to discover alternatives on their own. One way to do this involves the use of **Socratic questioning**, a technique that helps patients begin to view their problems in a new light. Together, patient and therapist **plan experiments** and **assign homework** that is designed to address the patient's problems. For example, one patient doubts her ability to deal with a family member in a new way. After **rehearsing** the new strategy in the session, perhaps in formal **role play**, patient and therapist agree to an experiment in which she tries out the new behavior between sessions and keeps track of what happens. Another patient believes that becoming more physically active will not improve his mood. Patient and therapist might design an experiment in which the patient adds 30 minutes of physical activity on alternate days of the week and keeps track of his resulting mood every day until the next therapy session. A somewhat insightful individual with psychosis might be asked to pay careful attention to the circumstances in which auditory hallucinations occur during the week. A common homework assignment early in treatment is for patients to keep track of their thoughts during the week when they notice that they are beginning to feel more anxious or depressed. Later in therapy, homework assignments might include filling out a structured form called a *thought record* that helps the patient analyze and challenge distressing ideas about a specific situation. At the end of a CBT treatment session the therapist asks the patient how the session was, what was helpful and what was not helpful, and whether therapist and patient should do something different in the next session.

CBT therapists adopt a style that is referred to as *collaborative empiricism*. This style requires that therapist and patient work together to determine "scientifically" the accuracy and utility of the patient's thoughts and ideas. Therapists do not impose their opinions on patients but instead suggest that it would be helpful to test certain beliefs to see whether they are true. Therapists may tentatively offer an hypothesis that differs from the one implicit in a patient's automatic negative thought, but they do so only to make the point that it might be worth questioning the associated belief. Therapists take the position that patients' automatic negative thoughts may in fact be correct, in which case therapist and patient will have to work together to remedy any associated deficit on the part of the patient, or the thoughts may not be accurate or useful, in which case it may be helpful to think in a different way. The only way to determine whether thoughts are accurate and useful—or not—is to test them, either in session or between sessions.

The CBT approach to patients' early life experiences differs rather sharply from that taken in models of psychotherapy that are more directly informed by psychoanalysis. In CBT it is accepted that patients' early life experiences influence who they are today and may be helpful in understanding why a certain core belief is prepotent. However, the main focus of treatment is on the patient's current thoughts, feelings, and behaviors. Early experiences are discussed only when required to help in developing a case conceptualization or—perhaps—in connection with core belief work.

Another significant point of departure from psychodynamic psychotherapies is the CBT approach to the concept of *resistance*. Obviously, CBT therapists recognize that patients may not progress quickly and may become "stuck" at various points in treatment. CBT therapists have four ways of thinking about the patient's difficulty moving forward. First, it may be that the patient isn't improving because the therapeutic alliance is weak. CBT places strong emphasis on maintaining a positive therapeutic alliance, and it is important to address any problems in this regard. Second, the patient may lack the skills required to make progress. For example, the therapist may not have inculcated a good understanding of the CBT model, may not have taught specific coping skills like assertive behavior, or may not have taught generic problem-solving skills. Third, a patient may fear the consequences of making changes in treatment. For example, patients may worry that if they become less symptomatic, family members will expect more of them, or they may view therapy as a kind of battle with the therapist over who is "right." If the patient harbors ideas like these, it is important for therapist and patient to investigate the associated cognitions; it may be possible to undertake experiments to determine whether those cognitions are accurate and useful. A final reason that patients fail to make changes in treatment is that the therapist has made a significant error, such as by applying the wrong set of treatment techniques in a given case.

Some newer variants of CBT are beginning to incorporate third-wave features, including mindfulness. We review one such group-based treatment, called mindfulness-based cognitive therapy, in a later section.

Research Findings
Since the early 1980s there has been a veritable explosion of research demonstrating the effectiveness of CBT in the treatment of a wide variety of disorders. Such research has typically involved adapting CBT principles to the details of a specific disorder, as a consequence of which there are now rather detailed CBT manuals available for a range of behavioral disorders. Many of these manuals are available commercially, and one such series of manuals is called *Treatments That Work*. (A few manuals in this series are based on psychotherapy models other than CBT.) The series, which generally pairs treatment manuals with patient workbooks, is available through Oxford University Press and is detailed at this website: http://global.oup.com/us/companion.websites/umbrella/treatments/series/

Empirical support has been established for variants of CBT in the treatment of adults with panic and agoraphobia (Siev & Chambless, 2007), depression (Driessen & Hollon, 2010), generalized anxiety disorder (Siev & Chambless, 2007), insomnia (Riemann & Perlis, 2009), opiate dependence (McHugh, Hearon, & Otto, 2010), obsessive-compulsive disorder (Olatunji, Davis, Powers, & Smits, 2013), posttraumatic stress disorder (Seidler & Wagner, 2006), social phobia (Gil, Carrillo, & Meca, 2001), somatoform disorders (Taylor, Asmundson, & Coons, 2005; Williams, Hadjistavropoulos, & Sharpe, 2006), and (adjunctively) schizophrenia (Zimmermann, Favrod, Trieu, & Pomini, 2005), among other conditions. There are empirically supported versions of CBT for the treatment of children with anxiety (Seligman & Ollendick, 2011), binge eating disorder (Rutherford & Couturier, 2007), depression (Harrington, Whittaker, Shoebridge, & Campbell, 1998), and distress regarding medical treatments (Powers, 1999). The use of CBT is also empirically supported in the treatment of a range of health behaviors related to chronic pain (Hofmann, Asnaani, Vonk, Sawyer, & Fang, 2012), childhood obesity (Wilfley, Kolko, & Kass, 2011), and other conditions.

The availability of CBT treatment manuals and patient workbooks with empirical support in the treatment of specific disorders clearly represents a major step forward in making demonstrably effective treatment available to a larger group of mental health patients. However, some therapists have complained that it is difficult to keep up with the proliferation of empirically supported treatments and associated manuals, and some have suggested that this fact limits the use of manuals by therapists. Several authors have begun to think about developing variants of CBT that can be applied across a range of diagnoses. One such principle-driven variant of CBT is that espoused in 2010 by Barlow and colleagues in their Unified Protocol, which can be applied to unipolar depression and a range of anxiety disorders. This "transdiagnostic" variant of CBT aims at increasing the patient's understanding of emotions, decreasing avoidance and ineffective self-regulation, and changing cognitions. These are considered to be the fundamental components of treatment for unipolar depression and anxiety, and the Unified Protocol assists the therapist in deciding which components are most likely to be helpful for a given patient. It will be interesting to see whether CBT research continues to focus on specific disorders or moves in the direction of the Unified Protocol. RCTs of the Unified Protocol are now beginning to appear (e.g., Farchione et al., 2012).

Case Example
We offer here four case examples from the files of a fictional Dr. Brown, illustrating the application of CBT principles in the treatment of depression, social anxiety disorder, a personality disorder, and psychosis. Case A (depression) is described at length, but to avoid redundancy the other cases are described in less detail and the general features of CBT are not repeated. Of course, there are many other conditions to which CBT can be applied; some of these are covered in the subsequent sections on cognitive-behavioral interventions with obsessive-compulsive disorder, panic disorder, and posttraumatic stress disorder.

Case A. George is a 43-year-old, married father of two children. He reports that for the past three months he has had low mood much of the day nearly every day. He indicates that he feels tired a lot, and some days he can hardly make himself go to his job as an accountant at a large industrial concern. His concentration is impaired at work, he has made some minor mistakes on the job, and he believes that he may be in danger of being fired, even though he has been a good worker over the course of his ten years with this employer. At night he comes home, somehow gets through dinner, and then watches television until he falls asleep on the couch. Later in the evening he may experience sleep-onset latency of up to an hour. He sometimes awakens during the night, and many mornings he lies awake worrying in bed for 30 to 60 minutes before his alarm goes off. He believes that his wife is becoming fed up with him, and the frequency of their lovemaking has declined precipitously. He is pretty certain that the children are avoiding him. Lately he has been thinking that it might be better if he weren't even in the picture anymore. Sometimes he thinks about how he could kill himself, but he doesn't have a definite plan and has never tried to hurt himself before.

George reports that he is generally in good physical health, and he denies current or past substance abuse. He admits that he has gained some weight since his twenties, such that he is now a little overweight. He reports that his energy is very poor, and he didn't put in a vegetable garden this summer. He was beginning to feel down in the spring, and he decided that the garden just wasn't worth the effort this year. He has also stopped exercising on the treadmill, and he no longer goes for walks in the neighborhood. George notes he says he has never felt like this before, and he says that until this year he always felt himself to be a pretty stable person.

Upon interview George presents in a somewhat flat, slightly worried manner. He makes adequate eye contact and relates in a socially appropriate manner.

Dr. Brown concludes that George is in a first episode of major depressive disorder. She doesn't find evidence of any other mental disorder. She explains to George that his condition is one that is marked by negative cognitions about himself, the world, and the future and that these thoughts prevent him from accessing necessary supplies of positive reinforcement. George agrees that he seems to view the world differently now, and he says that lately he has been worrying about things that never used to bother him. He then asks if there might be something wrong with his thyroid, or could "low iron" in his blood be causing problems? Dr. Brown asks if he has talked with primary care physician about this, to which George responds, "Well, yeah, I guess he did say that my blood work was normal when I saw him a couple of weeks ago." When Dr. Brown comments on this concern about health, despite the reassurance from his family doctor, George replies that he's noticed that his thinking often gets "stuck," and he says he has a hard time "talking sense" to himself.

Dr. Brown asks George what goals he would like to set for himself in therapy. He replies that he just wants to feel better. After they discuss it some more, however, he is able to say that he wants to improve his sleep pattern, to improve his concentration at work, to become more active around the house, and to spend more time doing things with his family. He also says he would like to decrease his ruminative worry, and he wants his mood to improve.

George and Dr. Brown decide to begin working on his sleep. They agree that he will keep track of his sleep during the upcoming week and will also track his evening naps. Dr. Brown asks George to read a short pamphlet on CBT and depression, and she also asks him to notice during the week when his mood drops. She asks that he keep track of what was happening just before his mood dropped and what he was thinking just as it began to drop. As the session ends, Dr. Brown invites George's feedback regarding the session and specifically asks if there was anything that he didn't understand or didn't like about it. George replies that the session seemed okay, although he admits that he's not all that optimistic that treatment will help.

When George comes in the following week, Dr. Brown explains the idea of setting an agenda for the session. She and George agree that they'll check in on his mood, briefly discuss any major events in his life since the last session, review the homework, and then address any problems George would like to discuss. However, George indicates that nothing special has happened in the past week that he wants to talk about. Dr. Brown says that they'll then agree on some homework, and just before the hour is up they'll discuss how the session went.

During this session Dr. Brown and George discuss his sleep at length, and she provides written information regarding sleep hygiene, asking that George try to cut down on the evening naps. She suggests that after dinner he go for a walk around the neighborhood. George says he doesn't believe he will have the energy to do this, but he agrees to try at least once in the coming week and to keep track of his predictions about the walk (how far he can walk and how he will feel afterwards) and then to write down how the walk actually went.

George and Dr. Brown also discuss a couple of instances during the week when he noticed his mood dropping. George reports that in one instance his boss called him into his office in order to begin planning for the annual report, which will be due in a few weeks. George was aware of feeling very anxious at first, and he then began to feel hopeless, believing that he wouldn't be able to concentrate on what the boss was saying. He was overcome with a wave of fatigue and was pretty certain the boss would notice that he wasn't following very well. He thought his boss might therefore begin disciplinary procedures against him. In fact, the meeting went well enough, but George attributes this to the boss's unusually cheerful mood that morning.

Using this example, Dr. Brown explains the idea of automatic negative thoughts. She draws a picture of how the situation (called into boss's office) leads to a thought ("I won't be able to function and will probably get in trouble"), and that thought leads to certain reactions, which can be behavioral (feeling physically weak), cognitive (worries about being fired), and/or emotional (fear and hopelessness). Dr. Brown asks George to reflect on whether his automatic thought was accurate and/or useful in this instance. She asks about George's recent annual evaluation at work, and George admits that it was entirely satisfactory—about which he was amazed at the time. She also asks how George would have felt if he had instead had the thought, "I'm not feeling very good today, but I can probably manage this meeting all right." He replies that he would have felt much less frightened and hopeless. He adds, however, that he doesn't think he could have convinced himself to believe that. Dr. Brown asks George if he has made other catastrophic predictions about situations at work, and he replies that he frequently does this, adding that he even thinks this way about his home life. For example, he worries that his wife is going to leave him, even though she seems more concerned than upset with him.

At session's end, Dr. Brown and George agree that he will continue to monitor his sleep, will try to decrease the evening naps, will go for at least one walk (rating his predictions ahead of time and then his performance afterwards), and will continue to pay attention to his thoughts when his mood drops during the week. When Dr. Brown asks for feedback about the session, George comments that he learned a lot this week and is feeling a tiny bit hopeful.

During the next few sessions George begins to make some progress. He discovers that his predictions about the evening walks were unduly pessimistic, and because he now feels more energetic in the evening, in time he is able to drop his weeknight naps. His sleep pattern begins to consolidate, but he still suffers from early morning awakening. He begins to question his automatic negative thoughts, although he still suspects that he is a burden to others at home and at work. He comes to recognize that he often engages in "emotional reasoning," a pattern of reasoning in which he concludes that if he feels depressed or anxious, it must mean that his situation is dire. He also recognizes that he engages in "black-and-white thinking," imagining, for example, that if he's unable to concentrate perfectly at work, it means that he is worthless as an employee.

At the beginning of Session 6 George says that on today's agenda he wants to place discussion of his relationship with his wife. He tells Dr. Brown that he's sure his wife is disgusted with him. Not only has he been depressed for months, but yesterday his wife commented that he seemed to be feeling just a little better. Afterwards, he had the thought that now his wife must be even angrier, because she knows he could have gotten help sooner.

Using this example, Dr. Brown introduces a "thought record" form, which permits George to map out on paper the relationship between the situation (wife comments he looks better) and his subsequent thought, leading to more thoughts, feelings, and actions. They discuss several possible beliefs George might have had about the situation. It could be that George's wife really is angry with him, in which case they might need marital counseling. It could also be that she doesn't know what to think, because she doesn't understand his depression, in which case it will be important that she receive some education about depression. Or perhaps she is worried about him and still loves him.

George agrees with Dr. Brown that the only way to find out what his wife actually thinks is to ask her. He admits that he is afraid to do this, and Dr. Brown suggests that they practice in the session how he might talk to her.

In the first role play, Dr. Brown plays George, and George plays his wife. In this way Dr. Brown models for George how he might talk to his wife. Then, Dr. Brown and George switch roles, and he plays himself. After the role play Dr. Brown makes a couple of suggestions but confirms for George that he actually presented himself very well.

In Session 7 George reports that he talked with his wife, and she reassured him that she wasn't at all angry. She told him she was well aware of how bad he felt, and she was actually upset with herself for not knowing how to help him. She said she was very happy he had found a treatment that seemed to be helping. George and Dr. Brown talk about what it might mean that he was unduly pessimistic about his relationship with his wife, and he agrees that this is certainly a pattern for him.

In Session 9 George reports that his mood has begun dropping again, and he doesn't know why. However, he happens to mention that his wife has had a big argument with her mother and has become a little irritable around the house. He also notes that work is becoming more pressured, because the annual report will be due in a few days. Dr. Brown uses Socratic questioning to help George reach the conclusion that he might be experiencing increased anxiety because of problems at home and at work. He seems genuinely surprised about this conclusion, and he comments, "I just thought I was getting worse again for no reason."

Dr. Brown then reviews with George what do when his mood drops like this, and together they decide that he can increase his physical activity, spend more time with friends, and remind himself to be patient. They also agree he can jog his memory about how to respond to a dip in mood by reading some three-by-five cards they compose together in today's session. George and Dr. Brown decide to write a card that says, "If my mood drops, I should ask myself how my situation has changed. Maybe the change in my mood represents a normal reaction to stress." Another card says, "If my mood drops, I should increase my physical activity, spend more time with friends, and remind myself that after a while I'll feel better again." George admits that he doesn't fully believe the second card, but he says he'll try reading it three or four times every day.

At the next session George reports that he is feeling better again, particularly since the annual report has been turned in at work, and his wife seems to have worked out whatever it was with her mother. He and Dr. Brown think about some other cards they can write out for George to read every day. One says, "If I'm feeling scared about something, I need to ask myself whether I'm engaging in black-and-white thinking." Another one says, "I have to be careful not to conclude that my circumstances really are dire, just because I feel anxious."

At the end of this session George and Dr. Brown review the status of his goals. They agree that his sleep and mood are improved, and he is concentrating better at work. He has become more active around the house and is now doing more things with his wife and also with the kids. He still engages in ruminative worry, however. George indicates that he wants to focus on the ruminative worry but doesn't feel the need to add any new goals.

In the next several sessions George and Dr. Brown experiment with some techniques to manage his ruminative worry. George keeps track of when he worries during the day, and he notices that he is more likely to worry when he is at loose ends or is feeling tired. He worries a lot while driving to and from work. Dr. Brown suggests to George that he might be afraid that if he doesn't plan carefully, he won't be able to handle the problems that arise in his life. George agrees that this is so. They agree to work toward limiting his ruminative worry to the drive home at the end of the workday, and they develop strategies to prevent ruminative worry at other times. For example, Dr. Brown suggests that George sing in the car on the way to work, and he is to remind himself at other times that he doesn't need to worry right now, because there's a special time every day when he can do all his worrying at once. Further, he's to remind himself that his ruminative worry doesn't solve problems but really just consists of spinning his wheels.

By Session 14 George indicates that he is feeling well enough to consider decreasing the frequency of treatment. He and Dr. Brown agree to meet every other week for two sessions and then every month for another four months, and they set about to review the course of treatment, with the intent of identifying strategies that have been helpful or might help in the future, as well as to predict the clues that might herald another drop in mood.

As therapy gradually fades out, George reports that he generally continues to feel good, although in one session he reports a drop in mood related to his son's behavior problems at school, resulting in the boy's suspension. He and Dr. Brown spend a little time discussing how he might handle this problem from a practical perspective, but they focus primarily on what George says to himself about the situation that causes his mood to drop. In particular, using Socratic questioning Dr. Brown helps George to see that there may be many reasons his son is misbehaving at school, other than that George has been an inadequate parent.

At the last session George and Dr. Brown again review the course of treatment, they plan for future dips in mood, and they agree that if George begins to feel depressed again, he can always call for another appointment.

Case B. Helene is a 33-year-old, single, childless woman who says that she wants help to overcome her shyness. She indicates that she enjoys spending time with two close friends, but she usually feels very anxious at the prospect of meeting new people or even when she must interact in an unstructured way with people she knows casually. She comments, however, that she is able to function all right in her job as a legal secretary, even though this not infrequently involves interacting with clients. Helene adds that because of her shyness, she is unable to date much. She had a steady boyfriend when she was in her twenties, but she hasn't dated often in the last four or five years. She indicates that on those rare occasions when she does go out with a man, she becomes so anxious that she may throw up ahead of time, and during the date she excuses herself repeatedly to visit the ladies' room. She denies symptoms of any other mental disorder, including particularly generalized worry, obsessive-compulsive symptoms, or other phobias.

Helene states that she has been shy as long as she can remember. She says her mother was also shy, although her father was normally outgoing. She has an older and a younger brother, whom she doesn't view as shy. When asked to say more about her shyness, Helene comments that she doesn't know what to do in social situations, and she is hopeless about making small talk, especially with people she doesn't know well. She has noticed that when she converses with strangers, they sometimes look as if they think that she's "weird or something."

Upon interview Helene speaks softly, makes little eye contact, and appears to be anxious. While her affect appears to be somewhat constricted, her mood is not depressed, and she makes occasional self-deprecating jokes. She seems to have more difficulty at the beginning and end of the session. By contrast, she responds directly and competently to the questions Dr. Brown poses.

Dr. Brown concludes that Helene has social anxiety disorder. She explains that Helene is likely to have incorrect beliefs about social interactions and about the meaning of certain social cues. For example, Helene may incorrectly believe that others pay very close attention to her behavior in social interactions, and she may believe that when an interlocutor glances away for a moment, he or she is having the thought that there is something wrong with Helene. Further, Dr. Brown notes that Helene's avoidance of social interactions and failure to exhibit certain behaviors, such as normal eye contact, are likely to increase symptoms of social anxiety. Finally, Dr. Brown suggests that in scripted social interactions, such as at work, Helene feels less vulnerable and isn't nearly as worried about her interlocutor's negative judgment, because she believes that she knows how to conduct herself at such times.

Over the course of the next several sessions Helene and Dr. Brown construct a hierarchy of 12 social situations that cause her to feel anxiety. Helene assigns a score of 10 (on a scale of 1 to 100) to "talking with my girlfriend, Mindy," while she assigns a score of 30 to going for a walk at lunch with a co-worker, and she says going out on a date with a handsome guy would be a 90. Dr. Brown and Helene also talk about how she can tell what people might actually be thinking of her, and they discuss whether other people might also feel anxious in social situations. Finally, Dr. Brown teaches Helene some breathing techniques to induce relaxation so as to lower her anxiety before social interactions.

Although Helene states that she is fearful about exposing herself in sequence to the items on her anxiety hierarchy, she says she is willing to try, particularly if she doesn't have to advance too quickly to the more difficult items. Dr. Brown asks Helene to start with the least anxiety-inducing item on the hierarchy (talking with Mindy). Helene is to predict ahead of time how much anxiety she will feel and how Mindy will react, and she is then to rate the interaction afterwards on the same scales. Helene also agrees to report evidence that Mindy judges her negatively during the interaction, by tracking such behaviors as long pauses, an irritated expression on Mindy's face, or Mindy's sudden termination of the conversation. Helene is also to rate her own social skills, such as making good eye contact, asking questions, and smiling pleasantly. Finally, Dr. Brown discourages Helene from using any "safety behaviors," such as rehearsing ahead of time what she will say or excusing herself to go to the ladies' room. However, if she does utilize a safety behavior, Helene is to report that she did so.

During the next few sessions Helene gradually advances up to a rating of 50 on her hierarchy. As she and Dr. Brown discuss these exposure experiences, they identify Helene's particular struggle maintaining appropriate eye contact, and they practice eye contact in the session. Helene gradually begins to change her view of the opinions that others hold of her, and she concludes that others may not think all that much about how she acts in social situations. After all, she says, "Most of the time I act pretty normal."

As Helene continues to make progress on her hierarchy, Dr. Brown raises the possibility of her participation in a CBT group for social anxious people. At first Helene says she doesn't want to consider this, but several sessions later she says she would be willing to try it. She and Dr. Brown agree that if the group goes well, they will discontinue individual sessions, and Helene can continue to work on her social anxiety in the group.

In the end, Helene finds that she enjoys the social anxiety group, which involves discussion of social anxiety and support for group members to undertake exposures in the coming week. Helene remains in the group for six months, after which she begins dating a young man from work and establishes a relationship with him. She remains a little uneasy in unscripted social relationships, but her life is no longer affected nearly as often by her shyness.

Case C. Ian is a 37-year-old, never-married, childless computer programmer who indicates that he doesn't feel as satisfied in life as he wishes he were. While his mood is not actually depressed, he says that the only things he really enjoys are his job and his bonsai collection. Ian reports some degree of irritability about careless coworkers, and he says that he doesn't like it when management pushes him to finish a project before he has thoroughly tested it. Ian indicates that he would like to have a girlfriend, but he finds women confusing and after several dates finds it difficult to know how to react to their moods. Ian denies symptoms consistent with a disorder of mood or anxiety.

Upon interview Ian presents as a somewhat pedantic man who describes his situation in careful detail. When Dr. Brown tries to ask a question or otherwise interrupts Ian, he becomes a little flustered and quickly returns to what he was saying just before she interrupted. His mood is a little constricted, but he is basically euthymic. Ian presents in the interview as slightly tense or irritable.

Dr. Brown asks if Ian has always valued precision and self-control, in response to which he smiles and says that it's nice to think that she might understand him. He talks about the various rituals he employs to keep his home in order and his desk uncluttered at work. He denies that anything bad would happen if he were unable to follow these rituals, stating instead that he just likes order, and wouldn't the world be a better place if others were as orderly as he is? Dr. Brown concludes that Ian may have obsessive-compulsive personality disorder.

Dr. Brown asks Ian to identify goals for treatment, in response to which he states that he would like to consider this more carefully and will bring in a list at the next session. At the next session Ian does indeed bring a list of goals for treatment, 27 in all, and he is somewhat reluctant to say which goals are the most important ones. With encouragement he finally states that he would like not to feel so irritated with "careless" people (including every one of his neighbors and all but two work colleagues), and he would like to figure out how to cope with the moods of the women he dates.

Over the course of the next ten or so sessions Dr. Brown and Ian work on managing his irritability, and he goes out on several dates that don't work out very well. It becomes increasingly evident that Ian lives life according to the belief that if things aren't just so, disaster might occur. He feels upset when he makes minor mistakes or notices others making minor mistakes, and when others express their emotions, Ian has difficulty understanding why, logically, they feel as they do. He tends to view those who express emotions as weak, foolish, and unpredictable. Finally, it becomes evident in therapy that Ian is actually quite frightened of his own feelings and of acting in an irrational or ineffective manner.

In Session 20 Dr. Brown offers the conceptualization that Ian fears lack of order in his life and is also worried about losing control of his feelings. Ian replies that this is obviously true and goes on to state that anyone who thinks about matters carefully would arrive at the same conclusion. Dr. Brown describes the idea of a core belief, likens it to a prejudice against oneself, and then ties Ian's beliefs about emotions and orderliness into his experience growing up in his family, when his overcontrolled father praised Ian for behaving well, particularly in comparison to his emotional sister. Dr. Brown asks Ian to identify a time in his early life when he was not so worried about logic and order, and they conclude that he started to become more rigid when he was in the fourth grade. Dr. Brown asks how he would feel about experimenting with the boundaries of his beliefs about emotions and control, in order to see if a slight change in his view of the world might yield some benefit. Ian replies that he doubts this is a good idea but is willing to try once or twice in order to prove his point.

In the next few sessions Dr. Brown targets several of Ian's specific beliefs, including, "I must never make mistakes," "It is dangerous to permit myself to have feelings," and "Other people cannot be trusted to make good decisions." She asks Ian to keep a record of the situations in which he has these thoughts during the week but to document this in ink, rather than to make his typically neat and very detailed charts using the computer. She asks him not to recopy this monitor but to give it to her, mistakes and all. She also suggests that he not leave detailed instructions for his cleaning lady at her next visit but simply suggest that she do whatever she thinks needs to be done. Ian subsequently reports that these experiments did not lead to catastrophic results and actually saved some time, although he says he doesn't like how he feels when he doesn't maintain control. In one session Ian expresses real sadness about the end of a short dating relationship with a woman he particularly liked, and Dr. Brown asks him to reflect on what it was like to express this sadness in the session.

Over the course of the next 20 sessions, Ian gradually begins to shift his core belief. He and Dr. Brown work together to describe some new intermediate beliefs, and they write them on cards that Ian is to look at every morning. The cards say, "In many situations the cost of perfect performance is greater than its benefit," "My own emotions are sometimes confusing but also give my life color and meaning," and "Other people usually make acceptable decisions, even if they don't do exactly what I would have done." He keeps a log of small instances in his daily life that are either consistent with his old core belief or with the new one. At first Ian finds this task very difficult, but with assistance from Dr. Brown he is over time more readily able to identify occurrences that are consistent with his new belief.

After 60 sessions Ian reports that he is feeling less irritable at work and no longer thinks so much about the behavior of other people. He demonstrates increased range of affect in the therapy sessions, tolerates Dr. Brown's interruptions much more readily, and reports that he has been dating the same woman for three months. However, he and Dr. Brown conclude that he is likely to benefit from continuing psychotherapy, albeit with less frequent sessions, and they agree to meet every two or three weeks for the foreseeable future.

Case D: Juanita is a 48-year-old, never-married, childless woman who in her late twenties and early thirties had four psychiatric hospitalizations following suicide attempts. She has long carried a diagnosis of schizoaffective disorder. For the past 15 years she has held a clerical position in a steel plant. She is fairly stable on psychotropic medications, although she continues to report daily auditory hallucinations, often involving voices that tell her to kill herself because she is unworthy. Every few months or so she has the thought that the people around her might be talking about her or conspiring against her, and she sometimes wonders whether the songs she hears on her car radio have been selected with her in mind.

Juanita reports that she never feels very good, even when the hallucinations and delusions are relatively quiescent, and when she was in her early twenties she had periods in which she was constantly depressed but was not troubled for months at a time by psychotic symptoms. She is physically healthy, other than that she is markedly overweight and has hypertension. Juanita states that the clinician managing her psychotropic medications referred her to psychotherapy with the goal of decreasing her suicidal ideation.

Upon interview Juanita presents as a cooperative but emotionally distant woman. Her conversation is generally unremarkable, other than that she is not particularly forthcoming. She does not report psychotic symptoms until directly asked about them. Mood is flat, and eye contact is limited.

Asked about her goals for treatment, Juanita replies that she would like to avoid becoming ill again, and she wants the voices to leave her alone. She adds that she doesn't like it when she becomes frightened about the possibility that unknown people might be watching her.

Dr. Brown encourages Juanita to describe her hallucinations in more detail. Somewhat reluctantly, Juanita states that the voices are unknown people, both men and women, who harass her by listing her many faults and defects. The voices tell her that she doesn't belong on this earth, because she doesn't contribute to society, and everyone would be better off if she were dead. Juanita indicates that she is most likely to hear the voices when she is alone, although she sometimes hears them at work, where they encourage her to jump into the steel furnace.

Dr. Brown explains that auditory hallucinations are actually much more common than many people think, and the key in dealing with hallucinations is not to engage them or to take them seriously. She tells Juanita that every hallucination will simply dissipate if she ignores it. She then asks Juanita if she would be willing to monitor the hallucinations using an appropriate form, on which she is to indicate for every hour that she is awake whether she heard voices and how upset she felt about them. There is also space on the form to make notes about any unusual hallucinations. Juanita seems a little uncertain but says she will try to do this. Dr. Brown also demonstrates some simple relaxation techniques, including a focus on her breathing, that she suggests Juanita practice at home.

At the next session Juanita states that she practiced the relaxation technique twice, but she forgot to fill out the form. Upon further discussion, she admits that the voices have discouraged her from cooperating with Dr. Brown. Juanita says she is unsure about whether to continue talking about these matters, but she then does comment that during the last few days at work she noticed the voices were most bothersome when she was going to work, just after lunchtime, and at the end of her shift. Dr. Brown suggests that these might be times when Juanita feels more anxious or fatigued, and Juanita replies that she finds this interesting, as it suggests that her physical and mental state have an effect on the voices. She then mentions that the voices have varied in volume over the course of the current session. Dr. Brown explores with Juanita what she thinks might have caused that. They conclude that Juanita's engagement in the discussion and also level of self-doubt may have co-varied with the strength of the hallucinations.

At the next session Juanita reports that she has continued to practice the relaxation technique, and she brings in two days of data regarding the voices. She comments that she's noticed that the voices don't bother her as much when she reminds herself that other people hear voices, too. Dr. Brown now suggests to Juanita that the voices may serve the purpose of expressing doubt about Juanita's competence, adding that almost everyone has such doubts. She suggests that doubts like these are socially beneficial, in that they help people remember to stay humble and to avoid doing foolish things. Dr. Brown asks Juanita if this might be why the voices say what they do to her. Juanita thinks about it but then says she doesn't believe other people have thoughts about killing themselves. Dr. Brown agrees that this is largely true but then suggests that perhaps the voices' punitive tone simply reflects Juanita's depression.

Over the next few sessions Juanita and Dr. Brown continue to discuss the voices, and Dr. Brown discloses to Juanita that she herself feels self-doubt and is at times troubled by personal disappointments and weaknesses. This surprises Juanita. Dr. Brown wonders with Juanita whether some of her acquaintances might also be troubled by self-doubts, and she encourages Juanita to ask one of her coworkers with whom she eats lunch whether the other woman also thinks about her faults and defects. However, Juanita replies that she wouldn't feel comfortable doing this.

Even so, two sessions later Juanita reports that she did find out from a lunch mate, a rather shy woman, that the other woman often experienced self-doubts. Juanita further reports that she has recently noticed that the voices don't come quite as often, and when they do, she doesn't worry about them as much. "I know what they are now," says Juanita. "I don't pay as much attention to them as I used to."

After congratulating Juanita for learning to accept the voices without reacting negatively to them, Dr. Brown raises the possibility that Juanita's paranoid fears might also operate in a way similar to the voices. In this regard, they discuss the fact that most people worry about how others see them. Dr. Brown suggests that just as Juanita's auditory hallucinations are in a way "normal," so, too, might her anxiety and suspiciousness reflect a normal human phenomenon. Dr. Brown adds that if Juanita doesn't engage the paranoia, it is likely to dissipate.

Over the course of the next half-dozen sessions Juanita reports that she is less troubled by all of her psychotic symptoms, and she no longer feels nearly as suicidal. Dr. Brown now wonders whether Juanita can apply what they have discovered about her psychotic symptoms to her problems with mood. However, Juanita points out that she feels sad all the time and that her sadness doesn't really come and go. She indicates that she doesn't believe she can make much progress on her mood right now. Nevertheless, she and Dr. Brown agree that it is helpful to meet from time to time to talk about these things, and they decide to get together once a month to continue monitoring her progress.

Exposure and Response Prevention (ERP)

Model of Psychopathology

ERP is a second-wave behavioral treatment for obsessive-compulsive disorder (OCD). In this treatment OCD is conceptualized in cognitive-behavioral terms. According to ERP, individuals with OCD misinterpret the meaning of upsetting thoughts. They fail to make a clear distinction between upsetting thoughts and upsetting physical events; that is, they believe that if they have upsetting thoughts, some sort of upsetting event is likely to follow. This is referred to as *thought–action fusion*. People with OCD take various actions to prevent upsetting events from occurring. First, they try to suppress the upsetting thoughts; however, this has the paradoxical result that the thoughts occur with greater frequency and intensity. Second, they engage in mental or physical rituals (referred to as *safety behaviors*) they believe will "neutralize" the thought. When the feared external event does not occur, they feel greatly relieved and conclude that the rituals prevented the thought from becoming a reality. This negative reinforcement makes it more likely that they will engage in rituals the next time around, and they may never have the opportunity to learn that even if they take no action at all following an upsetting thought, disaster will not follow.

Treatment Strategies

ERP consists of multiple exposure trials in which the patient is negatively reinforced for facing fears without invoking safety behaviors. That is, patients are encouraged to tolerate disturbing thoughts or situations repeatedly without engaging in neutralizing rituals. Eventually, patients learn that the events they fear do not occur, even though they take no action whatsoever. Therapy begins with the therapist providing **psychoeducation** regarding ERP, OCD, and the associated cognitive errors. Therapist and patient then **construct hierarchies** for each feared thought or situation. For example, in the case of a man who engages in compulsive hand washing, hierarchy items might range from touching his own clothes, at one end, to touching the sink, counters, towel dispenser, and door in a poorly maintained public restroom, at the other end. Having chosen the hierarchy corresponding to one feared thought or situation on which to start, the patient engages in **exposure** by working through each item in vivo. In the case of the hand washer, the patient would begin with the lowest item in the hierarchy: he might be asked in the therapist's office to rub his hands on his own clothing for thirty seconds without taking any subsequent action to disinfect himself. When the patient is able to do this without feeling very uncomfortable, he then moves to the next hierarchy item, which might require that he run his hands over the top of the therapist's desk for sixty seconds without engaging in any subsequent neutralizing behavior. Ultimately, the patient progresses to the last of the hierarchy items, although it may be necessary to repeat some hierarchy items several times before anxiety drops sufficiently to permit him to move to the next item. Having completed one hierarchy, therapist and patient then move on to the next hierarchy. When all hierarchies have been completed, the therapist works with the patient on **relapse prevention**, so that if the patient becomes symptomatic again, he will know how to undertake a course of exposure and response prevention without the therapist.

It is best for patients to do exposures in vivo, but it is sometimes necessary for patients to do them in their imagination. Some patients are extremely frightened and can only tolerate imaginal exposures until they build up the courage to try exposures in vivo. Other patients have obsessions than can't be done in vivo, such as fantasies about burning in hell. In the case of imaginal exposures, therapist and patient work together to create a vivid written scenario, and at the time of the exposure the therapist reads the scenario to the patient, who concentrates steadily on it for 30 to 60 minutes at a time.

ERP can be difficult to conduct, most often because of two specific problems. First, ERP is a treatment that requires a strong commitment on the part of patients, not only because they are asked to do things that they find very frightening, but also because treatment is time-intensive, with therapy sessions often occurring more than once a week and often lasting longer than an hour. Incidentally, therapists are sometimes reluctant to undertake ERP, because it often means that they have to leave their offices in order to conduct the exposures. Second, patients may need quite a bit of encouragement to refrain from *all* neutralizing behaviors after exposing themselves to a feared thought or situation. The therapist may not have inquired in sufficient detail to identify every neutralizing ritual. If patients expose themselves to feared thoughts or situations but still engage in subtle or covert neutralizing rituals, treatment will fail. One way to make sure that patients fully expose themselves to feared thoughts and situations is to track their distress level at frequent intervals during the exposure. If the distress level seems low, it may be that the patient is engaging in a covert neutralizing ritual, such as focusing attention elsewhere.

Research Findings

RCTs of ERP have generally shown it to be superior to a number of other approaches, including placebo medication and various general treatments for anxiety (Abramowitz, 1997). A high percentage of OCD patients who complete ERP achieve remission and maintain gains for a period of years. Evidence suggests that discussion of the patient's cognitive errors confers benefit beyond the improvement that results simply from exposure and response prevention itself (van Oppen et al., 1995). However, cognitive therapy without exposure and response prevention appears to be less effective than ERP itself (Olatunji et al., 2013).

Case Example

Kevin is a 42-year-old, married father of three children who works as a high school math teacher. He reports that he has lately had difficulty driving to and from school because he worries that he might strike a pedestrian along the way. He also states that he worries about the possibility that he might say or do something to one of his female students that is sexually inappropriate. Asked if he has ever struck a pedestrian or attempted to engage a student sexually, he replies, "Not that I can remember." However, he indicates that he can't stop thinking about the possibility that something like this *could* happen, and he wonders if he might actually have done something without recalling it. He states that these worries began about two years ago, when he read a couple of newspaper articles describing similar events in another city.

Asked how his worries affect him, Kevin replies that he limits the risk of hitting a pedestrian by driving to work very early in the morning and coming home well after suppertime, when there are fewer pedestrians around. Otherwise, he says, he has to drive the route twice to make sure that he hasn't hit anyone. Once at work, he says he repeats the Rosary under his breath off and on during the day (and usually straight through third period, in which his calculus class includes three very attractive young women), in the belief that God will shield him from sinful behavior. He says, however, that the constant prayer is distracting and has interfered with his ability to teach. Asked to assign a probability that either of his fears might actually come to pass, Kevin hesitates and finally says that he thinks his risk for hitting a pedestrian or behaving in a sexually inappropriate way is about 1%. However, as he says this, he appears to tense up and is noted to move his lips silently for a few moments.

Kevin otherwise denies significant problems in his life, and he specifically denies that he has additional fears or that he engages in other ritualized behavior to ward off catastrophe.

Upon interview Kevin presents as a pleasant and cooperative middle-aged man who describes his problems with some embarrassment. His mood appears to be euthymic, and he does not seem to be especially anxious, other than in connection with his fears.

Kevin's therapist, Dr. Chu, diagnoses him with obsessive-compulsive disorder. She explains the cognitive-behavioral model of this condition, and Kevin readily agrees that he has become dependent on his safety behaviors (driving at odd hours, checking his route, prayer) to cope with the anxiety. However, he exclaims, "I'd go crazy if I had to face those things any other way! I wouldn't be able to get to work or function once I'm there." Kevin appears to be quite interested in the idea of thought–action fusion, however, and he agrees that just because he thinks of something doesn't make it likely to occur.

As Dr. Chu explains the plan for treatment, Kevin appears to become increasingly anxious. However, he seems a little reassured when Dr. Chu tells him that they'll only proceed as fast as he can tolerate it. Kevin agrees with her suggestion that they begin with his fears about driving.

Dr. Chu comments that, given the nature of his fears, they should be able to limit their meetings to one 60-minute session per week.

In the next couple of sessions Kevin and Dr. Chu construct a hierarchy of 15 driving items, and they rate each item on a scale from 1 to 100. Kevin rates sitting in his garage in the morning at 10 and driving home from work when the school buses are out at 90, with the other items in between. They also discuss whether Kevin engages in other safety behaviors, and it develops that he prefers to drive to and from work along country roads, he drives slowly, he constantly checks his rear-view mirror to see if he has hit anyone, and he prays.

Toward the end of Session 3 Dr. Chu suggests that Kevin start with the easiest item on his hierarchy. Kevin comments that he can probably complete the first two items, particularly sitting in his garage in the morning, without invoking any safety behaviors (in this case, prayer), but he doubts he can do anything else. Dr. Chu asks if it would help if someone else were in the car with him for some of the more difficult items, and Kevin replies that it would.

The following week Kevin reports on the three exposures he completed for each of the first two items on the hierarchy, and he reports that they actually went well. He comments that it was hard not to pray, but he was able to stop himself from doing so after a few seconds. However, Kevin predicts that he won't be able to accomplish the next item on the hierarchy (driving along a country road in the early morning) without relying on safety behaviors. He and Dr. Chu decide to make this item easier by asking his wife to accompany him.

In Session 5 Kevin reports that having his wife in the car made the next exposure easy, because he decided that she would know if he had hit anyone. Therefore, Kevin and Dr. Chu agree that he is to repeat the hierarchy item, this time without his wife, but he'll pull over to the side of the road every five minutes (and later on every ten minutes) to talk to his wife for one minute on his cell phone.

Over the course of several more sessions Kevin makes gradual progress on his hierarchy, and at each level after several trials he is able to reduce his anxiety level to "below 50%," by his report. Kevin states that he hasn't driven slowly, retraced his route, or checked the rear-view mirror too often, but he has a harder time preventing himself from praying. He and Dr. Chu finally hit on the idea of programming some alarms on his phone to remind him not to pray.

After ten sessions Kevin reports that he has progressed to the highest hierarchy item. He says he still worries sometimes about hitting a pedestrian, but the thought doesn't bother him nearly as much as it did before, and he says he has learned that his safety behaviors were unnecessary. With encouragement from Dr. Chu, Kevin acknowledges that through his own efforts he has overcome a problem that caused him tremendous anxiety prior to treatment. She asks him if he is ready to tackle the next fear, that he might behave inappropriately with one of his students. Kevin replies that he is ready to create a new hierarchy and to begin exposure trials.

During the next five sessions Kevin and Dr. Chu work together on his second fear. He makes more rapid progress this time, lengthening the amount of time that he can go without prayer during the day. He does this by relying on unobtrusive cues in the classroom that remind him to stop praying, including colored dots in various places and a note card on his desk. Finally, Kevin reports that he is able to limit saying the Rosary to lunchtime and prep periods. He makes it clear that this is not a problem and that he would not wish to change this behavior.

At the end of treatment Kevin and Dr. Chu review the course of their work together, and they again discuss the principles involved in overcoming obsessions and compulsions. Dr. Chu encourages Kevin to contact her in the future if he has any other problems.

Brief Cognitive Therapy for Panic Disorder

Model of Psychopathology

This is a cognitive-behavioral treatment in which panic is thought to result from inaccurate beliefs about the meaning of physiological arousal. Patients who experience panic attacks believe that they are in grave physical danger. This idea causes them to become even more anxious and therefore physiologically more aroused, which creates a vicious cycle. Individuals with panic disorder may develop hypotheses about which environmental stimuli trigger a panic attack, and they work hard to avoid such situations. For example, they may avoid crowds in buildings or may only leave home when accompanied by someone they trust to take care of them, should a panic attack occur. Treatment involves changing the patient's belief about the meaning of physiological arousal, as a consequence of which the patient comes to learn that such arousal is benign and will simply dissipate after a short period of time. Treatment also involves overcoming the patient's phobic avoidance of certain environmental stimuli.

Treatment Strategies

Brief cognitive therapy for panic disorder begins with rather extensive **psychoeducation** about the nature of panic, the associated avoidance, and the way in which thoughts or appraisals color one's experience of the world. The patient is asked to document every panic attack that occurs over the course of treatment and for this purpose is given a supply of forms on which to record the situation, symptoms, thoughts, and feelings associated with each attack. Inasmuch as a minority of individuals with panic disorder experience physiologically verified hyperventilation, the patient may or may not be taught to breathe differently. Patients are generally provided some form of **relaxation training** (although a few individuals may respond adversely to this intervention, as noted by Lilienfeld, 2007). Patients are encouraged to use relaxation training to manage their anxiety during **exposure** trials later on in treatment. They are encouraged to question their appraisals of the panic symptoms, perhaps by identifying which cognitive distortions are operative. These might include catastrophizing, emotional reasoning, overestimating of the probability of negative events, and others.

It is at this point in treatment that the exposure trials begin. These trials usually take two forms. In preparation for *interoceptive exposure,* the therapist will have determined the patient's precise physical symptoms of panic, which might include tachycardia, dyspnea, diaphoresis, shakiness, vertigo, or other symptoms. Following medical clearance, interoceptive exposure involves the induction of such symptoms in the therapist's office. For example, tachycardia and diaphoresis might be induced by having the patient engage in vigorous physical exercise, while dyspnea might be induced by having the patient breathe through a straw. Before engaging in such exposure, therapist and patient discuss any *safety behaviors* the patient uses to decrease anxiety in the face of panic symptoms. Such safety behaviors might include keeping a bottle of water available, seeking reassurance, or grasping a certain object, such as a pill bottle or Rosary beads. Patient and therapist agree that such safety behaviors will not be utilized during the exposures. The patient then goes through a series of exposure trials until he or she demonstrates the ability to tolerate fairly intense exposure without panic for about a minute. After each exposure trial, patient and therapist discuss the experience, and the therapist underscores any changes in the way that the patient is interpreting panic symptoms.

In vivo exposure involves helping the patient overcome fears of situations formerly believed to trigger panic. In this portion of treatment, which may or may not be undertaken concurrently with the interoceptive exposure, the patient undergoes exposure to phobic situations that are arranged along a **hierarchy** that the therapist and patient have devised. In the case of a patient with marked agoraphobia, the lowest hierarchy item might involve standing alone in one's front yard for five minutes. The last hierarchy item, after perhaps 10 to 12 steps, might involve walking alone in the city's central business district. Again, it is important to ensure that the patient does not utilize safety behaviors to decrease any associated anxiety. In this instance, safety behaviors might include talking to shopkeepers, silent prayer, holding one's cell phone, carefully memorizing a map ahead of time, and so forth.

Brief cognitive treatment for panic usually requires 8 to 15 sessions. In the last treatment session, therapist and patient review the patient's progress, and the therapist spends some time talking about **relapse prevention**. It may also be necessary to plan for the patient to undergo a few more exposure trials after the end of formal treatment in order to complete any remaining hierarchy items.

Research Findings
Brief cognitive treatment for panic has been shown to be very effective in the treatment of panic, with or without agoraphobia. Well over half of patients are essentially panic-free following treatment (Barlow, Craske, Cerny, & Klosko, 1989), and these gains are maintained for at least two years following treatment (Craske, Brown, & Barlow, 1991). There is evidence that comorbid conditions, such as mood disorders and other anxiety disorders, are favorably affected for at least one year following treatment (Tsao, Mystkowski, Zucker, & Craske, 2005). It does appear that in cases of severe agoraphobia, rates of improvement may not be as impressive, although in this population treatment is also clearly beneficial. Brief cognitive treatment for panic has been shown to help individuals with nocturnal panic attacks as well (Craske, Lang, Aikins, & Mystkowski, 2005).

Case Example

Lou Ann is a 20-year-old college junior who reports that she has been having "heart attacks or something." She indicates that a cardiac workup was normal, and she was told that her symptoms were probably due to panic. She says she finds this hard to believe and doubts that psychotherapy can help what manifestly seems to her to be a physical problem of some kind.

Lou Ann explains that her first attack was six months ago, when for no obvious reason she began feeling hot and sweaty, and her heart started to race. Within five minutes she was feeling very frightened, her heart was beating as fast as it ever had, and she thought she was going to die. She asked her roommate to help her get to Student Health, but by the time she got there, she had begun to feel a little better, and the doctor didn't find anything wrong. Lou Ann indicates that since the first attack she has had attacks every week or two. Most recently, she had an attack two days ago in the dining hall. All of a sudden her heart began to speed up, and she thought she was going to faint. On this occasion she forced herself to sit quietly and to wait it out, and after about half an hour her symptoms resolved, although she did feel tired afterwards. Lou Ann says she remains concerned that something is very wrong with her heart, and every morning she worries about whether she will have an attack today. Lou Ann otherwise denies symptoms of emotional problems or diagnosed medical illness. She does note that when she leaves her dorm, she prefers to do so in the company of a friend, just in case she has another attack and needs help. She denies, however, that she completely avoids going anywhere or doing anything in particular.

Upon interview Lou Ann presents as a pleasant young woman who appears to be healthy and cheerful. She does not appear to be particularly anxious, other than when she discusses her health concerns.

Dr. Dennison confirms that Lou Ann appears to have panic disorder, with mild symptoms of agoraphobia. He then describes the CBT model of panic and agoraphobia. Lou Ann admits to doubts about the idea that she may be misinterpreting the meaning of her physiological arousal, and Dr. Dennison finally proposes that they simply give treatment a try for half a dozen sessions. If, after giving it "a college try," Lou Ann doesn't notice a change, they'll reconsider the diagnosis. Lou Ann laughs, commenting that her family hails from Missouri, and she likes the idea that Dr. Dennison is planning to "show me."

At Session 2 Lou Ann and Dr. Dennison review the nature of her panic symptoms in more detail. It develops that Lou Ann generally experiences tachycardia and diaphoresis, as well as anxious thoughts. Dr. Dennison asks Lou Ann if she does anything special to decrease her anxiety about the panic attacks (apart from having a friend with her when she leaves her dorm room). Lou Ann replies that she when she leaves her dorm, she ensures that she has a full bottle of water and her smart phone with her all the time.

Dr. Dennison advises that they will be inducing symptoms in the office in order to demonstrate to Lou Ann that such physiological arousal is not dangerous. When Lou Ann states that she would be afraid to do this, Dr. Dennison volunteers that he will go first, so that she sees that he isn't asking her to do something that is dangerous. He gives her a sheet that explains how they will induce symptoms and asks that Lou Ann check with Student Health to make sure that she is physically able to participate in this treatment. He also introduces her to a relaxation technique that involves visualizing a pleasant scene and asks that she practice it daily during the next week.

At Session 3 Lou Ann returns with a permission slip from Student Health, and she reports on her relaxation homework. She admits that she forgot to do it several days but found it helpful when she did remember to do it. Dr. Dennison then models for Lou Ann what he will ask her to do. He moves the furniture out of the way and proceeds to do 50 jumping jacks. Lou Ann comments afterwards that Dr. Dennison appears to be out of breath. He asks if she would be willing to take his pulse at the wrist. Lou Ann declines to do so, but Dr. Dennison takes his own pulse and reports that his heart is beating 114 times per minute.

Now it's Lou Ann's turn. Dr. Dennison asks that she give him her water bottle and her smart phone (both of which he places in the next room) and then relax for a moment. He then asks that she do 20 jumping jacks. She complies and reports that she feels uncomfortable but not out of control. He next asks her to do 35 jumping jacks and in a third trial 50 jumping jacks. After the third trial Lou Ann reports that her heart is beating very fast, and she feels afraid. Dr. Dennison encourages her to use the visualization to relax herself but to stay focused on her body and to observe while her heart rate drops back to normal. They discuss the possibility that Lou Ann may have been engaging in emotional reasoning, responding fearfully to her physiological arousal and then concluding that if she felt afraid, there must be something real that is threatening her. At session's end Lou Ann comments that Dr. Dennison does seem to be "showing me." He asks her to practice the exposures three times during the week but to limit herself to 35 jumping jacks at a time.

By Session 5 Lou Ann is able to tolerate the physical consequences of 60 jumping jacks in Dr. Dennison's office, and she has increased her home practice to 50 jumping jacks. Dr. Dennison suggests that they now address the agoraphobia. He and Lou Ann construct a hierarchy of seven items, each rated along an anxiety scale from 1 to 100, ranging from sitting in her room with a friend, at the low end, to going to the library alone, studying for an hour by herself, and returning to her dorm alone, at the high end. Dr. Dennison asks that Lou Ann expose herself to the first two items on the hierarchy prior to their next session. He asks that she not rely on any safety behaviors but encourages her to use the visualization as a way to relax herself enough to face the exposure. Lou Ann is reluctant not to have her phone with her when she is out of her room but with encouragement agrees to give it up for a brief period.

The following week Lou Ann reports that she was in fact able to accomplish the first three items on her hierarchy, and she expresses optimism that she will be able to get through the rest of the items. She indicates that she is feeling fairly optimistic about her ability to manage her panic symptoms. Dr. Dennison asks that she continue to work on exposing herself to hierarchy items without relying on safety behaviors.

By Session 8 Lou Ann and Dr. Dennison agree that she is doing well, and they decide that this will be their last session. They discuss what to do if Lou Ann experiences a relapse, and Dr. Dennison encourages her to contact him if in the future she experiences any symptoms that she can't manage on her own.

Prolonged Exposure for Posttraumatic Stress Disorder (PE-PTSD)

Model of Psychopathology

PE-PTSD is a cognitive-behavioral treatment in which the therapist helps the patient overcome avoidance and correct mistaken beliefs about thoughts and situations that the patient finds upsetting. After experiencing a traumatic event, it is at first normal to respond fearfully to memories of the event. Such memories can occur spontaneously, or they may be triggered by environmental cues. Over time, the fear response diminishes, because after thinking through the event and talking about it with others, traumatized individuals learn that the memories are themselves not dangerous; individuals begin to make a clear distinction between the trauma and their current everyday lives. In the normal course of recovery from a traumatic event, people develop an idea about the meaning of the event that permits them to move on in life.

It is hypothesized that individuals who develop PTSD fail to "heal" from the trauma because they do not follow the normal path of recovery. These individuals do not think about the trauma in a detailed, coherent manner, as a consequence of which they may draw incorrect conclusions about the trauma, such as, "I should have done more," or "I am responsible for what happened." Moreover, people who develop PTSD engage in cognitive and behavioral avoidance to such an extent that they don't have the opportunity to learn to distinguish between the event and their current lives. This further fuels their avoidance, as does the negative reinforcement of the short-term decrease in anxiety following avoidance. Over time these individuals develop two core beliefs: "Everything in the world is dangerous" and "I can't cope with anything." Such core beliefs have the effect of "locking in" individuals with PTSD, and they become unable to function in many areas of their lives.

Treatment Strategies

Both *imaginal* and *in vivo exposure* are used in PE-PTSD to help the patient decrease avoidance, with the goal that he or she begin to make a clear distinction between the trauma and everyday life. As well, the therapist utilizes discussion following exposure trials gently to challenge beliefs about the trauma that may lack accuracy or utility. Following **psychoeducation** about the nature of PTSD and the value of **exposure** in its treatment, the therapist begins **relaxation training** with the patient and asks the patient to practice this at home several times a day. Patients are taught to relax quickly and efficiently with the expectation that in time they will begin using this skill as a coping strategy in everyday life. The patient is also asked to describe his or her trauma in detail, and patient and therapist then **construct a hierarchy** of situations that the patient avoids in everyday life in an attempt to manage his or her painful memories.

From this point treatment proceeds along two tracks. Outside the therapy session, the patient steadily works through items on the hierarchy of avoided situations, remaining in each feared situation until the associated anxiety has decreased by about 50%. In therapy sessions, the patient engages in imaginal exposure by recounting the traumatic experience in detail, with eyes closed and in the present tense, for a period of 45 to 60 minutes. The therapist pays careful attention to ensure that the patient is focusing directly on the trauma and may help the patient to stay engaged, if necessary. If the patient fully recounts the trauma in less than 45 minutes, he or she is asked to start over again. Following each period of imaginal exposure, therapist and patient discuss the experience, and the therapist emphasizes the patient's developing insight that anxiety symptoms naturally dissipate, as well as to underscore any shifts in the patient's view of the trauma itself, which may be based in part on the patient's recall of previously forgotten details. To the extent possible, the therapist supports the patient in re-evaluating core beliefs that the world is dangerous and the patient cannot cope with it. The patient continues to undergo imaginal exposure in therapy sessions until he or she can complete an exposure without experiencing more than a limited amount of anxiety. Prior to this time, the patient also practices imaginal exposures at home by listening to an audiotape of the exposure done in the session.

PE-PTSD usually requires 10 to 15 sessions to complete. At the last session, patient and therapist review the course of treatment, discuss issues related to **relapse prevention**, and agree on continued exposures that the patient might need to conduct after treatment has ended.

Research Findings

PE-PTSD and similar CBT-based approaches to the treatment of PTSD have been shown to be effective in reducing symptoms of PTSD in numerous studies, most of which offered the treatment to traumatized soldiers or victims of sexual assault. In many studies only a minority of those treated still met criteria for PTSD at the end of treatment (Foa & Meadows, 1997). Active treatments have been shown to be more effective than nonspecific treatments of PTSD, but no consistent pattern has emerged to suggest that one CBT approach to PTSD is clearly more effective than another (e.g., Resick, Pallavi, Weaver, Astin, & Feuer, 2002). However, there are some data to suggest that changes in relevant cognitions may play an important role in treatment efficacy (Kleim et al., 2013).

Case Example

Mark is a 66-year-old, married father of four adult children. He has recently retired from his job as truck driver at an industrial plant, where he worked for 40 years. He reports that he now finds himself increasingly troubled by a recrudescence of memories from his experiences as a soldier in Vietnam nearly 50 years ago. He admits that he is puzzled and alarmed that his sleep has gotten worse due to frequent nightmares. He indicates that he is generally more irritable than he used to be, and he has begun to feel alienated from his wife and other family members. Mark says that after he retired, he began volunteering at the local VA hospital, but he finds that he becomes upset when he sees medical staff who appear to be of Asian descent. He has increased his gun collection, and he admits that while he tells his family he's buying more guns because he likes to hunt, in fact he is buying them because he feels safer with more guns in the house. Mark says he has begun to think that he may not live much longer, even though he is in physical good health. Indeed, part of him has begun to think that he doesn't *deserve* to live much longer.

Mark indicates that as an Army draftee, at the age of 20 he was sent to Vietnam for 12 months. He was assigned to the infantry and for much of his time in-country he saw action three or four times per month. He says his worst memory from Vietnam relates to an incident in which his outpost was nearly overrun by enemy soldiers, and several men in his unit died in the firefight. He comments that all these years later he still wonders if he could have done more to prevent their deaths. Mark adds that this is only the third time that he's told someone who wasn't a veteran about this event. He says he has gone decades without even talking about it.

Mark states that after he returned from Vietnam, he felt "lost" for six months or so but then set about to get his life together, especially with the support of his father, who had seen action during World War II. For many years Mark stayed busy working and raising a family. He was involved in his children's sports activities, he participated in two bowling leagues, and he worked long hours, took on many shifts, and made a good living, such that he is now comfortable in retirement. He says he never imagined he would have to face the memories from Vietnam in this way again. He comments, however, that his wife isn't so surprised. She tells him that he hasn't slept well for years, and she thinks he kept himself together by staying busy. Now he has time on his hands, and it's all coming back.

Mark states that he has never sought mental health treatment before, and he denies other significant problems. He does note that he has recently increased his use of alcohol and marijuana, but he denies that he uses either substance more than twice a week—and then only in limited amounts. Still, he admits to some concern about this, if only because his brother is alcoholic. Mark notes that he is in good health, apart from some generalized arthritis, particularly affecting his back and knees. He comments that, sadly, he no longer bowls.

Upon interview Mark presents as a pleasant and cooperative gentleman. Mood is mostly euthymic, although Mark seems to become sadder and more distracted when talking about Vietnam. Mark appears to be mildly anxious and comments that he has never talked with a therapist before.

Dr. Evans suggests that Mark is having a recurrence of PTSD, and she offers the view that Mark's wife may be right—he has engaged in (perfectly understandable) avoidance over many years while living his life, but now there is less to distract him, and the memories are coming back. Dr. Evans presents the CBT model of PTSD, emphasizing the ideas that Mark needs to "make sense" of the firefight experience in a new way, that he needs to learn to tolerate the memories from Vietnam without becoming so aroused, and that he needs to make the distinction in his mind between his life today and his life in Vietnam nearly 50 years ago. Mark says he would like to make these changes, but when he starts to think about Vietnam, it's like he's watching a film loop, and he ends up feeling sad, guilty, and angry.

Dr. Evans lets Mark know that they will work together to help him tolerate memories of the firefight more comfortably. She states they will also work on decreasing the degree to which daily experiences remind him of Vietnam. Mark replies that he hopes treatment will help.

During the next session Mark and Dr. Evans develop a hierarchy of situations in Mark's daily life that cause him discomfort because they remind him of Vietnam. These include entering a room in his house that doesn't have a gun in it, seeing a person of Asian descent, hearing a helicopter overhead, and watching certain television programs. Mark and Dr. Evans assign anxiety levels to each hierarchy item, using a scale from 1 to 100. Dr. Evans then spends about 15 minutes teaching Mark how to relax himself by following his breath, and she asks that he practice this at home every day.

Dr. Evans asks Mark if he would be willing to tell her a little more about the firefight, and she takes careful notes. He is somewhat vague about the details and does appear to become very uncomfortable during this portion of the session. For homework Dr. Evans asks that Mark write down his memory of the firefight, providing as much detail as he can, and she asks him to bring it in next week.

At the beginning of Session 3 Mark comments that he is definitely feeling worse, and he attributes his drop in mood to the assignment that he write down his experiences in the firefight. He says he tried to relax himself every day by following his breath, but this wasn't as successful as he hoped, at least in part because he knew that he had the task of describing the firefight hanging over him. Dr. Evans reassures Mark that such distress is not uncommon in this kind of treatment.

Dr. Evans then asks if Mark would be willing to read to her what he wrote about the firefight. Mark replies that he doesn't think he can do this. Dr. Evans and Mark then agree that he'll only read the first page of what he's written, after which he can stop. However, Mark eventually reads all five pages of his account. Along the way Dr. Evans encourages Mark to use his breathing to settle himself, but even so Mark appears to be on the verge of tears by the time he has completed his account. Afterwards, Dr. Evans asks Mark about why in his account the other men in his unit are portrayed much more as victims than Mark portrays himself. Mark begins to defend himself on this point but then stops and comments, "I've just always thought about what I didn't do for them. Maybe they worry about what they didn't do for me."

During the next four sessions Dr. Evans asks Mark to walk her through the firefight without the script. She asks that he speak in the present tense and that he keep his eyes closed so that he can concentrate on the memory. At intervals she asks him about his anxiety level, and in the first couple of sessions if it drops below 70% during the account, she helps him refocus and experience the anxiety more directly. After each in-session exposure trial Mark and Dr. Evans talk about how his memory of events is gradually shifting, and she helps Mark to identify any logical errors he may be making, particularly in terms of self-blame. She asks that Mark do exposures at home on his own every other day.

By Session 7 Mark reports that he is feeling better and that the exposures don't bother him as much as they did at first. Dr. Evans carefully inquires to determine whether there are any *other* memories from Vietnam that upset him as much or more than the firefight they have been discussing. Mark replies that there are not. At this point Mark and Dr. Evans agree that he is ready to begin exposing himself outside of session to situations that remind him of Vietnam. They decide that he will start with the first item on his hierarchy and slowly work through all the items, until he finds that he can tolerate the anxiety fairly well for each item.

During the next three sessions Mark continues to do in-session exposures to memories of the firefight, and he exposes himself in his everyday life to other upsetting situations. He makes steady progress and reports that he is feeling better. He no longer becomes upset in response to his hierarchy items, as a consequence of which, for example, he enjoys his volunteer work at the hospital and has begun locking up all his guns in the gun safe in his bedroom. He states that his sleep has improved (although he still has occasional nightmares), he feels closer to his family, and he is generally less irritable.

As treatment draws to a close, Mark and Dr. Evans review the course of their work together and discuss how Mark can recognize if he is having a relapse, as well as to list the steps he can take to cope with any return of symptoms. Dr. Evans encourages Mark to call for further sessions if he feels the need.

Dialectical Behavior Therapy (DBT)

Model of Psychopathology

DBT was developed by the American psychologist Marsha M. Linehan as a way to address self-injurious behaviors in patients, most of whom are diagnosed with borderline personality disorder (BPD). It is one of the third-wave behavior therapies, which are distinguished from standard CBT by their reliance on of the construct of **mindfulness**.

DBT is based on a theory regarding the development and maintenance of BPD. According to Linehan, people with BPD have a fundamental deficit of emotional regulation. From a very young age they are highly sensitive to emotional stimuli, they react strongly to feelings, and they return to baseline slowly. Moreover, children who later develop BPD do not learn to attend effectively to emotions or to manage arousal and behavior appropriately when their feelings are engaged. Linehan suggests that a young child with a biological predisposition to emotion dysregulation may develop BPD if he or she grows up in an environment in which the adults respond ineffectively to the child's emotions by negating them ("There's no reason for you to feel that way"), by meting out punishment in response to certain emotions ("How dare you feel that way!"), or by reacting erratically to the child's emotions. Linehan refers to this as an *invalidating environment*: it is the child's internal experience that is invalidated. The result is that a child who has always had powerful emotions is prevented from learning how to manage feelings effectively and grows up doubting that he or she can even label feelings correctly in the first place. If one doesn't acknowledge and accept one's own internal experience, how can one develop a stable identity?

Linehan suggests that throughout their lives people with BPD struggle to manage their feelings, but they lack the skills to do so effectively. She believes that people with BPD view emotion as a problem to be solved. However, the solutions they attempt often lead to more serious problems. These people swing between overcontrol and undercontrol of emotions, because they don't have the flexibility to self-regulate in a more nuanced way. Given their early histories, adults with BPD are acutely sensitive to invalidation, which can be a major problem for psychotherapists, who often communicate to patients that the patients would feel better if only they changed the way they view the world and how they behave in it. Moreover, most people with BPD focus their attention on managing their social environments, because they find that this helps them to manage themselves. However, it requires a great deal of energy to manage other people's feelings and behaviors, and the emotional liabilities of BPD make it difficult for affected individuals to treat others in a consistent manner. This leads to considerable interpersonal conflict. The fact that people with BPD try to manage themselves by managing others has as one consequence the fact that their behavior is inconsistent across situations.

Finally, Linehan suggests that individuals with BPD compound their emotional distress by failing fully to resolve losses and other setbacks in life. Because they can't process feelings effectively, they are likely to suppress painful emotions that cannot be resolved quickly, as a consequence of which crises pile on top of crises. One overreacts to the current crisis when previous crises still linger.

Linehan suggests that self-injury represents a strategy that people with BPD can use to regulate their emotions. There is no doubt that self-injury does effectively regulate affect in many instances. Of course, self-injury often has the effect of regulating one's environment, too, and it has obvious negative consequences in terms of physical health, self-image, and relationships. Linehan suggests that people can learn alternatives to self-injury through **building skills** in four areas: *core mindfulness, distress tolerance, emotion regulation,* and *interpersonal effectiveness.*

Core mindfulness represents the ability to integrate opposites without reacting ineffectively. This is the "dialectical" part of DBT. Linehan derived core mindfulness skills from the practice of meditation. Core mindfulness involves attending nonjudgmentally to apparently opposite ideas about a single thing. For example, individuals with BPD come to accept that their difficulty regulating affect is entirely understandable and could not be otherwise, given their history, but they must also commit themselves to making a change. It is through the skill of core mindfulness that therapists help individuals with BPD to work on problems without triggering a feeling of invalidation. Core mindfulness skills aim toward observing, describing, and participating in experiences in a manner that is nonjudgmental, one-minded, and effective. Linehan also talks about the idea that "wise mind" integrates "reasonable mind" and "emotion mind." This is a particularly helpful idea for people with BPD, who so often swing between overcontrol and undercontrol of affect.

Distress tolerance skills are designed to help patients tolerate painful circumstances that can't be resolved right away. They include a number of distracting strategies, self-soothing skills, strategies to "improve the moment," and the admonition to consider the pros and cons of deciding to cope with distress instead of taking the position that the distress is intolerable.

Emotion regulation skills include identifying and labeling emotions, acknowledging the reasons that one might not want to modify one's feelings (such as the fact that powerful expression of affect causes others to comply with one's wishes), decreasing vulnerability to excessive emotionality through balanced nutrition, sleep, exercise, and so forth, increasing positive emotional events, increasing **mindfulness** regarding one's current feelings, and engaging in behaviors that foster an opposing emotion.

Interpersonal effectiveness skills include promptly dealing with problems in relationships, balancing one's own needs against the needs of others, balancing what one does out of obligation against what one does for fun, and building mastery and self-respect. These skills depend in large measure on the patient's learning a rather sophisticated version of **assertiveness training** developed specifically for this population.

Treatment Strategies
Formal DBT is extremely labor-intensive, and it comprises four components, none of which is optional. First, each patient meets with an individual therapist once a week for 60 to 90 minutes. During periods of crisis, individual sessions may occur more frequently. Second, patient and therapist work out guidelines that require the patient to telephone the therapist

under specified circumstances outside of session. Third, the patient attends a weekly skills training group lasting two to two and a half hours. Fourth, all therapists on the treatment team hold a formal weekly meeting to discuss problems, to support one another, and to maintain compliance with the DBT format. The initial treatment contract between patient and therapist usually lasts one year and includes the patient's overt commitment to remain alive during that period.

Individual therapy in DBT aims to help the patient utilize DBT skills consistently in daily life. The topic of discussion in each session is selected from among the following items, which are listed in order of descending priority: behaviors that are life-threatening, behaviors that interfere with therapy (irregular attendance, inappropriate behavior vis-à-vis other skills group members, repeated and inappropriate crisis calls, and the like), behaviors that interfere with quality of life (substance abuse, financial crises, criminal behaviors, serious medical illness, and so forth), and behavioral skill deficits. The therapist utilizes the full range of cognitive-behavioral strategies within each session to help the patient apply DBT skills to his or her problems. In addition, the therapist adopts a dialectical stance, which includes a focus on synthesizing opposites in the patient's life and avoiding either/or positions, among other strategies.

DBT patients are given to understand that they are expected to telephone their individual therapist between sessions, based on the time guidelines that have been negotiated between therapist and patient, in order to seek crisis intervention prior to self-injury, to obtain coaching on use of the skills, and to repair problems in the therapy relationship. Calls are expected to be reasonably short and should focus on use of skills. They should not be a continuation of or a substitute for face-to-face individual therapy sessions. If the patient calls too often or not often enough, this is addressed as a therapy-interfering behavior in individual therapy.

Skill building occurs in the skills group, which is led by two DBT therapists, neither of whom provides individual therapy to any of the group members. The leaders present a different skills module each week from Linehan's (1993) skills training manual. It takes about six months to work through the skills manual, after which the cycle starts over. Patients generally remain in the skills group through two cycles. Sessions are highly structured and are generally split between a review of homework and teaching the next skill in the sequence. While patients are encouraged to participate actively in each week's group, there is limited therapeutic focus on interaction among group members.

Every therapist who participates on a given DBT treatment team participates on the consultation team, which meets weekly. Team meetings may involve discussion of particularly challenging patients, or they may involve shoring up one or several therapists who are feeling overwhelmed and fear burnout. Team members help one another to remain within the DBT framework so that no one drifts into some other style of treatment.

Research Findings

There is extensive evidence that formal DBT leads to decreased self-injury in individuals with the diagnosis of BPD (Kliem, Kröger, & Kosfelder, 2010). DBT also decreases general distress in BPD but has not yet been shown to be effective in addressing the full range of BPD diagnostic criteria (Kröger & Kosfelder, 2007). DBT has been shown to be helpful in the treatment of individuals with comorbid BPD and substance abuse (e.g., Linehan et al., 1999) and in individuals with binge-eating disorder who do not meet diagnostic criteria for BPD (Telch, Agras, & Linehan, 2001).

This treatment model has excited a great deal of interest among mental health practitioners, and many clinicians now utilize DBT skills in individual psychotherapy with patients with other symptoms or diagnoses. Such treatment may or may not involve participation in a DBT skills group, and the individual therapist generally does *not* participate on a consultation team. Obviously, this is not formal DBT. Indeed, it is unusual for therapists to treat more than a handful of patients at a time with individual psychotherapy as part of the full DBT package. While it seems reasonable to imagine that DBT strategies should be helpful to many patients, there is as yet only limited research that has demonstrated the effectiveness of a "DBT lite" package. Most such studies have focused on the addition of DBT skills groups to treatment as usual, rather than on the addition of specific skills modules to individual psychotherapy.

Case Example

Nancy is a 44-year old, divorced mother of two adult children. She has had five psychiatric hospitalizations in 20 years in the context of suicidal ideation or attempts. During the past six years she has worked as registration clerk at a local hospital, although during this period she has taken extended leave during two major depressive episodes. At present she is receiving intensive outpatient services in the hope that she can continue to work during what is now a third depressive episode. In addition to a long history of cutting herself, Nancy reports other persistent symptoms of BPD, including significant abandonment issues, chaotic relationships, impulsivity regarding sex, shopping, and gambling, feelings of emptiness, and difficulty managing her anger. She has been in and out of outpatient treatment for years, and when asked how many individual therapists she has had, she shrugs her shoulders and sighs, "What does it matter, anyway?"

Nancy's childhood was chaotic. She is one of four children to her mother by three different men. She reports that her mother drank a lot and usually ignored Nancy when she sought reassurance as a child. Shortly after Nancy experienced menarche, her stepfather began abusing her sexually, and this continued for two years until he was arrested for abusing Nancy's younger sister. Nancy married in her late teens to get out of the house, and she has had two marriages and two other long-term relationships with men.

When first seen by Dr. Fratelli, Nancy presents as an irritable, unhappy woman, who expresses general frustration with her life and offers mild complaints about other treatment staff. She is nicely dressed, but beneath her long sleeves is evidence of healing scabs, apparently from recent self-cutting. Eye contact is variable, and social manner is rather self-focused. She doesn't seem very interested in or involved with her interviewer. She doesn't present as particularly anxious, and there is no evidence of psychotic ideation.

Dr. Fratelli explains to Nancy that he has been asked to evaluate her for DBT. He explains that this is a very intensive treatment for individuals who struggle with self-injury, most of whom have a diagnosis of BPD. He says that in order to begin DBT, Nancy will have to commit to a year of treatment, with weekly psychotherapy sessions and also group sessions. Dr. Fratelli states that DBT has been shown to help people with problems like Nancy's, and he says that the goal of treatment is to help Nancy develop a life worth living. He admits that DBT asks a great deal from patients, and he notes that some patients don't feel they can commit to sticking with it for a year.

Nancy replies, somewhat offhandedly, that she's tried everything else, so why not try this? Dr. Fratelli again asks if Nancy can she commit to coming in for sessions twice a week for a year, and he points out that in order to keep her promise, she will need to remain alive during the next year. Can she promise not to kill herself during the next year? Nancy is surprised about this question but then more thoughtfully replies that she thinks she can stay alive for another year.

Dr. Fratelli makes arrangements for Nancy to begin seeing him on a weekly basis and also arranges for her to participate in the weekly DBT skills group affiliated with the intensive outpatient program. He tells Nancy that a major goal of treatment is to decrease parasuicidal activity, including cutting her arms, and he asks that Nancy call him at the office anytime between 7 a.m. and 11 p.m. if she is having difficulty inhibiting the impulse to harm herself. He explains that the purpose of the call is to help her implement the skills she has learned so she can avoid injuring herself. He adds that she should not call him *after* she has harmed herself but should instead simply tell him about it at their next regularly scheduled session. He adds that if she is admitted to the hospital because of self-harm, he won't be able to visit her on the inpatient unit. Nancy argues with him on the latter point, but Dr. Fratelli makes it clear that this is a condition of treatment, explaining in direct terms that some people with BPD find hospitalization to be reinforcing, as a consequence of which they may act in such a way as to ensure that they are admitted to the hospital. Dr. Fratelli says he doesn't want to encourage such behavior on Nancy's part.

Dr. Fratelli also states that Nancy should call him if she feels something has gone wrong in the therapy relationship and she doesn't want to wait until the next session to address it. However, she shouldn't call him to talk about life problems or as a substitute for their weekly individual session together.

When Nancy comes in for her first formal individual therapy session, Dr. Fratelli explains how they will choose the topic of discussion each week. Inasmuch as Nancy doesn't report any life-threatening or therapy-interfering behavior, he suggests that they discuss her recent pattern of dating many men sequentially, usually going out with them only once or twice. Nancy comments that she doesn't think much of men, and she glances meaningfully at Dr. Fratelli.

Nancy also starts the skills group during this week. At present the group is working on emotion regulation skills, but every week the group leaders make some reference to the value of integrating reasonable mind and emotion mind. Nancy asks Dr. Fratelli to say more about this in one of their early sessions.

During the next few weeks Nancy's mood begins to lift, and she skips an individual therapy session. Dr. Fratelli immediately focuses in on this therapy-interfering behavior, noting that while Nancy continues to attend the skills group regularly, she must also attend individual sessions, as well. At first Nancy refers to situational difficulties, in response to which Dr. Fratelli reminds her of her promise to attend sessions faithfully. Eventually, they are able to talk about Nancy's anxiety over her developing feelings of dependency on Dr. Fratelli. He responds by saying how impressed he is that Nancy is willing to discuss this matter. He acknowledges that such feelings can be painful and suggests that, given Nancy's early background, it is absolutely to be expected that she would have such feelings. However, they do have to abide by their contract, and this leads to discussion of how Nancy might cope with her feelings in other ways. They identify some self-soothing skills to lower her distress, and they decide that she can experiment by speaking up about her feelings vis-à-vis Dr. Fratelli, rather than to run away from them.

Two weeks later Nancy calls Dr. Fratelli at 9 one evening to say that she has the urge to cut herself, having had an argument earlier in the day with her daughter. During their ten-minute telephone call Nancy and Dr. Fratelli discuss the strategies she has tried to help cope with this impulse, and Dr. Fratelli encourages her to go for a walk and then to take a hot shower. If that doesn't work, she can try squeezing an ice cube in her hand for one minute. At the next session Nancy reports that she was in fact able to avoid cutting herself. She and Dr. Fratelli review step by step what led up to the thoughts of self-harm and what happened when the impulse began to weaken.

Over the course of the next few months Nancy continues to learn new skills in the group, and in individual sessions she works on relationship issues with family members and even with Dr. Fratelli. She says she finds the interpersonal effectiveness skills to be as helpful as anything else she has learned in the skills group.

Nancy continues to call Dr. Fratelli once or twice a month for coaching but then stops doing so, after which she cuts herself superficially on two occasions. Each time this occurs, in the next individual session she and Dr. Fratelli review the sequence of events in great detail, talking about what skills she might have used at various points to stop the sequence. Dr. Fratelli makes it very clear that he expects Nancy to telephone him outside of session at the very least every two weeks, as long as she continues to feel the way she does.

> In about Month 8 of treatment Nancy begins complaining about what she perceives as a dismissive attitude on the part of one of the skills group leaders, an older woman. Dr. Fratelli reflects sympathetically on the fact that Nancy is necessarily very aware of dismissive behavior from women like her own mother, and they then rehearse what Nancy might say to the older therapist in order to clear the air between them.
>
> By the end of the first year, Nancy has not engaged in self-harm for six months. Her mood is reasonably stable, and she reports less chaos in her relationships. She isn't dating around as much as she used to, and her financial situation is beginning to improve. She and Dr. Fratelli acknowledge that their agreement is now up for renewal, and he asks Nancy if she would like to consider addressing her history of sexual abuse by her stepfather. This then becomes the next focus of treatment.

Applied Behavior Analysis (ABA)

Model of Psychopathology

ABA is a first-wave behavioral treatment that could in theory be applied to the modification of any observable behavior in any person but is most commonly utilized in the treatment of individuals with diagnoses in the autism spectrum. ABA does not attempt to modify cognitions, nor does it rely on the individual's conscious understanding of changed contingencies. Rather, ABA utilizes principles of classical and especially operant conditioning to change the frequency of very carefully defined target behaviors, primarily through the use of positive reinforcement and **extinction**. According to the learning theory that underlies ABA, the frequency of *this* behavior in *this* specific setting depends on the previous reinforcement schedule for the behavior in this setting. While it may be useful to consider an individual's diagnosis in trying to understand the presence or absence of certain behaviors, ultimately it is the previous reinforcement schedule that accounts for the current behavior frequency in a given setting, and if the behavior is to change, the associated reinforcement schedule must also change.

In ABA a new behavior is taught by breaking it into discrete pieces. The frequency with which each constituent behavior occurs is increased by an appropriate reinforcement schedule, and the pieces are then chained together in order to produce the new behavior in toto. Conversely, decreasing the frequency of a problematic behavior can be accomplished by analyzing the behavior into a chain of discrete behaviors and then simply disrupting the chain by decreasing the frequency of a crucial link. In changing behavior, the ABA therapist considers which prompts might help the individual start each discrete behavior in the chain, as well as to plan later to modify therapist behavior by offering less intrusive prompts ("fading") and decreasing the frequency of reinforcement ("thinning"). ABA therapists may also "shape" behaviors, which involves the gradual modification of old behaviors into new behaviors.

Treatment Strategies

When ABA is used to *increase* the frequency of a desirable behavior, the behavior may be broken down into discrete components in a sequence.

Contingent reinforcement is utilized after effective reinforcers are identified for each link in the chain. For example, the sequence of behaviors required to use the bathroom appropriately would include tolerating the bathroom environment, the ability to grasp and move one's clothing, the ability to sit independently on the toilet, and so forth. After each component behavior is mastered, the behaviors are chained together. Utilizing principles of **stimulus control**, the individual is prompted to initiate the chain of behaviors or to continue to execute specific behaviors, although sometimes one link in the chain is automatically prompted by the previous link. Teaching complicated skills may also require the identification of a sequence of increasingly difficult behaviors, such that each behavior can be shaped into the next, more difficult one. For example, the first step in using the pencil appropriately in the classroom might be to grasp any object, then to grasp a pencil, then to scribble with the pencil anywhere, then to scribble with the pencil on a piece of paper, then to scribble within some boundary on the paper, and so forth.

When ABA is used to *decrease* the frequency of an undesirable behavior, it may or may not be helpful to break down the behavior into discrete units. A *functional behavior assessment* is used to identify the reinforcers for the problematic behavior—or its chain of sub-behaviors. Reinforcers may include environmental factors, sensory input, interpersonal attention, escape from something unpleasant (i.e., negative reinforcement), and others. The ABA therapist may decide to work directly to decrease the frequency of an undesirable behavior by changing the reinforcement schedule for some or all links in the behavior chain. For example, to decrease tantrum behavior, it may be helpful to reorganize the daily routine so that the individual doesn't become too hungry or tired, conditions the individual had previously modified through tantrum behavior. The ABA therapist may, however, prefer to train the individual to emit a different, competing behavior, again using ABA technology. For example, to decrease the tendency to hit others in frustration, the ABA therapist may teach the individual to communicate frustration in a more socially acceptable manner.

Research Findings

In most research studies ABA has demonstrated efficacy in changing behavior among individuals with autism spectrum disorder, with specific benefits including improved intellectual functioning, language skills, school performance, adaptive behavior, and social skills. Response to ABA interventions varies across patients and does require an ability to learn new behaviors (Warren et al., 2011).

> **Case Example**
> Oleg is a rather large, nine-year-old child adopted eight years ago from an institution in Eastern Europe. Minimally verbal, he is diagnosed with autism and attends a special school. His adoptive family is relatively stable and economically comfortable, although they are challenged by Oleg's many behavioral, educational, cognitive, and social deficits. Of late his full-time aide and the classroom teacher have identified Oleg's

tendency to strike other students as an increasing problem. They consult with Dr. Gaston about how to modify this behavior.

Dr. Gaston asks that staff gather careful data regarding the hitting behavior, including the circumstances under which the hitting occurs, the time of day, and the precise sequence of events that leads up to and then follows the hitting behavior. She and treatment staff review a week's worth of data, and they conclude that Oleg is most likely to hit other students when the class is changing activities, particularly just before and after lunchtime. Oleg typically strikes any child who happens to be within easy range, and he sometimes strikes the aide. After Oleg hits someone, he is consistently taken to time out for five minutes in a quiet corner of the room, after which his behavior is generally more easily managed.

Dr. Gaston and staff decide that Oleg may not know how to manage feelings of agitation from stimulus overload, and they wonder if he actually finds time out to be rewarding, because he can calm down there. They decide to attack this problem along several fronts. First, they will experiment by seeing whether Oleg benefits from a couple of minutes of peace and quiet prior to and after lunchtime (i.e., *before* he hits). They decide that the aide will take him from the classroom and also from lunch a few minutes early and sit quietly with him in the hallway prior to the next activity. Second, Oleg's aide will begin monitoring the child's level of agitation more closely and will consistently respond to behavioral indicators of discomfort by asking Oleg, "Feel bad?" If Oleg responds affirmatively to this query, the aide will reinforce socially and will remove him from the activity and sit with him in the hallway for two minutes. Third, if Oleg initiates a break by saying "Bad," the aide will reinforce socially and remove him briefly from the activity. Fourth, if Oleg appears to become agitated at lunch, the aide will speak softly to him and, if necessary, move his seat away from the other children. Finally, the aide will manage Oleg's portions more closely by increasing his midmorning snack and slightly decreasing the amount of food he gets at lunch.

Dr. Gaston and staff decide to implement these steps in sequence so as to determine which intervention is most helpful. Having determined that Oleg can in fact say "Bad" when he feels agitated, they begin fading the social reinforcement for this verbalization but continue to remove him briefly from the activity, gradually decreasing the amount of time that he is out of the classroom at one time. The aide also begins modeling slow breathing as a way to teach Oleg to self-regulate without having to leave the classroom. The aide gradually shapes this behavior with social reinforcement for any shift in breathing rate and then differentially reinforcing for longer, slower breaths. Oleg is in fact able to learn to signal his distress and to self-regulate by managing his breathing, although he still hits other children on rare occasion.

Other Individual Psychotherapies

Interpersonal Psychotherapy (IPT)

Model of Psychopathology

IPT was developed in the late 1960s by the American psychiatrist Gerald L. Klerman (1928–1992) and his future wife, Myrna M. Weissman (1935–), then employed as a social worker. Its structure and content are based on the supportive psychotherapy in vogue at that time. In designing IPT, Klerman, Weissman, and colleagues were influenced by the neo-Freudian Zeitgeist, and they were also strongly influenced by writings of the interpersonal school, which emphasized the importance of relationships in understanding psychopathology, and by attachment theory, including particularly the writings of British psychiatrist John Bowlby (1907–1990). Originally formulated as an adjunctive treatment for antidepressant drug trials, IPT was designed as a time-limited psychotherapy. When, somewhat unexpectedly, the first version of IPT turned out to be helpful in its own right, its progenitors formalized its procedures and created a treatment manual, which they then used in formal tests of IPT's efficacy.

In IPT mental disorders are viewed through the lens of interpersonal relationships. In this regard IPT stands in contrast to CBT, in which problems are viewed in terms of ineffective cognitions and behaviors, and it also differs from psychodynamic treatments, in which problems are understood as manifestations of intrapsychic conflict. In IPT interpersonal problems and particularly mood disorders are thought to be correlated, but no hypothesis is offered to the effect that one precedes the other. The focus of treatment is to clarify the relationship between symptoms, on one hand, and the individual's interpersonal relationships and social roles, on the other hand. The IPT therapist places emphasis on repairing and strengthening the patient's relationships and helps the patient to accommodate to current social roles, in the expectation that this will lessen symptoms.

Since about 1990 adaptations of IPT have appeared for use with specific populations and for disorders other than major depression. Longer-term maintenance formats have also been developed to decrease the risk of relapse/recurrence. In most adaptations of IPT the underlying model of psychopathology has remained largely unchanged. However, a version of IPT targeted at the treatment of bipolar disorder, called Interpersonal and Social Rhythm Therapy (IPSRT), does add a significant component to the IPT model. According to IPSRT, individuals with bipolar disorder are at risk to become destabilized if their daily routines become disrupted. Thus, while IPSRT continues to emphasize the examination and amelioration of relationships and social roles, it also focuses on maintaining a regular sleep–wake cycle, regulating activity levels, taking medications regularly, and so forth.

Treatment Strategies

The individual receiving IPT for major depression is told at the outset of treatment that the course will last from 16 to 20 sessions. However, if at the end of treatment there are still major problems to be resolved, patient and therapist may discuss other treatment options. The initial phase of treatment lasts from one to three sessions. In this phase the therapist provides

psychoeducation by reviewing the diagnosis and treatment options and by providing some information about the IPT model. The therapist also assigns the patient the *sick role*. In so doing, the therapist attempts to decrease the patient's guilt over failing to perform all his or her normal responsibilities in a fully competent manner, while at the same time making the point that the patient will have to devote considerable energy to the task of recovering. In this phase of treatment patient and therapist also complete a comprehensive review of the important relationships in the patient's life, past and present. This is referred to as an *interpersonal inventory*, and it provides the therapist important data to use in conceptualizing the case. The patient may or may not be referred for a medication evaluation at this point. Given that IPT was first designed for use in drug trials, the treatment model is designed to be fully compatible with the use of psychotropic medications.

The middle phase of treatment usually lasts 10 to 14 sessions and begins with the task of agreeing on a focus for treatment. In IPT for major depression there are four possible problem areas: grief, role disputes, role transitions, and interpersonal deficits. It has long been known that the failure to complete the normal mourning process following the death of a significant other places one at risk to become depressed. Patients are therefore assigned *grief* as the IPT problem area if they have not fully mourned the death of someone very close to them. The *role disputes* problem area refers to ongoing conflict with a significant person in the patient's life, such that there is a failure to agree on how the patient is expected to act or how the patient is expected to relate to the other person. It is hypothesized that such nonreciprocal role expectations are often correlated with mood disorders. The *role transitions* problem area targets the difficulty a patient may be experiencing as a consequence of a significant role change, such as leaving home, marrying, starting work or retiring, becoming a parent, and so forth. It is hypothesized that such periods of significant change can be destabilizing, particularly in terms of the availability of social supports, and they may leave the patient vulnerable to becoming depressed. The final problem area, *interpersonal deficits*, is identified when the patient has limited social contacts and/or social skills. It is thought that such people are at risk for depression, because they don't have much social stimulation and are likely to be lonely.

After therapist and patient have agreed on the primary problem area, the therapist refers to the IPT manual, in which session topics and activities are suggested for each problem area. For example, in the treatment of an individual with role transition as the main focus, the therapist helps the patient realistically evaluate the old role and grieve its loss. The therapist also helps the patient evaluate the new role, identify advantages and disadvantages of the new role, and plan to accept it realistically but also optimistically.

In the middle phase of treatment, the therapist actively works to keep the focus on the chosen primary problem area, reminding the patient that their time together is limited and that it is more helpful to make substantial progress in one area than to make a little progress in several areas. Such increased focus is one of the advantages of **setting time limits for treatment**. At every opportunity the therapist draws the connection between the patient's mood and relationship issues in the patient's life. When the patient talks about changes in mood, the therapist asks about what is happening in the patient's relationships. Contrariwise, when the patient talks about relationship changes, the therapist asks about accompanying mood changes. Discussion in the session focuses on the patient's current daily life, rather than to spend a great deal of time talking about history. The therapist encourages the patient to describe in detail current problematic interactions with significant others, and patient and therapist may engage in **role plays** to practice new interpersonal behaviors. When the patient needs to solve a difficult problem, patient and therapist undertake *decision analysis*, which is an IPT-specific form of **problem solving**. The therapist strives to maximize the therapeutic alliance and engages in "cheerleading" to encourage the patient to make changes outside the session and also to ensure that the patient takes credit for any resulting symptomatic improvement. The therapist directly encourages the expression of affect in session, not only as a way to help patients to understand fully their feelings about important issues, but also as a way to help patients learn to deal with emotions in a less avoidant manner.

The final phase of treatment lasts one to three sessions. It involves a review of the gains made in treatment, as well as discussion of issues related to relapse prevention. At this point therapist and patient may decide that further treatment would be helpful, either psychotherapeutic or psychopharmacological, and the available options are reviewed. Finally, the therapist encourages the patient to discuss feelings related to the impending loss of the therapeutic relationship.

Research Findings

There are extensive research data that show IPT to be effective in the treatment of acute depressive episodes (Cuijpers et al., 2011). As well, a once-a-month variant of IPT, called Maintenance IPT, has been shown to decrease the likelihood of relapse/recurrence in individuals with chronic depression (O'Hara, Schiller, & Stuart, 2010). Variants of IPT have also been shown to be helpful with depressed adolescents (Curry & Becker, 2008), with young mothers in the postpartum period (Miller, Gur, Shanok, & Weissman, 2008), and with older people (Reynolds et al., 2010). IPT has been applied to the treatment of DSM-IV dysthymia, but it appears that it may be less effective as a monotherapy than when used in conjunction with psychopharmacological treatments (Markowitz, Kocsis, Bleiberg, Christos, & Sacks, 2005). IPSRT has shown promise as a helpful adjunctive treatment for bipolar disorder in both adults and adolescents (Sylvia, Tilley, Lund, & Sachs, 2008).

There have been attempts to modify IPT for treatment of various anxiety disorders, including panic, social phobia, and PTSD. Research data are thus far mixed on the effectiveness of these modifications. IPT has generally not been effective in treating substance abuse that is comorbid with mood disorders (Markowitz, Kocsis, Christos, Bleiberg, & Carlin, 2008). By contrast, IPT has been shown to be moderately helpful in treating individuals with bulimia (Fairburn, 1998) and binge-eating disorder (Hilbert et al., 2012). There is some suggestion in the literature that in these populations the beneficial effects of IPT may take longer to appear than the effects of CBT, however.

Case Example

Paula is a 35-year-old, separated mother of two children who reports that since her husband left her four months ago, she has been feeling depressed. She notes that she has custody of both children and works part-time, and there is conflict regarding financial support for the children. Paula reports that for months she has felt sad and worried most of the day every day, and she indicates that she has crying spells at least daily. She has the thought that she may be entirely responsible for this separation, even though it develops that her husband is now dating a female colleague at work and may well have been doing so for the past year. She states that she feels inadequate to manage the role of single parent. She adds that she can't fall asleep or stay asleep very well, and she is so anxious that she sometimes can't hold her food down, as a consequence of which she has lost 12% of body weight in the past six months without intending to. At present she is on the thin side. Paula denies that she has ever felt this way before, although she comments that she has long doubted her ability to manage life on her own. She denies other symptoms of a mental disorder, and she says she is in good physical health.

Upon interview Paula presents as a pleasant but anxious woman who seems to be "smiling through tears." Paula makes good eye contact but sometimes has an expression almost as if she were pleading for help.

Dr. Heller tells Paula that he believes she is in a first episode of major depressive disorder. He discusses treatment options and the fact that this condition has a good prognosis. He recommends that Paula consider a course of IPT, explaining that this is a well-researched technique that in 16 sessions is often successful in helping people with depression. He tells Paula that one of the problems depressed people have is that they expect too much of themselves. He points out that if Paula had pneumonia, she would be content to stay in bed until she got better and would not chastise herself for failing to keep house perfectly. Similarly, since Paula now has the medical condition of depression, she needs to decrease the pressure she feels to adhere to her old standards and instead redirect her energy toward getting well. Paula comments that she finds this suggestion very helpful, because for some time she has been upset with herself about the fact that she isn't getting everything done that she thinks she should.

Now Dr. Heller conducts an interpersonal inventory, asking that Paula tell him briefly about the important relationships in her life, past and present. When Paula fails to mention anything about her relationship with her older brother, Dr. Heller specifically asks her about him, and it comes out that Paula has always had a difficult relationship with this sibling. Dr. Heller notices but does not comment on the fact that Paula consistently describes herself as less able than many of her acquaintances, and she seems to lean on others quite a bit.

Near the middle of Session 3 Dr. Heller suggests to Paula that her main problem right now seems to be the need to adapt to a new role in her life, and he says that such role transitions often accompany depressive disorders. He points out that Paula had consistent social involvement when she and her husband were still living together, but the end of her marriage has disrupted many relationships, and she has avoided old friends, because she feared that they might side with her estranged husband. Dr. Heller suggests that he and Paula work on becoming comfortable in her new role as a single parent who now depends less on the children's father and relies more on her own skills and abilities.

During the next few sessions Paula and Dr. Heller discuss the advantages and disadvantages of Paula's old role and begin to think about how she might feel her way into the new role. Dr. Heller points out the relationship between variations in Paula's mood and her contacts with other people. For example, when Paula has lunch with a friend from church, her mood rises, but when she spends the weekend at home while the children are visiting their father, her mood drops. Paula cries frequently in session, and Dr. Heller encourages this expression of affect as a way to help Paula sort out exactly why she feels as she does. Paula begins to discover that she is actually angrier at her husband than she realized, and sometimes when she feels like crying, she is actually feeling frustrated and irritated with him.

Dr. Heller provides encouragement and support to Paula as she begins to explore ways in which to meet her social and more practical needs as a single parent. She joins a divorce support group at church, and in therapy she talks with Dr. Heller about how she can deal with her mother more effectively, particularly in that she believes her mother is angry with her about the end of the marriage. Dr. Heller and Paula role play how she can talk to her mother, and after Paula is successful in securing more emotional support from her mother in this way, Dr. Heller tells her how impressed he is that she was able to speak up to her mother. Along these same lines, he and Paula discuss whether and under what circumstances she might wish to consider dating.

Paula and Dr. Heller discuss how to solve practical problems in her new role, such as how she might go about finding a more remunerative job. They utilize the technique of decision analysis to think through the options available to her to solve this problem, as well as to consider the pros and cons of each option. Dr. Heller is careful always to point out when Paula has done something on her own, and in this way he works toward shifting her view of herself toward a more self-sufficient person.

Over the course of treatment Paula's mood gradually rises, and she begins to make her peace with the next phase of her life. She is able to see more clearly some of the disadvantages of the old role (particularly in terms of how her husband treated her), and she is pleased at the prospect of becoming more self-sufficient in the new role. In Session 14 she and Dr. Heller begin to discuss the fact that treatment will soon end. Paula expresses sadness about the impending loss of Dr. Heller's support, but they discuss how this loss will offer Paula another opportunity to test her ability to manage on her own. She and Dr. Heller discuss the course of treatment, review what was helpful and what was not, and plan what to do if Paula notices that her mood is dropping in the future. At the end of Session 16 she and Dr. Heller bid one another goodbye, but he encourages her to contact him if in the future she notices that her mood is beginning to dip.

Motivational Interviewing (MI)

Model of Psychopathology

MI is gaining increasing acceptance in many medical disciplines. Residents in psychiatry and primary care are encouraged to learn motivational interviewing skills to help patients with behavioral change. MI was originally developed by American psychologist William R. Miller (1947–) as a brief intervention to help individuals who are ambivalent about committing to work on addictive behaviors. In recent years, however, MI techniques have been increasingly used to help individuals who are ambivalent about making *any* behavior change. MI is now used both as a brief stand-alone procedure with individuals who are considering whether they wish to take steps toward a particular behavior change (e.g., curtailing alcohol use or learning new parenting skills) and as a therapeutic module that is dropped into another ongoing treatment when the patient expresses ambivalence regarding some clearly defined issue (e.g., undertaking exposure in anxiety treatment or becoming more physically active in treatment of depression). The model that underlies MI has to do with the nature of ambivalence, what is required to help an individual to overcome it, and what is needed for an individual actually to make a change in behavior.

In MI *ambivalence* is viewed as a universal phenomenon that is fundamentally nonpathological. Ambivalence can take the form of approach–approach conflicts and avoidance–avoidance conflicts, but the most challenging kind of ambivalence is the approach–avoidance conflict, in which the individual is simultaneously attracted to and repelled by the object of ambivalence. In MI the approach–avoidance conflict is usually related to the prospect of changing a behavior. There are costs and benefits associated with changing a behavior, and there are costs and benefits associated with continuing to behave as before. The salience of these costs and benefits is affected by a number of factors, including the individual's deeply held value system, his or her beliefs about what will occur with or without the behavior change, the individual's social milieu, issues of self-esteem (including the effect on self-esteem of acceding to social pressure), and the individual's ability to reason and to exert self-control.

A second important construct in MI has to do with the idea of *resistance*, which is now referred to in MI as *sustain talk*. In MI this phenomenon is viewed as an interpersonal process rather than as a psychological state that resides within the patient. In fact, when someone is stuck on the horns of a dilemma and is pushed in one direction or the other, the natural reaction is to push back, to resist, which maintains the status quo. In the context of psychotherapy, certain actions on the part of the therapist are known to increase sustain talk (e.g., teaching and confronting), and other actions are likely to decrease it (e.g., facilitating and supporting). Inasmuch as the presence of sustain talk prevents useful discussion regarding behavior change, the therapist must work to decrease it when it becomes apparent. The therapist must stop and do something different.

A final aspect of the model underlying MI has to do with the psychological characteristics of people who go on to make behavior changes. According to MI, when individuals are "ready, willing, and able," they are likely to make a behavior change. More specifically, this means that an individual must attach priority to making the change, must view the change as important because of its effect in his or her life, and must be confident that the change can in fact be made. Research has demonstrated that when patients engage in *change talk* in MI, it does in fact lead to behavior change. In particular, there is evidence that individuals with substance abuse diagnoses are most likely to maintain abstinence during the next year when they express increasing levels of commitment to change over the course of a treatment session. In other words, the best predictor of actual behavior change is the degree to which the patient expresses a strong commitment to change at the end of the session. This is a better predictor of change than any other pattern of speech during the session (Amrhein, 2004).

Treatment Strategies

MI seldom lasts longer than one or two sessions and often takes up only a portion of a single psychotherapy session. A longer, formal, and manualized version of MI is called Motivational Enhancement Therapy, and it may last four sessions. In any of its variants, MI consists of both relational components and technical components. The relational components of MI are largely based on the tenets of client-centered psychotherapy, with a strong emphasis on the therapist's empathic behavior. The MI therapist focuses on communicating acceptance to the patient, rather than any pressure to change. The therapist works to make the patient feel safe in the relationship, since this promotes self-focus and self-disclosure on the part of the patient.

The technical components of MI include developing discrepancy, rolling with resistance, and supporting self-efficacy. Generally, therapists should speak in such a way that the patient is likely to argue against the status quo. This sometimes means that therapists articulate (without endorsing) the position that is *opposite* to the one they hope the patient will eventually adopt. *Developing discrepancy* involves providing patients with objective information about their condition and emphasizing the difference between patients' current circumstances and their deeply held values and goals in life. It also involves making the point that patients' circumstances are most likely to change if they change their own behavior. However, it is important that the therapist not advocate for a particular change in the patient's behavior; any such suggestions should come from the patient. When therapists engage in *rolling with resistance*, they avoid arguing with the patient. They communicate respect for the patient and provide support as the patient tries to sort out the ambivalence. They consistently utilize the fundamental MI skills of asking *open* questions, *affirming* the patient, *reflecting* the content of the patient's verbalizations, and offering *summaries* ("OARS"). MI therapists respond to sustain talk mostly by agreeing with it, although they may slightly modify these kinds of patient verbalizations in such a way that the patient is likely to react against them. For example, therapists may amplify the patient's statement ("I see your point. Actually, life without alcohol would hardly be worth it"), agree with a twist ("That's exactly right. It doesn't make sense to single out your actions and ignore your wife's contribution to the problem. Drinking affects everyone in the family"), **reframe** resistance ("The fact that you're feeling hopeless is evidence of how hard you've worked at managing your drinking. That tells me you're about to try an entirely new strategy"), or invoke a number of other specific techniques. *Supporting self-efficacy* is important, because patients who don't believe they can actually make changes in life cannot tolerate the thought that such changes are important. Therapists must communicate that they believe in their patients' ability to change and can also take steps to help patients recognize that they have the resources to change.

Research Findings
Notwithstanding its brevity, MI has been shown to be surprisingly effective in the treatment of substance abuse. In a large, multisite RCT, individuals with alcohol dependence participating in the four-session Motivational Enhancement Therapy had generally positive outcomes. In a 2010 meta-analysis Lundahl, Kunz, Brownell, and Burke found a mean effect size of $g = .21$ for MI in the treatment of alcohol, marijuana, and other drugs when compared with nonspecific treatments, waitlist control, and so forth. The g statistic is very similar to the d statistic we have previously cited in discussing the effectiveness of psychotherapy as a whole ($d = .87$) and the relationship between therapeutic alliance and outcome ($d = .57$). When 119 studies covering a wide range of substance abuse, health-related behaviors, gambling, and engagement in treatment were lumped together, MI showed an effect size of $g = .28$ in comparison with nonspecific treatments, waitlist control, and so forth.

Case Example

Quinn is a 28-year-old, divorced, childless man who drives a forklift in a warehouse. He is referred to the plant physician, Dr. Ito, after slipping on wet concrete at work and spraining his wrist. It quickly becomes evident that Quinn was hung over on the day of the accident. Moreover, Dr. Ito notes that Quinn has frequently called in sick following long weekends. She engages Quinn in discussion regarding his drinking habits and learns that on each of his days off he consumes about half a case of beer, and while he drinks less on workdays, his average weekly intake is 40 standard drinks.

In a comfortable and slow-paced way, Dr. Ito asks Quinn how he views his drinking, and he admits that other people have suggested that he might have a problem. Dr. Ito provides information about how his drinking pattern compares with that of most males his age. She asks about the advantages and disadvantages of his drinking pattern and, feigning uncertainty, leads him to repeat his admission that he has twice been arrested for DUI.

When Dr. Ito asks Quinn to list his options regarding drinking, he replies that he could keep drinking, or he could "just stop." Dr. Ito asks about the advantages of continuing to drink, but fairly quickly Quinn begins to talk about the disadvantages of this. As they then discuss Quinn's idea that he "just stop," Dr. Ito asks Quinn about his attempts to quit in the past. She repeats Quinn's idea that a decision to cut down or stop will work out differently this time, but she further suggests that he won't mind the discomfort involved and the lack of support in quitting on his own. Dr. Ito is careful to communicate that she understands Quinn's point of view, and she doesn't offer an opinion about what she thinks he should do.

Picking up on an earlier comment by Quinn, Dr. Ito then steers the discussion to a consideration of whether Quinn might benefit from the support available through Alcoholics Anonymous meetings or counseling. Dr. Ito asks Quinn's thoughts about getting help to quit, and, in particular, she asks Quinn what the disadvantages would be in seeking assistance. When he denies that there are meaningful costs, she asks him about the time required, the expense, the opinions of his friends, and the possibility that Quinn will think less of himself. Dr. Ito then permits Quinn to argue against her suggestions regarding the costs of seeking assistance.

Finally, Quinn says that he thinks he should at least look into getting help, but another part of him doesn't want to do this. Dr. Ito carefully reflects Quinn's ambivalence without offering her opinion on the matter. She communicates her trust in Quinn's ability to make the right decision, points out that he has given serious thought to the matter for a long time, and gently asks how he will decide what to do. Quinn finally says that he wants to think about it some more and asks if he can return to talk to Dr. Ito again about his drinking. She responds that she is impressed by his thoughtfulness on the matter, and she assures him that her door is always open to discuss it with him anytime.

Three weeks later Quinn returns for another visit. He reports that he has tried to stop drinking but has once again had little success. He expresses the wish to get some help and asks Dr. Ito for a referral for outpatient counseling. However, when she provides this information, Quinn again expresses doubt about whether it's necessary to seek help. Dr. Ito carefully reflects his ambivalence and then suggests that he could try again on his own. Perhaps this time it will be different. Quinn responds that he knows it won't be different, but he doesn't want to commit himself to treatment. Dr. Ito reflects his worry that if he had an intake at the counseling center, he would feel duty-bound to continue in treatment, and it would be extremely difficult to drop out. Quinn replies that that sounds silly, and perhaps he really should give therapy a try.

Dr. Ito then asks Quinn to rate, on a scale from 1 to 10, how important it is to him that he get counseling. Quinn rates this a 6. Dr. Ito asks why it's not a 5, and Quinn responds that he's tired of drinking the way he does and wants to change. She then asks him to rate how likely he thinks it is that he will actually call for an appointment. Quinn also rates this as a 6. Dr. Ito asks what would be needed to make the likelihood rating a 7, and he replies that if he knew Dr. Ito were going to ask him about it the following week, it would increase his motivation. Dr. Ito asks Quinn directly if he wants her to check in with him next week, and he replies that he would like her to do so.

At this point the session ends. When Dr. Ito contacts Quinn the next week, he confirms that he is now scheduled for an intake at the counseling center.

Twelve-Step Facilitation

Model of Psychopathology

This is a 12- to 15-session manualized psychotherapy to treat individuals early in recovery from substance abuse. Treatment is aimed primarily at encouraging the patient to become actively involved in an appropriate Twelve-Step program, such as Alcoholics Anonymous, Narcotics Anonymous, or other similar groups. These Twelve-Step programs advocate that substance abusers adopt a goal of complete abstinence. They take the position that willpower alone cannot overcome addiction and that substance abusers must become less self-centered by depending on the program and by developing themselves spiritually. The programs are organized around activities that have the effect of bringing about cognitive, behavioral, and spiritual changes that are supportive of recovery from addiction.

Alcoholics Anonymous (AA) was the first Twelve-Step program. It was founded in the 1930s; after that other programs followed, such as Narcotics Anonymous, with only very minor adaptations in form and structure. The structure and philosophy of AA are based in part on the tenets of the Oxford Group, a popular religious movement in the early 1900s that encouraged its members to work toward self-improvement through performing self-inventory, admitting one's faults and making amends, maintaining spiritual awareness through prayer and meditation, and "carrying the message" to others. The founding of AA was set in motion by none other than the Swiss psychiatrist Carl G. Jung, who was consulted in the early 1930s by an American man regarding his alcoholism. Jung concluded that only a profound spiritual experience would help this individual. He encouraged the American to return home and to attend meetings of the Oxford Group. The American found the Oxford Group meetings helpful, and through a network of friends two other men with alcohol problems, a stockbroker (Bill W.) and, shortly thereafter, a surgeon (Dr. Bob), began attending Oxford Group meetings, as well. Both were able to achieve sobriety through practicing its principles. Wishing to make such an experience more accessible to others with alcohol problems, Bill W. and Dr. Bob began in 1935 to make adaptations to the Oxford Group program, and over the course of the next several years AA came into being.

The AA program is based on Twelve Steps to recovery, which include admitting powerlessness over alcohol, committing to a spiritual program of one's own choosing, acknowledging personal deficiencies in the form of a "searching and fearless moral inventory," working to overcome these personal deficiencies, making amends to others where appropriate, maintaining an active spiritual program through prayer and meditation, and carrying the message to other alcoholics. Major emphasis is placed on regular participation in AA meetings, where group members discuss the tenets of the program, provide support to one another, and offer advice about how to cope with the difficulties encountered in recovery. Many AA members believe that their sobriety is largely dependent on participation in the program and on their relationships with other AA members, including especially their "sponsors," who assume primary responsibility for acculturating them to the program, and their "sponsees," whom they in turn help.

AA and other Twelve-Step programs maintain a strong tradition of anonymity and have not encouraged research regarding their effectiveness. However, over time it has become clear that Twelve-Step programs are enormously helpful to individuals who are recovering from addiction, and for many years professionals providing services to individuals with substance use disorders have tried to smooth the way for patients to become as involved as possible in Twelve-Step programs. The Twelve-Step facilitation treatment model is fundamentally just a formalization of that practice.

Treatment Strategies

In Twelve-Step facilitation the therapist does an assessment of the patient's substance use and encourages the patient to adopt the goal of abstinence. The therapist discusses the format and content of the appropriate Twelve-Step program and provides support for the patient to begin attending as many regular meetings as possible, subject to the patient's willingness and ability to participate. The therapist explains the difference between psychotherapy and regular attendance at a Twelve-Step program and underscores the point that these do not serve the same function. Later in treatment, the therapist works with the patient on issues related to the first three of the Twelve Steps. In particular, the rather challenging concepts of acceptance and powerlessness are discussed. The therapist may also encourage the patient to begin working on a moral inventory and may discuss other relevant issues, as well. Therapist and patient review some of the AA literature, and they may discuss how to make use of helpful phrases ("Easy does it," "Turn it over," "HALT: Hungry, Angry, Lonely, Tired," and so forth). The therapist encourages the patient to get the most out of Twelve-Step program participation by committing to one meeting per week as a "home group," obtaining a sponsor, and contacting other group members when the patient becomes aware of urges and cravings.

Research Findings

In a large, multisite RCT, individuals with alcohol dependence participating in Twelve-Step facilitation therapy had generally positive outcomes. In fact, individuals receiving this form of treatment had fewer drinking days for up to three years posttreatment and participated in more AA meetings than those receiving CBT or Motivational Enhancement Therapy, a four-session variant of Motivational Interviewing. As well, individuals with less psychiatric comorbidity did better in Twelve-Step facilitation therapy than in CBT, and individuals whose social networks *supported* drinking had better outcomes from Twelve-Step facilitation therapy than from CBT (Stout et al., 2003).

Case Example
Rona is a 40-year-old, divorced mother of two children referred for outpatient treatment of her alcohol use disorder. She is currently unemployed and has lost her license for a year due to multiple DUIs. She is estranged from her family of origin because of her alcoholism. Until a few days ago Rona was consuming an average of four standard drinks daily, with occasional binges, and she has been told that she has early signs of peripheral neuropathy. She has been abstinent for periods of weeks or months in the past (particularly during incarceration following her third DUI), and she now admits that she doesn't believe she can drink without greatly risking adverse consequences. Still, it is only following the recent breakup with her boyfriend of four years that she has been willing once again to seek treatment for her drinking.

Rona also reports some anxiety and low mood at present. However, she says that she usually feels emotionally stable after she has been abstinent for a few weeks. In this connection, she says she is perplexed about why in the past she has eventually returned to drinking. She reports that in her teens and twenties she frequently experimented with various street drugs but states that she has rarely used these in recent years. She has had peripheral involvement with AA in the past but has never committed herself to a home group or had a permanent sponsor.

When first seen by Dr. Johnson, Rona presents as a pleasant woman who appears to be a few years older than her stated age. Her cognitive and mnemonic functions appear to be generally intact. Mood is euthymic.

Dr. Johnson congratulates Rona on her insight that she is unlikely to be able to drink in a controlled manner, and he says they will work together to help her achieve sobriety. He says that getting sober isn't too hard, but living sober can be much harder, and he indicates that the AA program is specifically designed to help people work out the problems that arise in life without alcohol. Rona expresses surprise that there *are* problems in life without alcohol, to which Dr. Johnson replies that such problems, while sometimes subtle, may explain why Rona has relapsed in the past.

Rona states that AA never appealed much to her. Dr. Johnson indicates that he will work with Rona to help her get the most out of the program, and he asks that she be willing to give the program an honest try. Rona replies that she will try to keep an open mind. Dr. Johnson gives Rona a list of the local AA meetings and explains the difference between open and closed meetings (the latter are only for self-identified alcoholics) and between speaker and discussion meetings (the latter have no speaker and instead consist of group discussion on a particular topic). Dr. Johnson asks that Rona try to attend at least three meetings in the coming week, and he urges that in the meetings she think about the ways in which she is similar to the others present, rather than to focus on how she is different from them.

The next week Rona returns to discuss her experiences, and she indicates that she liked two meetings but disliked a third. Dr. Johnson encourages her to attend the meetings at which she feels most comfortable, and he points out that there are many more local meetings for Rona to try.

Dr. Johnson then begins discussion of the First, Second, and Third Steps of AA, which have to do with the concepts of acceptance (of one's addiction) and surrender (to the need to seek assistance from the AA program and also in a spiritual sense). This discussion continues over the next session. Dr. Johnson provides written material and gives Rona homework assignments at the end of each session.

In Session 4 Dr. Johnson discusses in more detail how to make use of AA. He talks about the basics of the AA program, including readings, sponsors, working the Steps, alcohol-free social activities sponsored by AA groups, the ability to contact group members in order to cope with urges and cravings, and other matters. He also talks about how AA is different from psychotherapy, in that AA is a mutual self-help organization focused specifically on recovery from alcoholism, while psychotherapy involves the provision of personalized support for any mental health problem Rona might have that is related to her alcohol problem. Indeed, she and Dr. Johnson spend time in the current session discussing some of the practical problems she is facing right now, and he encourages her to tolerate current discomfort as she continues to detoxify and to adjust to life without the ability to avoid through drinking.

In the next couple of sessions Dr. Johnson continues to provide Rona practical support in early sobriety, and he encourages Rona to pick out a temporary home group and temporary sponsor. He explains how to make use of a sponsor, and he cautions Rona against choosing as a sponsor someone of the opposite gender or someone relatively new in the program. Dr. Johnson continues to discuss themes of powerlessness and surrender, and, having assessed Rona's particular needs, decides to discuss issues of managing feelings and changing habits. As he discusses these matters with Rona, he provides readings and worksheets, and he ensures at the end of each session that Rona is able to state how the material covered actually applies to her.

If Rona had been currently involved in a romantic relationship, Dr. Johnson would have asked her to bring in her partner for a couple of sessions to provide education and to ensure that Rona receives appropriate support and understanding from her partner early in sobriety.

In Session 7 Rona reports that she had three drinks the day after their last therapy session. Dr. Johnson reviews with Rona what led up to the drinking episode, what happened afterwards, and how she might avoid a similar slip in the future. Dr. Johnson makes clear that slips do occur in early sobriety, and he discusses the difference between a lapse and a relapse.

In subsequent sessions Dr. Johnson checks in each week with Rona about her attendance at AA meetings, and he encourages her as she involves herself more deeply in the local AA community. He also talks with her about what she has learned at the meetings she attends every week. He suggests that Rona gradually increase the number of meetings she attends each week, and he reminds Rona that AA members are glad to pick her up for meetings, since she can't yet drive again.

By the end of treatment, Dr. Johnson has worked with Rona on the basic themes of early recovery, and he has encouraged her to commit herself to a plan of attending 90 AA meetings in 90 days. However, if Rona doesn't want to or can't do this, Dr. Johnson will compromise so as still to optimize Rona's active participation in the program. Dr. Johnson gradually encourages Rona to rely more and more on her sponsor for assistance in adjusting to the program, and he encourages her to talk with her sponsor about working through all of the Steps. They spend some time discussing the importance of the Fourth Step, and Dr. Johnson provides Rona some written material on this topic.

At various points during treatment Dr. Johnson may ask Rona to obtain an alcohol test, usually right in his office. If Dr. Johnson believes that Rona is intoxicated at the time of a session, he will obtain an alcohol test and will end the session early if she is in fact intoxicated.

Eye Movement Desensitization and Reprocessing (EMDR)

Model of Psychopathology

Developed by American psychologist Francine Shapiro (1948–), EMDR is a novel treatment for PTSD that purports to speed the processing of emotional information during imagined **exposure** through the bilateral stimulation of the brain hemispheres. This is accomplished by having patients move their eyes rapidly back and forth between the left and right sides of the visual field during the therapy protocol. Alternatively, the therapist can stimulate first one ear and then the other with alternating clicks or can use a device that taps first one side of the patient's body and then the other in an alternating pattern. It has been pointed out by EMDR's developers that rapidly alternating eye movements are naturally produced during REM sleep, which is a time during which memories are thought to consolidate. Whether the eye movements contribute to the efficacy of EMDR, however, is the subject of research inquiry. There is little clear evidence of support for the hypothesis at this time. It is important to note that EMDR also contains many elements of CBT, and the treatment might be described as a variant of CBT, to which bilateral eye movements, clicks, or taps have been added.

Treatment Strategies

To treat one traumatic memory, EMDR usually requires four to six psychotherapy sessions, each lasting between 90 and 120 minutes. Treatment involves eight phases, the first of which involves taking a history and planning treatment. Interestingly, the patient is *not* obliged to reveal the nature of the trauma in this session. There follow two phases of treatment in which the patient is told what to expect during the desensitization and reprocessing segment of treatment, and the therapist ensures that the patient has access to a self-soothing strategy (sometimes requiring a brief course of **relaxation training**), that can be used later in treatment. Patient and therapist identify a specific visual image that represents the trauma, an associated negative cognition, and a positive cognition that the patient would rather believe in connection with the trauma. In the fourth phase of treatment, the patient is asked to visualize the trauma-related image, to think about and say aloud the associated negative cognition, and then to notice what emotions and physical sensations arise. Rating scales are used to quantify these experiences. Next the patient is asked simultaneously to hold in mind the trauma image, the negative words, the emotion, and its bodily representation while visually following a target (such as the therapist's forefinger) that moves rapidly back and forth across the patient's visual field. Alternatively, auditory or tactile stimulation may be used to help the patient focus first on one side of the body and then the other. Multiple trials are undertaken (possibly using new images spontaneously reported by the patient), until the patient reports a very low level of distress. In the fifth phase of treatment, the patient visualizes the target image and thinks about the positive belief he or she would like to acquire in connection with the trauma; at this time the patient again engages in the bilateral stimulation, either visual, auditory, or tactile. This continues until the patient reports acceptance of the positive belief as "completely true." In the sixth phase of treatment the patient engages in a body scan to identify any areas of tension. If any are discovered, the patient focuses on that body area while engaging again in bilateral stimulation. In the last two phases the therapist encourages the patient to use the earlier identified self-soothing technique if the patient is experiencing any tension, and some homework is assigned, such as keeping a **journal** of distressing thoughts and memories. Therapist and patient also re-evaluate their progress to date, after which they may decide to revisit a previously addressed trauma, or they may move on to a new target.

Research Findings

EMDR has been shown to be as efficacious as CBT in the treatment of PTSD (e.g., Power et al., 2002). There are data to suggest that EMDR is as effective without eye movements as is the full package, including the eye movements (Renfrey & Spates, 1994, but cf. Wilson, Silver, Covi, & Foster, 1996). Given that one of the major differences between CBT and EMDR is the eye movements, it is perhaps not surprising that CBT and EMDR are equivalently effective in the treatment of PTSD.

Case Example

Sam is a 68-year-old, widowed father of three adult children. He is a retired civil engineer who felt healthy and stable until he was involved in a car accident nine months ago. He was driving his car along a city street when another car darted out from a side street and plowed into the passenger side of Sam's car, when Sam was unable to brake and swerve sufficiently to avoid impact. Sam sustained a concussion and some bruises, but the only other passenger in the car, Sam's wife of 43 years, Mary, was killed. Sam's injuries resolved within a couple of weeks, but since the accident he has been tortured by nightmares and flashbacks of the accident. He limits his driving to a minimum, and he carefully avoids driving near the scene of the accident. He has trouble sleeping and feels much more irritable than usual. Some of his irritability is directed toward his children and grandchildren, as a consequence of which he limits his involvement with them. He prefers staying at home by himself, where he frequently ruminates about the accident and wonders what he could have done to avoid it. Sam has been treated with antidepressant medication, which has had a modest effect on his mood and energy level, but he remains quite distressed about the accident itself.

Upon interview Sam presents as a rather serious older gentleman who becomes tearful as he recounts the details of the accident that killed his wife. Dr. Knowles reviews Sam's history and determines that he is indeed a candidate for EMDR treatment. She then explains to Sam what will happen in the desensitization and reprocessing portions of treatment and teaches Sam to follow his breath as a means to decrease his arousal. She asks that Sam practice this relaxation technique at home twice daily prior to the next session. She also suggests that he might find that he can utilize the relaxation as a means to improve his sleep.

In Session 2 Sam and Dr. Knowles discuss the relaxation homework and then turn to the question of what visual image best represents the trauma. Sam recalls having watched as his wife was loaded onto the ambulance after the accident, worrying that she would die en route to the hospital (which is in fact what happened). After some discussion Sam is able to identify as his negative cognition the idea, "I am responsible for Mary's death." Sam has a much harder time coming up with a positive cognition that he would rather believe regarding the accident. With assistance from Dr. Knowles, however, he is finally able to settle on the idea, "I am competent; it was an accident that's over now." At the end of this session Dr. Knowles again asks Sam to practice focusing on his breath twice a day in the coming week.

In Session 3, which is scheduled for two hours, Dr. Knowles begins the desensitization and reprocessing trials. She asks that Sam fix the ambulance image in his mind and think about and say aloud his negative belief about himself (I am responsible for Mary's death). Next they review Sam's selected positive cognition (I am competent; it was an accident that's over now), and she asks him to rate on a scale how true that feels. Sam is then asked to focus on the trauma image plus the negative belief and identify and verbalize the emotion that is elicited. At this point, a rating scale is used to quantify Sam's level of distress. This is followed by guiding Sam to notice and identify what bodily sensation is associated with that emotion.

Dr. Knowles then asks Sam to simultaneously hold in mind the ambulance image, the negative belief, and the body sensation while following her right forefinger with his eyes as she rapidly moves her finger back and forth from one side of Sam's visual field to the other about 24 times. Sam has previously been instructed to permit the image to change on its own and to let new information arise without censorship during the eye movements. He has also been instructed that he may signal to stop at any time. After the end of the eye movements, Sam is told to "let it go" and just breathe. Following this, Dr. Knowles asks Sam to reveal what new images or information came up, and then the eye movements are repeated based on the newest image and associated material. Sam completes 15 trials before he reports that his distress is only 10 on a scale from 1 to 100. Of note, this is his distress rating following having been asked once again to focus on the original target.

Dr. Knowles now asks Sam if the positive statement previously selected continues to be the one he feels is best. After he confirms that it is, she asks him to think about the accident and bring up the positive words (I am competent; it was an accident that's over now) while once again doing eye movements. Afterwards she asks Sam to rate how true the positive words feel in his gut. The process is repeated for as long as each set results in improvement. After nine trials Sam reports that he entirely concurs with the positive cognition. Next Dr. Knowles asks Sam to close his eyes and bring to mind simultaneously the original traumatic memory plus the positive belief while he scans his body for any tension, sequentially focusing his attention on individual body parts from his head down to his feet. When he reports some tension in his shoulders, Dr. Knowles asks him to focus on this sensation in his shoulders while they do several additional sets of eye movements. After four sets, a repeat body scan fails to find any additional tension.

At the end of this session Dr. Knowles assigns Sam the task of keeping a journal during the next week, in which he is to briefly jot down any thoughts, feelings, or memories he has regarding the trauma, which will be used as targets in the next session. He is specifically instructed to avoid going into a great deal of detail with regard to new disturbing material and instructed instead just to take a representative snapshot.

At the beginning of Session 4 Sam reports that he definitely felt less distress during most of the week after the last session, but yesterday he was again troubled by his memories. He and Dr. Knowles decide that it might be helpful to undertake a few more desensitization and reprocessing trials in the current session. They do so, and Sam soon reports decreased distress, indicating after only two reprocessing trials that he completely concurs with his newest positive cognition, which is that he is a good husband and can honor his wife's memory by supporting the children and grandchildren. Afterwards, Dr. Knowles and Sam review the course of treatment and decide that they have met their goal. Dr. Knowles encourages Sam to follow up on his positive belief, and she tells him that if he experiences a return of symptoms, she will be happy to resume their work together.

Biofeedback for Mental Disorders

Model of Psychopathology

Biofeedback involves giving an individual real-time information about a body process of which the individual is not normally much aware. For example, one might be provided second-by-second information about hand temperature, skin conductivity, muscle contraction, EEG, heart rate, or other indicia of autonomic arousal. Having this information permits the individual to become efficient at modifying the body process through focusing attention, consciously relaxing or tightening the associated muscles, visualizing a relaxing scene, following one's breath, or other means. Biofeedback is used in behavioral medicine to help patients with various pain syndromes, insomnia, urinary incontinence, hypertension, Raynaud's disease, and a number of other conditions. It can be applied to the treatment of anxiety, as well. The idea is that most anxiety syndromes lead to increased muscle tension and general autonomic arousal, and anxious individuals often interpret such somatic changes as evidence that they are under threat, which sets up a vicious cycle of escalating anxiety and physical arousal. Many anxious people have limited awareness of how arousal manifests in their body or, if they are aware, don't know how to decrease the arousal. Biofeedback is used to help anxious people get control over body processes that contribute to their arousal. Once new skills are learned using biofeedback, individuals practice the skills without biofeedback, and in time they become able to generalize the skills to everyday life.

Treatment Strategies

Biofeedback can be offered as a separate service or in the context of more comprehensive psychotherapy. The therapist selects a body process to be monitored, such as tension in a specific muscle, and utilizes an appropriate sensor to provide feedback. In the case of muscle tension, electromyography is utilized to detect microvolt-level changes in muscle action potentials on the skin near the muscle in question. The therapist explains the procedure, connects the sensing device to the patient, and then switches on the machine, which provides visual feedback, auditory feedback, or both. The therapist may simply let the patient experiment to determine the best means to slow down the process in question. Alternatively, the therapist may suggest that the patient utilize a previously learned skill (e.g., from **relaxation training**) or may instruct the patient to undertake some action, such as paying attention to one's breath, that is likely to cause the biofeedback output to show decreased arousal. Over many trials the patient becomes adept at modifying the process on demand and then begins practicing this new skill without being connected to the machine.

Research Findings

Biofeedback has been shown to be efficacious in the treatment of many medical disorders. With regard to psychiatry, it has been shown to be efficacious in the treatment of attention-deficit/hyperactivity disorder (ADHD) and anxiety. Biofeedback is described as "probably efficacious" in the treatment of substance abuse, and there have been positive findings in studies that have used biofeedback to treat autism (now referred to as autism spectrum disorder in DSM-5), depression, and PTSD (Yucha & Montgomery, 2008).

Case Example

Tina is a 32-year-old, married, childless woman who is being treated in psychotherapy for generalized anxiety disorder. She and her therapist have become aware of Tina's frequently high level of physical tension, but they have difficulty figuring out how she can learn to relax, particularly her neck and shoulders. Tina is therefore sent to see Dr. Landon, who provides adjunctive biofeedback treatment.

After Dr. Landon reviews Tina's history, he explains how biofeedback might be helpful, and he places her in front of a monitor connected through a PC to a biofeedback device. He applies EMG electrodes to her left trapezius and switches on the program so that Tina can see a visual representation of the moment-by-moment level of tension in her trapezius, associated also with an auditory signal that is higher or lower, depending on the tension in that muscle. He suggests that Tina play around a little with the tension in her left trapezius and see what happens. Dr. Landon then turns to his desk, where he busies himself with paperwork for a few minutes. After a little while he asks Tina about her experience so far, and she says that she is able to control the output by relaxing her shoulders. However, after looking at the biofeedback output, Dr. Landon recognizes that Tina remains quite tense. He therefore explains that he would like to teach Tina a relaxation technique she can use to decrease her shoulder tension even more.

Dr. Landon disconnects the EMG electrodes and gives Tina two inexpensive alcohol-based thermometers and asks that she hold a thermometer between the thumb and forefinger of each hand. He explains that when people relax, their peripheral circulation increases, and their hands become warmer. He also notes that a normal consequence of anxious arousal is a decrease in peripheral blood flow. Tina and Dr. Landon note the current temperature on each thermometer. He then sets about to teach her a relaxation technique (visualizing a pleasant scene), and after 20 minutes they look again at the thermometers, noting that her hand temperature has increased by 5° and 8°F in her right and left hands, respectively. Dr. Landon advises Tina that many people demonstrate greater temperature variability in the non-dominant hand, and he asks that Tina practice this relaxation technique at home twice daily. He gives her both a form on which to track her practice as well as a copy of an audio recording he made while inducing relaxation in Tina earlier in the session.

At Session 2 Tina and Dr. Landon review her experience with the week's relaxation practice. Tina states that on one day she didn't practice at all, but on the other days she practiced at least once. She says she was consistently able to raise her hand temperature bilaterally. Dr. Landon suggests that they reconnect Tina to the EMG to see how a conscious attempt to relax herself will affect the tension in her shoulder. He again starts up the biofeedback program, with electrodes attached to her left trapezius, and this time Tina is able to decrease the level of tension in that muscle quite significantly. Tina comments that she likes the feeling of decreased tension in her shoulder, but she admits that it is unfamiliar to her. She and Dr. Landon discuss her thoughts and feelings about the increased relaxation of her muscles, and Dr. Landon encourages her to discuss it with her psychotherapist, as well. He asks that she continue to practice the visualization every day at home.

In Session 3 Tina and Dr. Landon discuss how she might shorten the visualization technique, with the goal that she implement it for five minutes four times a day and experiment with dropping the use of the thermometers. Dr. Landon connects Tina to the biofeedback, this time placing the EMG electrodes on other neck and shoulder muscles, and Tina is again able to decrease the tension by visualizing a pleasant scene.

In the next two sessions Tina and Dr. Landon continue to work on simplifying the technique she uses to relax herself, and Tina reports that she now routinely feels less physical tension in her body during the day. At the end of Session 5 she and Dr. Landon conclude that they have reached their goal in treatment. Dr. Landon encourages Tina to call in the future if she would like further assistance. After terminating with Dr. Landon, Tina continues to attend weekly psychotherapy sessions with the therapist who referred her to Dr. Landon for biofeedback.

Therapies from Complementary and Alternative Medicine

There are literally hundreds of specific psychotherapies in current use, and more are being developed all the time. Many of these approaches to treatment are likely to be at least somewhat effective, if only on the basis of the Dodo bird's conclusion: "Everybody has won, and all must have prizes." We have suggested earlier in the text that therapeutic alliance predicts to outcome across the range of psychotherapies. Similarly, we have suggested that psychotherapy is more likely to be effective to the extent that therapists expertly employ five basic psychotherapy skills: attending and listening, restatements, questions, empathy, and challenges. Since most varieties of psychotherapy involve the use of these skills and aim to establish a high level of therapeutic alliance, it is not surprising that various little-known or nonstandard psychotherapies help many patients. Moreover, many such psychotherapies include standard behavioral, psychodynamic, or other techniques for which research exists to attest to their effectiveness, and any new or unusual components of treatment may have little effect. Many have argued, for example, that the effectiveness of EMDR results from the fact that it consists of CBT plus benign but inert eye movements.

If one comes across a novel treatment for which there does not yet exist a body of research demonstrating effectiveness, how should one proceed? What advice can one offer a patient who asks about such treatment? One strategy would be to play it safe by adopting the position that one will only encourage the use of treatments that have been shown to be empirically supported. As an alternative, however, one might examine the novel therapy through three lenses. First, is there any research at all that suggests the therapy may be effective? Is there research that suggests it is *not* effective or even harmful? In this regard, it is helpful to review lists of possibly harmful psychotherapies, such as the one offered by Lilienfeld (2007). Second, to what extent does the novel therapy contain treatment elements that are known to be effective, such as exposure in the treatment of anxiety or behavioral activation in the treatment of depression? Conversely, to what extent does the therapy contain treatment elements that are truly novel or are *not* known to be effective? Finally, to what extent does the novel therapy contain elements that seem likely to boost therapeutic alliance? If the therapy involves confrontation or harsh **feedback**, this increases risk, since such behavior on the part of the therapist is known to increase the probability of negative outcomes.

Sometimes patients ask about psychosocial treatments that are intended to augment the effect of the individual psychotherapy they are already receiving. Such augmenting treatments might include hypnosis, guided imagery, **relaxation training**, and the like. These treatments are not new, and there is research that shows them to be helpful in the treatment of certain specified disorders. In this case, the best thing to do is to review the research to determine whether the addition of the augmenting treatment to the individual psychotherapy currently being offered is likely to be helpful—or, at least, not harmful.

One might be tempted to encourage the patient inquiring about an additional treatment simply to pursue such treatment at the same time that one continues to offer the patient the course of treatment currently being provided. However, this can be risky, because the patient may receive conflicting advice or may become confused about what advice is actually being offered. The risk is particularly significant in the case of stand-alone treatments that are intended to accomplish the same thing as the treatment the patient is already receiving, as contrasted with augmenting treatments, which may be less of a problem. Patients may work hard in one treatment and not so hard in the other or may switch attention back and forth between treatments. As a consequence, it becomes virtually impossible to assess the effectiveness of treatment, because one doesn't know what contributes to improvement or deterioration when the patient is receiving multiple services. It may be possible to miss treatment that actually harms the patient under these circumstances. If in the end the patient does elect to pursue simultaneously a second mode of treatment, it is very important that the treatment providers remain in regular contact with one another and that, in particular, they touch base whenever there is evidence that the patient's condition may be deteriorating.

Psychotherapy for Multiple Patients

Group Psychotherapy

Model of Psychopathology

Some commentators have suggested that psychotherapy conducted in a group format can be thought of as individual psychotherapy modified to a greater or lesser extent by special features peculiar to groups. Sometimes the special group features are of limited theoretical significance. For example, in DBT skills groups, psychopathology and treatment are understood primarily from a DBT perspective, with the addition of group support and some amount of **modeling** from other group members. Indeed, one important reason that patients are taught DBT skills in a group format is simply that it is convenient and efficient to do so. In other cases the special group features are of much more importance. For example, in many "process" groups informed by psychoanalytic theory, the main focus is on the interpersonal determinants of psychopathology, and the goal of therapy is to understand and ultimately modify relationships among group members. Thus, models of group psychotherapy can be situated along the continuum from individual therapy conducted in a group format, at one end, to treatment focused almost solely on the interaction among group members, at the other end.

Psychotherapy groups are used to teach skills (e.g., in DBT), to enhance the structured treatment of an acute episode of illness through the support of other patients (e.g., substance abuse groups), to provide support to patients during periods of relative remission (thus reducing treatment costs while offering patients the opportunity to help one another), and to modify ineffective relationship styles among individuals with significant personality pathology. Some individuals with personality disorders are better treated in groups than individually. In groups the interpersonal "data" are immediately available in the session, and the therapist's conceptualization can be informed by more than the developing transference and the patient's possibly distorted reports of interactions that occur outside of therapy. As well, the presence of multiple individuals in the therapy session makes it more likely that a particularly apt conflict (or transference) will develop.

More generally, groups have the advantage over individual psychotherapy that group members usually engage in less self-denigration after coming to recognize their own problems in other group members. Group members experience decreased isolation and benefit from a sense of solidarity with their peers. In this connection, group members are usually more tolerant of critical **feedback** from peers in the group than they are of similar criticism from therapists, and they are more likely to trust positive **feedback** from peers than from therapists, who, they think, "are just saying that because they're supposed to." Group members may be more inclined actually to make a behavior change they have discussed with the group than they would be if they had only committed to an individual therapist to make the change. Indeed, *group cohesion* can be viewed as the analogue to therapeutic alliance in individual therapy in its effect on outcome, in that cohesion and alliance predict to outcome at about the same rate. In a pair of meta-analyses published in 2011, the cohesion–outcome correlation in group psychotherapy was $r = .25$ (Burlingame, McClendon, & Alonso, 2011), and the alliance–outcome correlation in individual psychotherapy was $r = .275$ (Horvath et al., 2011).

Treatment Strategies

Psychotherapy groups are usually scheduled to last from 90 to 180 minutes. Groups can be open or closed. In open groups, which are not typically time-limited, one or two new members may be introduced at intervals, often around the time that an existing member or two leave the group. By contrast, once a closed group is started, no new members are admitted. Closed groups are usually time-limited, even if the length of the group may not be known from the outset. Psychotherapy groups may be run by a single therapist, but most group therapists prefer to work in pairs, given the multitude of member-specific issues that can arise and the complexity of members' interactions. Group psychotherapy may be the primary psychosocial treatment offered to a patient, or it may be a secondary treatment that is designed to augment other treatment modalities.

The exigencies of the group format lead to the use of treatment strategies that differ in certain respects from those used in individual psychotherapy. Almost all group therapists have the goal of encouraging cohesion among the members. Of course, group therapists offer responses to the verbalizations or other behavior of individual group members. However, they may also respond to the behavior of the group as a whole, for example by commenting on the group's apparent discomfort with silence, on members' willingness to challenge one another, on the effect on the group when members are absent, and so forth. In this sense therapists intervene with the entire group, rather than to direct each intervention to one member or another. Group therapists "hang back" more frequently than do individual therapists, which encourages group members to assume responsibility to help one another, rather than to depend solely on the therapist. Group therapists may also encourage one group member to respond to another's comments, as a way to encourage members to interact and, ideally, to cause group members to provide one another with useful feedback that the therapist would otherwise have to offer. If group therapists teach a specific skill, they do so to the entire group. The resulting discussion in the group is often more illuminating than would be the case if the therapist and an individual patient were the only ones talking about the skill.

Research Findings

In 1998 McRoberts, Burlingame, and Hoag published a meta-analysis that included 23 studies, each of which directly compared the outcome of group psychotherapy with the outcome of individual psychotherapy. They concluded that group and individual psychotherapy had essentially equivalent outcomes. Other meta-analyses of group psychotherapy alone have shown that its effectiveness is in the same range as that of individual psychotherapy. In two meta-analyses group psychotherapy based on the principles of CBT was more effective than groups based on other treatment models, but a third meta-analysis did not find such a difference. More generally, there has been little evidence to support the proposition that psychotherapy groups in which group-specific elements are of limited importance differ in effectiveness from groups that substantially emphasize member interaction and "group process." It is also important to recognize that certain individuals may have worse outcomes with group therapy, such as children with conduct disorder who may engage in worse behaviors due to negative peer influences.

Case Example

Ulrich is a 52-year-old, divorced father of one adult child. An actuary for a large insurance underwriter, Ulrich has received 92 sessions of individual psychodynamic psychotherapy for treatment of persistent depressive disorder and avoidant personality disorder. Over the course of treatment Ulrich and his therapist have identified the fear that if he permits himself to feel his emotions or to interact directly with others, he will be flooded with distress and is likely to be rejected by others. Ulrich and his therapist have concluded that this belief results from his childhood circumstances. The middle of five children, Ulrich was largely ignored by his harried, working-class parents, and when he did seek nurturance or other attention from his parents or siblings, he perceived that family members ignored him. If he pushed harder for attention, family members often responded with overt annoyance. Ultimately, Ulrich made his peace by asking little of others and by repressing awareness of his feelings.

After nearly two years of individual treatment Ulrich has begun to feel better. His mood has lifted somewhat, he has become more active in his free time, and he has begun to think about dating. However, he remains worried that he will again be disappointed in love, as happened in his marriage, and he says he isn't sure it's worth the risk. He and his individual therapist decide to end their work together, and Ulrich is referred to an open psychotherapy group that meets for two hours every Wednesday evening. The group has two leaders and consists of six other members, most of whom have some combination of depression, anxiety, and Cluster C personality disorders.

Before starting in the group, Ulrich meets with Dr. Morris, the primary therapist. She explains that an advanced graduate student will serve as her co-therapist but will rotate out at the end of this year, at which point another student will rotate into the group for a year's placement. Dr. Morris explains the format and expectations for the group, and she makes the point that Ulrich should plan to attend the group for at least three months before deciding whether it is likely to help him. As well, she stresses the importance of regular group attendance, noting that when Ulrich misses an individual appointment, the only cost is to him, but when he misses a group appointment, it adversely affects everyone in the group. Almost apologetically, Ulrich replies, "I'll try not to miss. I'm usually pretty organized about my appointments."

In his first group session Ulrich is introduced to the other group members and is told that he needn't speak in this session unless he wishes to. Ulrich decides not to speak up, but toward the end of the session he finds himself offering some practical advice to a group member who happens to bring up the topic of life insurance. Over the course of the next few sessions Ulrich becomes increasingly comfortable in the group. He is struck that neither Dr. Morris nor the student seems to do much in the group, and they certainly say less than his individual therapist did. For the most part, the group leaders encourage group members to talk to one another, and they occasionally comment on issues *between* group members, rather than to offer advice or interpretation regarding personal issues raised by any group member. Ulrich has the thought that the group might not help him so much with his thoughts and feelings but could be very helpful in working on relationship issues.

By his second month in the group Ulrich is surprised at his level of interest in the lives of the other group members, and he makes occasional supportive comments about the stories they tell. However, sometimes there is tension in the group between two particular members, and at such times Ulrich says nothing. Dr. Morris comments once or twice on the way Ulrich becomes quiet in the face of confrontation, and this leads to a discussion of what each group member feels when tension rises in the session. Ulrich is interested to learn that everyone reports feeling uncomfortable, much as he does, but some group members comment that they feel better if they engage irritable group members, rather than passively to hang back.

On another occasion, Ulrich talks about a minor conflict at work, and one of the group members disagrees with Ulrich's view of the matter, suggesting that Ulrich had unreasonable expectations of his coworker. Ulrich immediately agrees with the other group member and says he was probably too aggressive with the coworker. This leads to further discussion in the group when still another member points out that Ulrich didn't even tell his coworker how he felt. Again, the group discusses Ulrich's fear of unpleasant affect and avoidance of conflict.

In subsequent sessions group members urge Ulrich to speak up more, and when he seems to avoid conflict, they point it out to him. One group member begins going out of his way to argue with Ulrich, imagining that this is helping him, but Dr. Morris intervenes to suggest that it might be enough for group members just to say what they really feel, rather than to help one another "more actively."

Ulrich remains in the psychotherapy group for three years. Over the course of treatment he observes other group members speaking directly to one another and also letting the group know their feelings of pain, sadness, and fear. Gradually, Ulrich finds himself to be more willing to speak up about his most private thoughts and feelings. The group remains interested in and supportive of Ulrich throughout. He is surprised to recognize that when he talks about his fears and anxieties, he actually feels better afterwards.

Without particularly realizing it, Ulrich begins taking more risks outside of group to speak up and to acknowledge his own feelings, both to himself and to the people who are close to him. He begins dating a woman, and a few months later he decides that he is ready to take a break from treatment. After discussing this in the group for a month, Ulrich discontinues treatment. Afterwards, he very much misses the weekly group sessions and wonders what has happened to the other people he came to know so well. On the other hand, he's pleased to have back his Wednesday evenings.

Mindfulness-Based Cognitive Therapy (MBCT)

Model of Psychopathology

MBCT is a third-wave behavioral group-based treatment that emphasizes the use of mindfulness as a means to prevent relapse/recurrence in individuals with chronic depression. MBCT is based on the idea that the experience of repeated depressive episodes leads one to engage in self-devaluation in response to mildly depressed mood. While individuals who have never had a major depressive episode can usually distance themselves from dysphoric mood, those with a history of serious depression are likely to respond to a drop in mood by engaging in self-devaluation, which leads to worse mood and still more self-devaluation, until at last a full-fledged depressive relapse occurs. MBCT targets the interplay between low mood and self-devaluation. While CBT helps people to modify thoughts that are inaccurate or lack utility, MBCT aims to *change the individual's relationship to dysphoric thoughts*, teaching the individual to respond in a decentered manner to these thoughts. MBCT participants are also given extensive information regarding relapse in depression, with the instruction that they apply their newly acquired **mindfulness** skills to cope with potential relapse triggers.

Treatment Strategies

MBCT was adapted from mindfulness-based stress reduction, with the intent to increase its relevance for chronically depressed individuals in remission. Following an individual orientation session, MBCT participants attend eight weekly two-hour group sessions in which they are exposed to a variety of meditation techniques and are asked to practice meditation at home every day. Group leaders, who follow a treatment manual, are skilled in **mindfulness** and consistently model this for the group. MBCT group participants are encouraged to face and accept uncomfortable thoughts, even as they remain aware of the fact that these mental phenomena are transitory and lack palpable reality. Participants are urged to identify and to "nip in the bud" any signs of relapse/recurrence, including thoughts, feelings and physical sensations. They also devise individualized plans to deal with impending relapse; such plans might include seeking support from family members, increasing activities that improve mood, and the like. After the weekly group has ended, two to four follow-up meetings are arranged in the first 6 to 12 months after treatment.

Research Findings

There have been several RCTs from various laboratories that have shown MBCT plus treatment as usual to be more effective than treatment as usual alone in preventing relapse/recurrence among remitted individuals with a history of chronic depression (Godfrin & van Heeringen, 2010). However, individuals who have had only one or two previous episodes of depression do not appear to benefit from MBCT (Piet & Hougaard, 2011). Some findings suggest that MBCT is more effective with individuals who have a ruminative style (Ramel, Goldin, Carmona, & McQuaid, 2004). A recent meta-analysis concluded that individuals with a history of at least three depressive episodes have a 43% decreased risk of a future relapse as a consequence of participating in MBCT (Piet & Hougaard, 2011). However, there are a few data to suggest that relapses are simply *delayed* following MBCT participation (Bondolfi et al., 2010). Some recent studies have shown that MBCT may be helpful in the treatment of individuals with anxiety (Kim et al., 2009) and perhaps also with those with treatment-resistant depression (Eisendrath et al., 2008).

Case Example
Valerie is a 51-year-old, married mother of two children who has had six major depressive episodes in her life, beginning after her older child was born 26 years ago. Four of the depressive episodes have occurred in the last ten years, and most recently she attained remission eight months ago following a five-month episode. She is currently maintained on antidepressant medication, and although she reports episodic mild dysphoria on some days, she says that her general mood is euthymic. She works full-time on night shift as a licensed practical nurse at a long-term care facility.

Valerie had a difficult childhood. The eldest of four children, she grew up in straitened circumstances and was primarily responsible for raising her younger siblings, since her parents drank heavily and were often unavailable. In high school she was raped by one of her father's friends. As an adult, she has tended to ruminate about what she views as her shortcomings and inadequacies, and she avoids talking about her childhood. However, she has a good marriage, her children are doing reasonably well, and she has maintained consistent employment for many years.

Valerie has been referred for participation in an MBCT group as an adjunctive treatment to decrease her risk for relapse into depression. She is initially seen for an individual session by the group leader, Dr. Newell. He reviews Valerie's history and explains to her what to expect in the MBCT group.

In the first of eight two-hour group sessions Dr. Newell again explains to Valerie (and the seven other group members) the basic tenets of MBCT, stressing the idea that to decrease the risk of relapse, individuals with a history of depression can benefit from learning to experience their thoughts and feelings in a new way. At this session, and in each subsequent session, Dr. Newell introduces the group to a different meditation technique (body scan, various breathing techniques, compassion, and so forth), and he encourages group members to practice the newly introduced technique daily during the ensuing week. At each session Dr. Newell also discusses topics relevant to depression relapse, such as willingness to change, rumination, focus on pleasant/unpleasant events, coping with stress, viewing thoughts as thoughts, and others. These topics are linked back to the meditation practice, and direct reference is made to Buddhist concepts like suffering and impermanence. Dr. Newell encourages group members to respond to depressive ruminations in a decentered way, recognizing that they are just thoughts and don't necessarily reflect reality. Throughout treatment Valerie and other group members are encouraged to discuss the challenges they face in daily meditation practice, and group members provide support and advice to one another about overcoming barriers to practice. Toward the end of the group, Dr. Newell assists Valerie and other members in developing a specific and personalized relapse-prevention plan.

Following the eight weekly sessions, Dr. Newell schedules several follow-up sessions at three-month intervals. At those sessions group members discuss how they have coped with their mood, review relevant relapse-related topics, and practice meditation together.

Family Therapy

Model of Psychopathology

There are many models of psychotherapy in which services are provided directly to couples (once known as "marital counseling"), to families as a whole, or to the parents of children with behavior problems. Family therapies are similar to one another in that virtually all family therapists carefully consider the effect of the larger environment in which the family is situated, and these therapists usually consider the ways in which current family members are affected by previous family constellations. In particular, family therapists consider how parents may have been influenced by the families in which they themselves were raised. Family therapies differ according to the models on which they are based. Some family interventions are based rather directly on extensions of psychodynamic or behavioral principles to which we have already referred in this text. Other interventions for couples and families are based on a different theory altogether and are referred to as *systems therapies*.

System therapies take as their starting point the idea that families function as self-correcting systems. It is posited that families have something like a thermostat, as a consequence of which they return to a set point through a negative feedback loop. Thus, if one family member begins to behave in a new way, other family members will, without necessarily knowing why, act in such a way as to force the changing member to revert to the old behavior. The theory underlying systems therapies ties together individual symptoms, family structure, and communication patterns. Problematic behaviors and the network of family relationships are viewed as two sides of the same coin. The symptoms of family members preserve the network of relationships, and if family members begin relating to one another in a new way, the symptoms of individual family members will also change. Because relationships and communication patterns are closely tied, systems therapists pay careful attention to communication within the family. They believe that family power relationships may be difficult for the outsider to discern but can be understood by analyzing the structure of the participants' communication with one another. They further believe that family members transmit messages by overt communication and also when they fail to communicate.

Treatment Strategies

We provide here a few examples of family interventions, organized by their underlying theories. Among interventions strongly influenced by psychoanalytic theory is attachment-based family therapy, an intervention for the families of depressed adolescents. It emphasizes attachment issues and aims to build trust between adolescents and their parents. Object relations couples therapy, an example of psychodynamically informed couples therapy, is an intervention that generally lasts about two years in which the therapist takes a somewhat passive role but does offer **interpretations** of each partner's defenses against intimacy.

Interventions based on behavioral principles include various approaches to altering the environmental or interpersonal reinforcement of problematic behavior. The behavioral family therapist pays particular attention to self-reinforcing cycles, in which one family member behaves in such a way as to reinforce (often unintentionally) another family member's undesirable behavior, and that undesirable behavior has the effect in turn of reinforcing the first family member's behavior. For example, a parent may respond to an adolescent's wish for privacy by becoming suspicious and therefore more intrusive. Of course, the parent's behavior is likely to drive the adolescent further away, which in turn raises the parent's anxiety, causing the parent to become even more intrusive, thus creating a vicious cycle. The behavioral therapist also attends to the relevant cognitions of each family member; the therapist may challenge the beliefs or ideas that lead family members to behave ineffectively. Thus, when one parent undercuts the other parent's discipline as a way to maintain intimacy with the children, the therapist may suggest other ways to improve communication that are less likely to confuse and alienate the children.

Behavioral interventions have had particular success in the treatment of externalizing children through teaching parents better child-management skills. There are several manualized programs for this purpose, and they typically include modules on **behavior monitoring** to track problem behaviors, as well as modules on positive reinforcement to increase desirable behaviors and on **extinction** (e.g., time-out procedures) to decrease undesirable behaviors. Such treatment sometimes includes live coaching sessions, in which the therapist observes the parent implementing a new skill with a child and provides immediate suggestions about how to improve the parent's performance. Parent-Child Interaction Therapy is a widely accepted and well-researched behavioral intervention that involves such live coaching.

There are also a number of behavioral approaches to couples therapy. These typically involve teaching partners specific skills, such as assertive behavior, responding empathically, and negotiation skills. Couples may also be challenged regarding cognitions that have a negative effect on the relationship, such as one partner's belief that the other would rather win arguments than solve problems or a partner's belief that compromise means that no one will be happy in the end. Behavioral couples therapists pay attention to self-reinforcing negative cycles and attempt to replace these with positive cycles. For example, one partner may complain about the other's over-involvement in outside activities. It may develop that the over-involvement represents a kind of avoidance, and the wish to avoid is made worse by the frequent complaints. Therefore, the therapist might encourage the abandoned partner to decrease complaints about the other's outside activities and instead to reinforce the partner during the time that they do spend together.

Systems family therapies often involve attempts on the part of the therapist to strengthen the hierarchy within the family, either directly or through the assignment of behavioral tasks that lead to clearer structure within the family. Treatment focuses squarely on present (not past) interactions, and systems therapists employ a variety of techniques that are intended to destabilize family members' entrenched understanding of their problems— and, equivalently, the current power structure. The therapist may **reframe** undesirable behaviors in such a way that the family thinks differently about them—for example, describing heated arguments as evidence of intimacy within the family. In some instances paradoxical interventions are utilized, in which the therapist may ask family members to exhibit more of the problematic behavior or may discourage the family from using preferred methods to stop escalating conflict. Systems approaches have also been applied to interventions for couples. Again, the therapist's interventions may be paradoxical or may be designed to disrupt a current pattern of behavior. For example, when one partner accuses the other of dishonest behavior, the therapist asks the one being accused to exhibit more of the suspicious behavior (e.g., unexplained telephone conversations) between sessions, while the accuser keeps track of all such behavior and is then asked to guess which suspicious behavior is "real" and which feigned.

There are a number of family psychotherapies that are based on models integrating psychodynamic, behavioral, and/or systems approaches. For example, functional family therapy combines a psychodynamic understanding of family functioning with change techniques that are largely behavioral in nature. In this treatment, aimed primarily at the families of adolescents with externalizing behaviors, the therapist targets specific behaviors and environmental factors for change using standard behavioral interventions but does so in a way that is consistent with family members' understanding of their roles vis-à-vis one another.

One other family intervention of note combines behavioral interventions with substantial amounts of **psychoeducation**, with the intent of increasing periods of remission from schizophrenia. In this intervention, families with a member who has schizophrenia are given a great deal of specific information regarding the course of schizophrenia, in the hope that this will enable family members to respond more effectively to the target family member. Such programs often contain modules on expressed emotionality, in which family members are taught to interact with relatives diagnosed with schizophrenia without becoming overly angry or emotional.

Research Findings

Interventions for families have not been as extensively researched as have individual psychotherapies. However, such research as exists has demonstrated a record of efficacy. The psychodynamically informed attachment-based family therapy was shown to be effective in decreasing anxiety, suicidal ideation, and depressive symptoms on the part of adolescents (Diamond et al., 2010). Behavioral interventions, including particularly child-management training for parents, have demonstrated clear effectiveness in various research studies investigating the decrease of disruptive behavior in preteens (Serketich & Dumas, 1996). In particular, Parent-Child Interaction Therapy has shown probable efficaciousness in the treatment of disruptive behavior among preschoolers (Eyberg, Nelson, & Boggs, 2008). Several integrative family interventions have been shown to be effective with specified populations. In particular, functional family therapy is seen as an evidence-based program for the treatment of adolescents with conduct disorder, substance abuse, and delinquency (Kaslow, Bhaju, & Celano, 2011). Various psychoeducational/behavioral family interventions have been shown to lengthen periods of remission for family members with schizophrenia (McFarlane, Dixon, Lukens, & Lucksted, 2003). By contrast, limited research has investigated the effectiveness of family interventions based on systems theory.

In general, interventions for couples appear to be about as effective as individual psychotherapy, although the lion's share of this research has addressed behaviorally based interventions.

Case Example

Walt and Xenia, the parents of daughters aged one and three, are a married couple in their early thirties. Walt is a computer network technician, and Xenia works as a registered nurse. Married for five years, Walt and Xenia began to experience increased conflict with one another around the time that their younger child was born 15 months ago. They are now requesting couples counseling.

Dr. Philips, a couples therapist knowledgeable about communication skills training (e.g., Guerney, 2005), initially sees Walt and Xenia together for about 20 minutes, at which time he asks them their view of the problem (Xenia: "We stopped being kind to one another." Walt: "And we argue a lot"), and he gathers some background information about the relationship. Dr. Philips then meets with each partner for a 45-minute individual session, in which he gathers personal background information and determines whether either partner has another mental disorder in need of treatment. After he determines that Walt and Xenia are generally doing well, are committed to the relationship, but do have poor communication skills, he lays out a treatment plan to the couple in which he proposes to help them improve their communication skills, as well as to work on conflict resolution. He explains that he will not offer an opinion about how they should resolve their specific problems, because he is sure that they are quite capable of solving problems themselves. He suggests that they don't need advice but might benefit from assistance in knowing *how* to solve problems together. Walt and Xenia indicate that this treatment approach sounds good to them.

In the next session Dr. Philips lays out some communication ground rules. Among other rules, only one partner is to express his or her opinion at a time. The other partner's job is to listen carefully and to repeat back what the speaker said, in the listener's own words. If the speaker indicates that the listener has understood correctly, the speaker may choose to say more or may switch roles with the listener, who now becomes the speaker. The speaker is never permitted to speculate about the listener's state of mind, intent, or emotional experience, and neither speaker nor listener is to use words like "always" and "never." The listener is not permitted to express an opinion about or disagree with the speaker until the speaker indicates that he or she has nothing more to say, at which time the listener becomes the speaker and can express an opinion about the matter at hand.

Dr. Philips helps Walt and Xenia practice these skills over the course of three sessions, gradually moving from topics on which they agree to neutral topics, and then on to minor conflicts. He frequently coaches the couple and reminds them to remain within the speaker/listener framework. He explains that he doesn't expect Walt and Xenia routinely to communicate like this at home, but he does state that eventually they will acquire the habit of talking about serious problems in this way. He suggests they will find that their discussions are much more fruitful when they follow the rules they are learning in couples counseling.

Dr. Philips takes every opportunity to offer praise when the couple succeeds in executing their roles. From time to time he points out communication patterns he notices. For example, Dr. Philips notes that in the role of listener Walt often needs to be reminded not to express his own opinion, while in the role of speaker Xenia is at times difficult to follow. Dr. Philips also helps the couple to agree on several safety mechanisms, including the use of a limited time-out procedure.

In Session 5 Dr. Philips offers some rules about conflict resolution. He explains that this task should not begin until each partner believes that all of his or her feelings about the matter have been fully understood by the other. Then one partner can suggest a resolution, which the couple will modify several times until both partners agree on a solution to the problem, even as they continue to use the speaker/listener format they have employed up to now. Dr. Philips encourages the couple to discuss how the partner who does less to implement the solution can provide assistance to the partner who does more.

At the beginning of any session after which Walt and Xenia settle on a problem solution, Dr. Philips asks about how the solution was implemented. If there were problems, he asks the couple to discuss them within the speaker/listener framework.

Over time Walt and Xenia begin dealing with more and more difficult topics, until at last they are able to talk about issues of sexual intimacy, the interference of Xenia's mother in raising the children, and Walt's sense that Xenia has stopped caring about him.

After 15 sessions Walt and Xenia indicate that they are communicating better and are feeling closer to one another. They and Dr. Philips decide that they no longer need couples counseling sessions. Dr. Philips urges Walt and Xenia always to use the skills they have learned when they find themselves in serious discussions about problems, and they settle on a signal they can use to switch into their speaker/listener roles. Dr. Philips invites them to return for booster sessions in the future, should they feel the need.

Recommended Readings

Barlow, D.H. (Ed.) (2008). *Clinical handbook of psychological disorders: A step-by-step treatment manual* (4th ed.). New York: Guilford Press.

Beck, J.S. (2011). *Cognitive behavior therapy: Basics and beyond* (2nd ed.). New York: Guilford Press.

Frank, E., & Levenson, J.C. (2010). *Interpersonal psychotherapy (Theories of psychotherapy)*. Washington, DC: American Psychological Association.

Gabbard, G. (2005). *Psychodynamic psychiatry in clinical practice* (4th ed.). Arlington, VA: American Psychiatric Publishing.

Linehan, M. (1993). *Cognitive-behavioral treatment of borderline personality disorder*. New York: Guilford Press.

Miller, W.R., & Rollnick, S. (2012). *Motivational interviewing: Helping people change* (3rd ed.). New York: Guilford Press.

Weissman, M.M., Markowitz, J.C., & Klerman, G.L. (2000). *Comprehensive guide to interpersonal psychotherapy*. New York: Basic Books.

Chapter 6

Conclusions

Psychiatry, Psychotherapy, and the Future 250
Anticipations in Neuroscience 252
Anticipations in Psychological Theory 254
Next Steps: Further Training and Self-Study 256

Psychiatry, Psychotherapy, and the Future

The publication of DSM-5 may have some effect on the practice of psychotherapy, but much will remain unchanged. The diagnostic criteria for most major disorders of mood, anxiety, psychosis, and impulse control, as well as other conditions, are not much changed from DSM-IV. It is true that DSM-5 diagnostic criteria have become more specific for a number of disorders, and one expects that this will lead to better results in efficacy studies for psychiatric treatments applied to those conditions—to the extent that such treatments are specific to the conditions in question. However, much of the time psychotherapy targets symptoms rather than disease entities, and our basic understanding of those symptoms is little changed in the transition from DSM-IV to DSM-5.

Looking beyond DSM-5, it seems likely that over time psychiatry will continue to move away from phenomenology and toward biology, and in future diagnostic manuals one anticipates that disease states will be more precisely and biologically defined, yielding the possibility of clearer links between psychological and biological levels of analysis. As we saw in the section on the neurobiological correlates of psychotherapy, there is the potential of improved understanding and probably better psychotherapeutic treatments when the psychology and biology of mental phenomena are examined simultaneously.

Since the 1990s there has been increased focus in the field on the use of empirically supported models of psychotherapy. Notwithstanding objections from those who hold extreme positions favoring the Dodo bird hypothesis, most psychotherapists take the position that patients are more likely to benefit if one provides treatments that have been empirically supported, in comparison to the result one can expect from providing a treatment for which efficacy has not been demonstrated. In this book we have urged that clinicians rely primarily on such empirically supported models of treatment, although we acknowledge that it can be difficult to choose *between* empirically supported treatments for a given condition. Given our current state of knowledge, it is most likely not too important whether one chooses one empirically supported treatment rather than another for any particular condition. We expect that advocates of various psychotherapy models will continue to invest time, money, and energy in demonstrating the efficacy of their preferred treatments, which will serve to widen the choices available to responsible clinicians.

6 CONCLUSIONS

Anticipations in Neuroscience

The increased availability of a wide range of investigative techniques applied to neural function promises to yield some very useful research findings in psychiatry, and these are likely to expand significantly our understanding of mental disorders, leading to useful advances in their treatment. We expect that researchers will be particularly interested in focusing on the intersection between psychological and biological variables in an attempt to understand at a neurobiological level how learning works, the details of implicit memory (with implications for the concept of unconscious motivation), attention and meditative states, the neural representation of interpersonal relationships, and coping strategies such as avoidance, rumination, and the full range of ego psychological defenses. As well, it seems likely that further investigation of the neurobiology of disease states themselves, at all hierarchical levels of brain organization and function, will help in understanding the nature and interrelationships among symptoms of psychopathology, leading to useful speculation about further refinements in psychotherapeutic treatment.

A variable of particular interest is the neurobiology of attachment. In view of the long history of speculation about how this phenomenon affects both intimate and psychotherapeutic relationships, it will be useful to investigate attachment more fully at a neurobiological level. It seems likely that attachment plays a significant role in the placebo response in psychotherapy, in the sense that the patient's view of the therapist as sensitive and supportive, as a "secure base," has the effect of permitting the patient to consider his or her problems more calmly and carefully, even as the patient gains the courage to try out new problem-solving strategies. Some of these new strategies will prove effective, permitting the initiation of a "benign cycle" in the patient's life. We are just beginning to understand interpersonal variables from a neurobiological perspective (cf. the discovery of mirror neurons), and it seems likely that neurobiology can contribute substantially to this area of inquiry, a field on which psychiatrists and psychologists have been toiling for over a century.

Another set of psychological variables we expect will receive the attention of neurobiological researchers consists of the key components of treatment described in unified treatment protocols, such as the one espoused by Barlow and colleagues (2010). This protocol permits the psychotherapist to choose among the interventions of psychoeducation, exposure, increased self-regulation, and changed cognitions. If these targets, especially the last three, can be understood more clearly from a neurobiological perspective, one would expect that the associated interventions can be modified to make them more precise and effective, and the protocol can be expanded to include other psychotherapeutic and somatic interventions. For example, neurobiological findings may enable psychotherapists to optimize exposure trials and may offer useful insights about how to help patients achieve increased self-regulation, notwithstanding difficulties with attention and planning, motivation, and learning.

It bears repeating that psychiatric treatment can only benefit from an increasing rapprochement between psychology and neurobiology. To the extent that psychological variables can be understood neurobiologically and neurobiological variables can be understood psychologically, there is bound to be a more fruitful dialogue than has existed heretofore. The use of these two sets of constructs has led to the development of some very effective interventions in the treatment of mental disorders, and increased cross-fertilization between them will surely improve the quality of the treatments we offer patients.

Anticipations in Psychological Theory

While it is certainly reasonable to wish to relate psychological and psychotherapeutic phenomena to other explanatory variables, as occurs in neuroscience, it is also helpful to continue to investigate psychotherapy at the level of strictly psychological variables. Thus, researchers will continue to "look under the hood" of psychotherapy in an attempt to understand how it works at a psychological level. Some variables of current interest include chronicity, attachment (again), and the identification of coping strategies that are not hijacked in the service of avoidance. One more issue of current interest has to do with the relative virtues of disorder-specific versus principle-driven treatment.

There is increasing evidence that chronicity plays a role in the effectiveness of psychotherapeutic interventions. Many psychotherapies are as effective as somatic interventions in the treatment of first-episode nonpsychotic disorders. Chronic disorders are generally more difficult to treat, although there are now a few models of psychotherapy that are very helpful with these conditions. For example, Mindfulness-Based Cognitive Therapy has been shown to decrease depressive relapse among individuals with multiple previous episodes but has not been shown to be helpful for people who have had just one or two previous episodes. It is known that a subgroup of individuals with only one previous episode of depression, for example, will never have another episode, and it is probably the case that these individuals differ in important ways from those who go on to establish a course of relapse and remission. To the extent that a model of psychotherapy helps people to solve specific emotional problems in their lives, such treatment may be more useful with those whose mental disorders are basically reactive in nature. Thus, one would anticipate the development of treatments that are aimed at either first-episode or more chronic illness, but not both at once.

We return to the variable of attachment yet again, not only because it appears to be an important predictor of behavior over the lifespan, but also because of its similarities with and differences from the therapeutic alliance variable, which is of central interest in psychotherapy in its own right. Unfortunately, it appears that the interaction between the patient's and the therapist's attachment style has a complicated effect on outcome, and this effect may depend on the nature of the treatment in question. It is helpful that there are now data to show that the portion of the patient's attachment predicting to outcome is that which pertains to the expectation of rejection (as versus the desire for closeness), but there obviously remains much more to understand here. It seems likely that attachment may play a different role in different conditions, as a consequence of which the relationship between attachment and outcome will end up being rather complicated. This is an area in which further research is likely to yield valuable insights.

It is becoming increasingly clear that avoidance plays a major role in anxiety and obsessive-compulsive disorders, even if on their face anxiety symptoms, such as chronic rumination, often appear to involve exactly the opposite of avoidance. However, it is now evident that anxious rumination and similar symptoms do represent an avoidance of more distressing anxious thoughts and feelings. For example, it is certainly the case that anxious rumination keeps one in a state of high arousal, and some individuals may intuitively sense that they are "safer" when highly aroused, as if this will prevent them from being ambushed by problems. In other words, rumination can be thought of as a "safety behavior" that protects the individual from having to cope with an unexpected event. The centrality of avoidance in these conditions helps to explain why exposure treatments have been so effective. This represents something of a paradigm shift, since in the past psychotherapy for anxiety and obsessive-compulsive disorders was aimed at providing patients coping skills, such as relaxation techniques, thought stopping, and the like. The challenge now is to determine how to provide useful coping strategies, particularly those that decrease autonomic arousal, in a way that doesn't encourage the patient to use them in the service of avoidance.

Finally, we return to a question we raised earlier: Will future psychotherapists provide treatment based on diagnosis-specific manuals within each theoretical school (psychodynamic, behavioral, and so forth), or will therapists revert to the provision of service based on larger principles? Ultimately, the question is whether effective unified protocols can be developed for more than just a few groups of diagnoses, balancing specificity with generality. The development of such protocols will probably depend on researchers' better understanding of disease states and the psychological factors relevant to each.

Next Steps: Further Training and Self-Study

In Chapter 4 we laid out a plan for learning psychotherapy. To recapitulate, we encouraged you to begin by working to understand the theoretical basis, both psychodynamic and behavioral, that underlies most of psychotherapy, as it is currently practiced. You can obtain this information in this and similar texts. We then encouraged you to locate a partner with whom you could do brief role plays to practice the five basic psychotherapy skills: attending and listening, restatements, questions, showing empathy, and challenges. After that, we suggested that you do longer psychotherapy role plays and that you videotape them for review. At this point, we encouraged you to learn in more detail about one model of psychotherapy by reading an appropriate text. We encouraged that you start with a manualized treatment, such as interpersonal therapy or cognitive-behavior therapy. We suggested that you videotape your sessions (assuming the patient gives all necessary written permissions) and that you review the tapes with a supervisor who is expert in the model of psychotherapy you are delivering, as well as to review the tape with a peer. We encouraged the use of therapist compliance checklists and suggested you set specific behavioral goals for yourself, which you can monitor in every therapy session. After you have treated at least three or four patients using one model of treatment, we suggested you repeat the process for a second model of treatment—and then perhaps a third or fourth.

There are excellent overviews of specific psychotherapy models that cover the theory and practice of treatment in far more depth than is possible in a text like this one. We have listed these references elsewhere in the text. We would also encourage that you obtain copies of several treatment manuals, so that you gain a sense of the session-by-session progression of psychotherapy within several different schools.

References

Abramowitz, J.S. (1997). Effectiveness of psychological and pharmacological treatments of obsessive-compulsive disorder: A quantitative review. *Journal of Consulting and Clinical Psychology, 65*, 45–52.

Ackerman, S.J., & Hilsenroth, M.J. (2001). A review of therapist characteristics and techniques negatively impacting the therapeutic alliance. *Psychotherapy, 38*, 171–185.

Adler, A. (1911). *Zur Kritik der Freudschen Sexualtheorie des Seelenlebens/A critical review of the Freudian sexual theory of psychic life*. Retrieved from: http://www.textlog.de/adler-psychologie-kritik-sexualtheorie-seelenlebens.html

Alberti, R.E., & Emmons, M.L. (2008). *Your perfect right: Assertiveness and equality in your life and relationships* (9th ed.). Atascadero, CA: Impact Publishers.

Amrhein, P.C. (2004). How does Motivational Interviewing work? What client talk reveals. *Journal of Cognitive Psychotherapy, 18*, 323–336.

Andrusyna, T.P., Luborsky, L., Pham, T., & Tang, T.Z. (2006). The mechanisms of sudden gains in supportive-expressive therapy for depression. *Psychotherapy Research, 16*, 526–535.

Apfel, B.A., Ross, J., Hlavin, J., Meyerhoff, D.J., Metzler, T.J., Marmar, C.R., Weiner, M.W., Schuff, N., & Neylan, T.C. (2011). Hippocampal volume differences in Gulf War veterans with current versus lifetime posttraumatic stress disorder symptoms. *Biological Psychiatry, 69*, 541–548.

Baddeley, A. (2000). The episodic buffer: A new component of working memory? *Trends in Cognitive Science, 4*, 417–423.

Baldwin, S.A., Berkeljon, A., Atkins, D.C., Olsen, J.A., & Nielsen, S.L. (2009). Rates of change in naturalistic psychotherapy: Contrasting dose-effect and good-enough level models of change. *Journal of Consulting and Clinical Psychology, 77*, 203–211.

Baldwin, S.A., Wampold, B.E., & Imel, Z.E. (2007). Untangling the alliance-outcome correlation: Exploring the relative importance of therapist and patient variability in the alliance. *Journal of Consulting and Clinical Psychology, 75*, 842–852.

Barlow, D.H., Craske, M.G., Cerny, J.A., & Klosko, J.S. (1989). Behavioral treatment of panic disorder. *Behavior Therapy, 20*, 261–282.

Barlow, D.H., Ellard, K.K., Fairholme, C.P., Farchione, T.J., Boisseau, C.L., Ehrenreich May, J.T., & Allen, L.B. (2010). *Unified protocol for transdiagnostic treatment of emotional disorders: Workbook*. New York: Oxford University Press.

Bateman, A., & Fonagy, P. (2008). 8-year follow-up of patients treated for borderline personality disorder: Mentalization-based treatment versus treatment as usual. *American Journal of Psychiatry, 165*, 631–638.

Bateman, A., & Fonagy, P. (2009). Randomized controlled trial of outpatient mentalization-based treatment versus structured clinical management for borderline personality disorder. *American Journal of Psychiatry, 166*, 1355–1364.

Beck, A.T. (1979). *Cognitive therapy of depression*. New York: Guilford Press.

Beck, J.S. (2011). *Cognitive behavior therapy: Basics and beyond* (2nd ed.). New York: Guilford Press.

Blais, M.A., Malone, J.C., Stein, M.B., Slavin-Mulford, J., O'Keefe, S.M., Renna, M., & Sinclair, S.J. (2013). Treatment as usual (TAU) for depression: A comparison of psychotherapy, pharmacotherapy, and combined treatment at a large academic medical center. *Psychotherapy, 50*, 101–118.

Blomberg, J., Lazar, A., & Sandell, R. (2001). Long-term outcome of long-term psychoanalytically oriented therapists: First findings of the Stockholm Outcome of Psychotherapy and Psychoanalysis study. *Psychotherapy Research, 11*, 361–382.

Bondolfi, G., Jermann, F., van der Linden, M., Gex-Fabry, M., Bizzini, L., Rouget, B.W., Myers-Arrazola, L, Gonzalez, C., Segal, Z., Aubry, J.-M., & Bertschy, G. (2010). Depression relapse prophylaxis with mindfulness-based cognitive therapy: Replication and extension in the Swiss health care system. *Journal of Affective Disorders, 122*, 224–231.

Börne, L. (1840). *Gesammelte Schiften/Collected works*. Hamburg, Germany: Hoffmann & Campe.

Bratton, S.C., Ray, D., Rhine, T., & Jones, L. (2005). The efficacy of play therapy with children: A meta-analytic review of treatment outcomes. *Professional Psychology: Research and Practice, 36*, 376–390.

Breuer, J., & Freud, S. (1895/2000). *Studies on hysteria*. New York: Basic Books.

Buchheim, A., Viviani, R., Kessler, H., Kächele, H., Cierpka, M., Roth, G., George, C., Kernberg, O.F., Bruns, G., & Taubner, S. (2012). Changes in prefrontal-limbic function in major depression after 15 months of long-term psychotherapy. *PLoS ONE, 7*, Article e33745.

Burlingame, G.M., McClendon, D.T., & Alonso, J. (2011). Cohesion in group psychotherapy. In J.C. Norcross (Ed.), *Psychotherapy relationships that work: Evidence-based responsiveness* (2nd ed., pp. 110–131). New York: Oxford University Press.

Butler, A.J., & James, K.H. (2010). The neural correlates of attempting to suppress negative versus neutral memories. *Cognitive, Affective, & Behavioral Neuroscience, 10*, 182–194.

Casacalenda, N., Perry, J.C., & Looper, K. (2002). Remission in major depressive disorder: A comparison of pharmacotherapy, psychotherapy, and control conditions. *American Journal of Psychiatry, 159*, 1354–1360.

Castonguay, L.G., Goldfried, M.R., Wiser, S., Raue, P.J., & Hayes, A.M. (1996). Predicting the effect of cognitive therapy for depression: A study of unique and common factors. *Journal of Consulting and Clinical Psychology, 64*, 497–504.

Chiesa, A., Brambilla, P., & Serretti, A. (2010). Functional neural correlates of mindfulness meditations in comparison with psychotherapy, pharmacotherapy and placebo effect. Is there a link? *Acta Neuropsychiatrica, 22*, 104–117.

Clark, D.A., & Beck, A.T. (2010). Cognitive theory and therapy of anxiety and depression: Convergence with neurobiological findings. *Trends in Cognitive Science, 14*, 418–424.

Clarkin, J.F., Levy, K.N., Lenzenweger, M.F., & Kernberg, O.F. (2007). Evaluating three treatments for borderline personality disorder: A multiwave study. *American Journal of Psychiatry, 164*, 922–928.

Constantino, M.J., Glass, C.R., Arnkoff, D.B., Ametrano, R.M., & Smith, J.Z. (2011). Expectations. In J.C. Norcross (Ed.), *Psychotherapy relationships that work: Evidence-based responsiveness* (2nd ed., pp. 354–376). New York: Oxford University Press.

Craske, M.G., Brown, T.A., & Barlow, D.H. (1991). Behavioral treatment of panic disorder: A two-year follow-up. *Behavior Therapy, 22*, 289–304.

Craske, M.G., Lang, A.J., Aikins, D., & Mystkowski, J.L. (2005). Cognitive behavioral therapy for nocturnal panic. *Behavior Therapy, 36*, 43–54.

Cuijpers, P., Dekker, J., Hollon, S.D., & Andersson, G. (2009). Adding psychotherapy to pharmacotherapy in the treatment of depressive disorders in adults: A meta-analysis. *Journal of Clinical Psychiatry, 70*, 1219–1229.

Cuijpers, P., Driessen, E., Hollon, S.D., van Oppen, P., Barth, J., & Andersson, G. (2012). The efficacy of non-directive supportive therapy for adult depression: A meta-analysis. *Clinical Psychology Review, 32*, 280–291.

Cuijpers, P., Geraedts, A.S., van Oppen, P., Andersson, G., Markowitz, J.C., & van Straten A. (2011). Interpersonal psychotherapy for depression: A meta-analysis. *American Journal of Psychiatry, 168*, 581–592.

Cuijpers, P., Reynolds, C.F., Donker, T., Li, J., Andersson, G., & Beekman, A. (2012). Personal treatment of adult depression: Medication, psychotherapy, or both? A systematic review. *Depression and Anxiety, 29*, 855–864.

Cuijpers, P., van Straten, A., Schuurmans, J., van Oppen, P., Hollon, S.D., & Andersson, G. (2010). Psychotherapy for chronic major depression and dysthymia: A meta-analysis. *Clinical Psychology Review, 30*, 51–62.

Cuijpers, P., van Straten, A., van Oppen, P., & Andersson, G. (2010). Comparing psychotherapy and pharmacotherapy for adult depression: Adjusting for differential dropout rates. *Journal of Clinical Psychiatry, 71*, 1246.

Curry, J.F., & Becker, S.J. (2008). Empirically supported psychotherapies for adolescent depression and mood disorders. In R.G. Steele, T.D. Elkin, & M.C. Roberts (Eds.), *Handbook of evidence-based treatments of children and adolescents: Bridging science and practice. Issues in clinical child psychology*. (pp. 161–176). New York: Springer Science + Business Media.

De Maat, S., Dekker, J., Schoevers, R., & De Jonghe, F. (2006). Relative efficacy of psychotherapy and pharmacotherapy in the treatment of depression: A meta-analysis. *Psychotherapy Research, 16*, 562–572.

De Maat, S., Dekker, J., Schoevers, R., van Aalst, G., Gijsbers-van Wijk, C., Hendriksen, M., Kool, S., Peen, J., Van, R., & de Jonghe, F. (2008). Short psychodynamic supportive psychotherapy, antidepressants, and their combination in the treatment of major depression: A mega-analysis based on three randomized clinical trials. *Depression and Anxiety, 25*, 565–574.

De Maat, S., de Jonghe, F., Schoevers, R., & Dekker, J. (2009). The effectiveness of long-term psychoanalytic therapy: A systematic review of empirical studies. *Harvard Review of Psychiatry, 17*, 1–23.

DeRubeis, R.J., Gelfand, L.A., Tang, T.Z., & Simons, A.D. (1999). Medications versus cognitive behavior therapy for severely depressed outpatients: Mega-analysis of four randomized comparisons. *American Journal of Psychiatry*, 156, 1007–1013.

Diamond, G.S., Wintersteen, M.B., Brown, G.K., Diamond, G.M., Gallop, R., Shelef, K., & Levy, S. (2010). Attachment-based family therapy for adolescents with suicidal ideation: A randomized controlled trial. *Journal of the American Academy of Child and Adolescent Psychiatry*, 49, 122–131.

Diener, S.J., Wessa, M., Ridder, S., Lang, S., Diers, M., Steil, R., & Flor, H. (2012). Enhanced stress analgesia to a cognitively demanding task in patients with posttraumatic stress disorder. *Journal of Affective Disorders*, 136, 1247–1251.

Doering, S., Hörz, S., Rentrop, M., Fischer-Kern, M., Schuster, P., Benecke, C., Buchheim, A., Martius, P., & Buchheim P. (2010). Transference-focused psychotherapy v. treatment by community psychotherapists for borderline personality disorder: Randomised controlled trial. *British Journal of Psychiatry*, 196, 389–395.

Driessen, E., & Hollon, S.D. (2010). Cognitive behavioral therapy for mood disorders: Efficacy, moderators and mediators. *Psychiatric Clinics of North America*, 33, 537–555.

Eisenberger, N.I., Master, S.L., Inagaki, T.K., Taylor, S.E., Shirinyan, D., Lieberman, M.D., & Naliboff, B.D. (2011). Attachment figures activate a safety signal-related neural region and reduce pain experience. *PNAS Proceedings of the National Academy of Sciences of the United States of America*, 108, 11721–11726.

Eisendrath, S.J., Delucchi, K., Bitner, R., Fenimore, P., Smit, M., & McLane, M. (2008). Mindfulness-based cognitive therapy for treatment-resistant depression: A pilot study. *Psychotherapy and Psychosomatics*, 77, 319–320.

Elkin, I., Gibbons, R.D., Shea, M.T., & Shaw, B.F. (1996). Science is not a trial (but it can sometimes be a tribulation). *Journal of Consulting and Clinical Psychology*, 64, 92–103.

Erikson, E.H. (1964). *Insight and responsibility*. New York: Norton.

Eyberg, S.M., Nelson, M.M., & Boggs, S.R. (2008). Evidence-based psychosocial treatments for children and adolescents with disruptive behavior. *Journal of Clinical Child and Adolescent Psychology*, 37, 215–237.

Eysenck, H.J. (1952). The effects of psychotherapy: An evaluation. *Journal of Consulting Psychology*, 16, 319–324.

Fairburn, C.G. (1998). Interpersonal psychotherapy for bulimia nervosa. In J.C. Markowitz (Ed.), *Interpersonal psychotherapy. Review of psychiatry series* (pp. 99–128). Arlington, VA: American Psychiatric Association.

Farchione, T.J., Fairholme, C.P., Ellard, K.K., Boisseau, C.L., Thompson-Hollands, J., Carl, J.R., Gallagher, M.W., & Barlow, D.H. (2012). Unified protocol for transdiagnostic treatment of emotional disorders: A randomized controlled trial. *Behavior Therapy*, 43, 666–678.

Farsimadan, F., Draghi-Lorenz, R., & Ellis, J. (2007). Process and outcome of therapy in ethnically similar and dissimilar therapeutic dyads. *Psychotherapy Research*, 17, 567–575.

Felmingham, K., Kemp, A.H., Williams, L., Falconer, E., Olivieri, G., Peduto, A., & Bryant, R. (2008). Dissociative responses to conscious and non-conscious fear impact underlying brain function in post-traumatic stress disorder. *Psychological Medicine, 38*, 1771–1780.

Ferenczi, S. (1934). Thalassa: A theory of genitality. *Psychoanalytic Quarterly, 3*, 1–29.

Ferenczi, S., & Rank, O. (1925). *The development of psycho-analysis*. New York: Nervous and Mental Disease Publication Co.

Foa, E.B., Liebowitz, M.R., Kozak, M.J., Davies, S., Campeas, R., Franklin, M.E., Huppert, J.D., Kjernisted, K., Rowan, V., Schmidt, A.B., Simpson, H.B., & Tu, X. (2005). Randomized, placebo-controlled trial of exposure and ritual prevention, clomipramine, and their combination in the treatment of obsessive-compulsive disorder. *American Journal of Psychiatry, 162*, 151–161.

Foa, E.B., & Meadows, E.A. (1997). Psychosocial treatments for post-traumatic stress disorder: A critical review. *Annual review of psychology, 48*, 449–480.

Frank, E., Kupfer, D.J., Thase, M.E., Mallinger, A.G., Swartz, H.A., Fagiolini, A.M., Grochocinski, V., Houck, P., Scott, J., Thompson, W., & Monk, T. (2005). Two-year outcomes for Interpersonal and social rhythm therapy in individuals with Bipolar I disorder. *Archives of General Psychiatry, 62*, 996–1004.

Freud, E.L. (Ed.) (1970). *The letters of Sigmund Freud and Arnold Zweig*. London, England: The Hogarth Press.

Freud, S. (1895/1953). Project for a scientific psychology. In J. Strachey (Ed.), *The standard edition of the complete works of Sigmund Freud* (vol. 1, pp. 281–391). London, England: Hogarth Press.

Freud, S. (1896/1953). The etiology of hysteria. In J. Strachey (Ed.), *The standard edition of the complete works of Sigmund Freud* (vol. 3, pp. 189–224). London, England: Hogarth Press.

Freud, S. (1900/1954). Letter of 3.10.97. In *The origins of psycho-analysis: Letters to Wilhelm Fliess, Drafts and Notes: 1887-1902*. New York: Basic Books.

Freud, S. (1900/1955). *The interpretation of dreams*. New York: Basic Books.

Freud, S. (1905/1962). *Three essays on the theory of sexuality*. New York: Basic Books.

Freud, S. (1909/1953). Analysis of a phobia in a five-year-old boy. In J. Strachey (Ed.), *The standard edition of the complete works of Sigmund Freud* (vol. 10, pp. 1–147). London, England: Hogarth Press.

Freud, S. (1912/1953). The dynamics of the transference. In J. Strachey (Ed.), *The standard edition of the complete psychological works of Sigmund Freud* (vol. 12, pp. 99–108). London, England: Hogarth Press.

Freud, S. (1913/1953). On beginning the treatment (Further recommendations on the treatment of psycho-analysis, I). In J. Strachey (Ed.), *The standard edition of the complete psychological works of Sigmund Freud* (vol. 12). London, England: Hogarth Press.

Freud, S. (1916-7/1989). *Introductory lectures on psycho-analysis*. New York: Norton.

Freud, S. (1922/1953). Two encyclopaedia articles. Psycho-analysis. In J. Strachey (Ed.), *The standard edition of the complete psychological works of Sigmund Freud* (vol. 18, pp. 234–255). London, England: Hogarth Press.

Freud S. (1933/1965). *New introductory lectures on psycho-analysis*. New York: Norton.

Freud, S., Jung, C.G., & McGuire, W. (Ed.) (1974). *The Freud/Jung letters: The correspondence between Sigmund Freud and C.G. Jung* (pp. 3–122). Princeton, NJ: Princeton University Press.

Friedman, M.A., Detweiler-Bedell, J.B., Leventhal, H.E., Horne, R., Keitner, G.I., & Miller, I.W. (2004). Combined psychotherapy and pharmacotherapy for the treatment of major depressive disorder. *Clinical Psychology: Science and Practice*, 11, 47–68.

Gay, P. (2006). *Freud: A life for our time*. New York: W.W. Norton & Co.

Giesen-Bloo, J., van Dyck, R., Spinhoven, P., van Tilburg, W., Dirksen, C., van Asselt, T., Kremers, I., Nadort, M., & Arntz, A. (2006). Outpatient psychotherapy for borderline personality disorder: Randomized trial of schema-focused therapy vs transference-focused psychotherapy. *Archives of General Psychiatry*, 63, 649–658.

Gil, P.J.M., Carrillo, F.X.M., & Meca, J.S. (2001). Effectiveness of cognitive-behavioural treatment in social phobia: A meta-analytic review. *Psychology in Spain*, 5, 17–25.

Gilbertson, M.W., Shenton, M.E., Ciszewski, A., Kasai, K., Lasko, N.B., Orr, S.P., & Pitman, R.K. (2002). Smaller hippocampal volume predicts pathologic vulnerability to psychological trauma. *Nature Neuroscience*, 5, 1242–1247.

Godfrin, K.A., & van Heeringen, C. (2010). The effects of mindfulness-based cognitive therapy on recurrence of depressive episodes, mental health and quality of life: A randomized controlled study. *Behaviour Research and Therapy*, 48, 738–746.

Guerney, B. G., Jr. (2005). *Relationship Enhancement couple/marital/family therapist's manual* (4th ed.). Silver Spring, MD: IDEALS, Inc.

Guidi, J., Fava, G.A., Fava, M., & Papakostas, G.I. (2011). Efficacy of the sequential integration of psychotherapy and pharmacotherapy in major depressive disorder: A preliminary meta-analysis. *Psychological Medicine*, 41, 321–331.

Harrington, R., Whittaker, J., Shoebridge, P., & Campbell, F. (1998). Systematic review of efficacy of cognitive behaviour therapies in childhood and adolescent depressive disorder. *BMJ*, 316, 1559–1563.

Hatcher, R.L., & Gillaspy, J.A. (2006). Development and validation of a revised short version of the Working Alliance Inventory. *Psychotherapy Research*, 16, 12–25.

Hayes, J.P., LaBar, K.S., McCarthy, G., Selgrade, E., Nasser, J., Dolcos, F., Morey, R.A., & VISN 6 Mid-Atlantic MIRECC workgroup (2011). Reduced hippocampal and amygdala activity predicts memory distortions for trauma reminders in combat-related PTSD. *Journal of Psychiatric Research*, 45, 660–669.

Henry, W.P., Schacht, T.E., Strupp, H.H., Butler, S.F., & Binder, J.L. (1993). Effects of training in time-limited dynamic psychotherapy: Mediators of therapists' responses to training. *Journal of Clinical and Consulting Psychology*, 61, 441–447.

Hilbert, A., Bishop, M.E., Stein, R.I., Tanofsky-Kraff, M., Swenson, A.K., Welch, R.R., & Wilfley, D.E. (2012). Long-term efficacy of psychological treatments for binge eating disorder. *British Journal of Psychiatry, 200,* 232–237.

Hofmann, S.G., Asnaani, A., Vonk, I.J.J., Sawyer, A.T., & Fang, A. (2012). The efficacy of cognitive behavioral therapy: A review of meta-analyses. *Cognitive Therapy and Research, 36,* 427–440.

Hofmann, S.G., Sawyer, A.T., Korte, K.J., & Smits, J.A. (2009). Is it beneficial to add pharmacotherapy to cognitive-behavioral therapy when treating anxiety disorders? A meta-analytic review. *International Journal of Cognitive Therapy, 2,* 160–175.

Horvath, A.O., Del Re, A.C., Flückiger, C., & Symonds, D. (2011). Alliance in individual psychotherapy. In J.C. Norcross (Ed.), *Psychotherapy relationships that work: Evidence-based responsiveness* (2nd ed., pp. 25–69). New York: Oxford University Press.

Jacobson, N.S., & Hollon, S.D. (1996). Cognitive-behavior therapy versus pharmacotherapy: Now that the jury's returned its verdict, it's time to present the rest of the evidence. *Journal of Consulting and Clinical Psychology, 64,* 74–80.

Jones, E. (1953). *The life and work of Sigmund Freud.* New York: Basic Books.

Joyce, A.S., Ogrodniczuk, J.S., Piper, W.E., & McCallum, M. (2002). A test of the phase model of psychotherapy change. *Canadian Journal of Psychiatry, 47,* 759–766.

Jung, C.G. (1907/1909). *The psychology of dementia praecox.* New York: Nervous and Mental Disease Publishing Co.

Jung, C.G. (1921/1976). Psychological types. In R.F.C. Hull (Ed.), *The collected works of C.G. Jung* (vol. 6). Princeton, NJ: Princeton University Press.

Jung, C.G. (1954/1966). *The practice of psychotherapy: Essays on the psychology of the transference and other subjects* (2nd, augmented ed.). Princeton, NJ: Princeton University Press.

Jung, C.G. (1961/1989). *Memories, dreams, reflections.* New York: Vintage Books.

Kabat-Zinn, J. (1994). *Wherever you go, there you are: Mindfulness meditation in everyday life.* New York: Hyperion.

Kandel, E.R. (1999). Biology and the future of psychoanalysis: A new intellectual framework for psychiatry revisited. *American Journal of Psychiatry, 156,* 505–524.

Karremans, J.C., Heslenfeld, D.J., van Dillen, L.F., & Van Lange, P.A.M. (2011). Secure attachment partners attenuate neural responses to social exclusion: An fMRI investigation. *International Journal of Psychophysiology, 81,* 44–50.

Kaslow, N.J., Bhaju, J., & Celano, M.P. (2011). Family therapies. In S.B. Messer & A.S. Gurman (Eds.), *Essential psychotherapies: Theory and practice* (3rd ed., pp. 297–344). New York: Guilford Press.

Keller, M.B. (2001). Long-term treatment of recurrent and chronic depression. *Journal of Clinical Psychiatry, 62*(24), 3–5.

Keller, M.B., McCullough, J.P., Klein, D.N., Arnow, B., Dunner, D.L., Gelenberg, A.J., Markowitz, J.C., Nemeroff, C.B., Russell, J.M., Thase, M.E., Trivedi, M.H., & Zajecka, J. (2000). A comparison of nefazodone, the cognitive behavioral-analysis system of psychotherapy, and their combination for the treatment of chronic depression. *New England Journal of Medicine, 342,* 1462–1470.

Kennedy, S.H., Konarski, J.Z., Segal, Z.V., Lau, M.A., Bieling, P.J., McIntyre, R.S., & Mayberg, H.S. (2007). Differences in brain glucose metabolism between responders to CBT and venlafaxine in a 16-week randomized controlled trial. *American Journal of Psychiatry, 164*, 778–788.

Kim, Y.W., Lee, S.-H., Choi, T.K., Suh, S.Y., Kim, B., Kim, C.M., Cho, S.J., Kim, M.J., Yook, K., Ryu, M., Song, S.K., & Yook, K.-H. (2009). Effectiveness of mindfulness-based cognitive therapy as an adjuvant to pharmacotherapy in patients with panic disorder or generalized anxiety disorder. *Depression and Anxiety, 26*, 601–606.

Kleim, B., Grey, N., Wild, J., Nussbeck, F.W., Stott, R., Hackmann, A., Clark, D.M., & Ehlers, A. (2013). Cognitive change predicts symptom reduction with cognitive therapy for posttraumatic stress disorder. *Journal of Consulting and Clinical Psychology, 81*, 383–393.

Klein, M. (1919/1923). The development of a child. *International Journal of Psycho-analysis, 4*, 419–474.

Klein, M. (1924). The role of the school in the libidinal development of the child. *International Journal of Psycho-analysis, 5*, 312–331.

Kliem, S., Kröger, C., & Kosfelder, J. (2010). Dialectical behavior therapy for borderline personality disorder: A meta-analysis using mixed-effects modeling. *Journal of Consulting and Clinical Psychology, 78*, 936–951.

Knekt, P., Lindfors, O., Härkänen, T., Välikoski, M., Virtala, E., Laaksonen, M.A., Marttunen, M., Kaipainen, M., Renlund, C., & the Helsinki Psychotherapy Study Group (2008). Randomized trial on the effectiveness of long- and short-term psychodynamic psychotherapy and solution-focused therapy on psychiatric symptoms during a 3-year follow-up. *Psychological Medicine, 38*, 689–703.

Kröger, C., & Kosfelder, J. (2007). Eine Meta-Analyse zur Wirksamkeit der Dialektisch Behavioralen Therapie bei Borderline-Persönlichkeitsstörungen. / A meta-analysis of the efficacy of dialectical behavior therapy in borderline personality disorder. *Zeitschrift für klinische Psychologie und Psychotherapie: Forschung und Praxis, 36*, 11–17.

Kühn, S., & Gallinat, J. (2013). Gray matter correlates of posttraumatic stress disorder: A quantitative meta-analysis. *Biological Psychiatry, 73*, 70–74.

Kwan, B.M., Dimidjian, S., & Rizvi, S.L. (2010). Treatment preference, engagement, and clinical improvement in pharmacotherapy versus psychotherapy for depression. *Behaviour Research and Therapy, 48*, 799–804.

Lafferty, P., Beutler, L.E., & Crago, M. (1989). Differences between more and less effective psychotherapists: A study of select therapist variables. *Journal of Consulting and Clinical Psychology, 57*, 76–80.

Lambert, M.J., & Shimokawa, K. (2011). Collecting client feedback. In J.C. Norcross (Ed.), *Psychotherapy relationships that work: Evidence-based responsiveness.* (2nd ed., pp. 203–223). New York: Oxford University Press.

Leichsenring, F., & Rabung, S. (2008). Effectiveness of long-term psychodynamic psychotherapy: A meta-analysis. *JAMA: Journal of the American Medical Association, 300*, 1551–1565.

Leichsenring, F., Rabung, S., & Leibing, E. (2004). The efficacy of short-term psychodynamic psychotherapy in specific psychiatric disorders: A meta-analysis. *Archives of General Psychiatry, 61*, 1208–1216.

Lenzi, D., Trentini, C., Pantano, P. Macaluso, E., Lenzi, G.L., & Ammaniti, M. (2013). Attachment models affect brain responses in areas related to emotions and empathy in nulliparous women. *Human Brain Mapping, 34*, 1399–1414.

Levin, F.M. (2011). *Psyche and brain: The biology of talking cures.* London, England: Karnac.

Levy, K.N., Ellison, W.D., Scott, L.N., & Bernecker, S.L. (2011). Attachment style. In J.C. Norcross (Ed.), *Psychotherapy relationships that work: Evidence-based responsiveness* (2nd ed., pp. 377–401). New York: Oxford University Press.

Lilienfeld, S.O. (2007). Psychological treatments that cause harm. *Perspectives on Psychological Science, 2*, 53–70.

Linehan, M.M. (1993). *Skills training manual for treating Borderline personality disorder.* New York: Guilford Press.

Linehan, M.M., Schmidt, H., Dimeff, L.A., Craft, J.C., Kanter, J., & Comtois, K.A. (1999). Dialectical behavior therapy for patients with borderline personality disorder and drug-dependence. *American Journal of Addiction, 8*, 279–292.

Luborsky, L., Diguer, L., Seligman, D.A., Rosenthal, R., Krause, E.D., Johnson, S., Halperin, G., Bishop, M., Berman, J.S., & Schweizer, E. (1999). The researcher's own therapy allegiances: A "wild card" in comparisons of treatment efficacy. *Clinical Psychology: Science and Practice, 6*, 95–106.

Lundahl, B.W., Kunz, C., Brownell, C., Tollefson, D., & Burke, B.L. (2010). A meta-analysis of motivational interviewing: Twenty-five years of empirical studies. *Research on Social Work Practice, 20*, 137–160.

Manber, R., Kraemer, H.C., Arnow, B.A., Trivedi, M.H., Rush, A.J., Thase, M.E., Rothbaum, B.O., Klein, D.N., Kocsis, J.H., Gelenberg, A.J., & Keller, M.E. (2008). Faster remission of chronic depression with combined psychotherapy and medication than with each therapy alone. *Journal of Consulting and Clinical Psychology, 76*, 459–476.

Mann, J. (1980). *Time-limited psychotherapy.* Cambridge, MA: Harvard University Press.

Markowitz, J.C., Kocsis, J.H., Bleiberg, K.L., Christos, P.J., & Sacks, M. (2005). A comparative trial of psychotherapy and pharmacotherapy for "pure" dysthymic patients. *Journal of Affective Disorders, 89*, 167–175.

Markowitz, J.C., Kocsis, J.H., Christos, P., Bleiberg, K., & Carlin, A. (2008). Pilot study of interpersonal psychotherapy versus supportive psychotherapy for dysthymic patients with secondary alcohol abuse or dependence. *Journal of Nervous and Mental Disease, 196*, 468–474.

McFarlane, W.R., Dixon, L., Lukens, E., & Lucksted, A. (2003). Family psychoeducation and schizophrenia: A review of the literature. *Journal of Marital and Family Therapy, 29*, 223–245.

McHugh, R.K., Hearon, B.A., & Otto, M.W. (2010). Cognitive behavioral therapy for substance use disorders. *Psychiatric Clinics of North America, 33*, 511–525.

McRoberts, C., Burlingame, G.M., & Hoag, M.J. (1998). Comparative efficacy of individual and group psychotherapy: A meta-analytic perspective. *Group Dynamics: Theory, Research, and Practice, 2*, 101–117.

Meyer, B., Pilkonis, P.A., Krupnick, J.L., Egan, M.K., Simmens, S.J., & Sotsky, S.M. (2002). Treatment expectancies, patient alliance and outcome:

Further analyses from the National Institute of Mental Health Treatment of Depression Collaborative Research Program. *Journal of Consulting and Clinical Psychology, 70*, 1051–1055.

Mickleborough, M.J.S., Daniels, J.K., Coupland, N.J., Kao, R., Williamson, P.C., Lanius, U.F., Hegadoren, K., Schore, A., Densmore, M., Stevens, T., & Lanius, R.A. (2011). Effects of trauma-related cues on pain processing in posttraumatic stress disorder: An fMRI investigation. *Journal of Psychiatry & Neuroscience, 36*, 6–14.

Mikulincer, M., & Shaver, P.R. (2007). *Attachment in adulthood: Structure, dynamics, and change.* New York: Guilford.

Miller, L., Gur, M., Shanok, A., & Weissman, M. (2008). Interpersonal psychotherapy with pregnant adolescents: Two pilot studies. *Journal of Child Psychology and Psychiatry, 49*, 733–742.

Minami, T., Wampold, B.E., Serlin, R.C., Hamilton, E.G., Brown, G.S., & Kricher, J.C. (2008). Benchmarking the effectiveness of psychotherapy treatment for adult depression in a managed care environment: A preliminary study. *Journal of Consulting and Clinical Psychology, 76*, 116–124.

Munder, T., Flückiger, C., Gerger, H., Wampold, B.E., & Barth, J. (2012). Is the allegiance effect an epiphenomenon of true efficacy differences between treatments? A meta-analysis. *Journal of Counseling Psychology, 59*, 631–637.

Muran, J.C. (2002). A relational approach to understanding change: Plurality and contextualism in a psychotherapy research program. *Psychotherapy Research, 12*, 113–138.

Najavits, L.M., & Strupp, H.H. (1994). Differences in the effectiveness of psychodynamic therapists: A process-outcome study. *Psychotherapy: Theory, Research, Practice, Training, 31*, 114–123.

Nathan, P.E., Stuart, S.P., & Dolan, S.L. (2000). Research on psychotherapy efficacy and effectiveness: Between Scylla and Charybdis? *Psychological Bulletin, 126*, 964–981.

Nielsen, S.L., Smart, D.W., Isakson, R.L., Worthen, V.E., Gregersen, A.T., & Lambert, M.J. (2004). The *Consumer Reports* effectiveness score: What did consumers report? *Journal of Counseling Psychology, 51*, 25–37.

Nissen-Lie, H.A., Monsen, J.T., & Rønnestad, M.H. (2010). Therapist predictors of early patient-rated working alliance: A multilevel approach. *Psychotherapy Research, 20*, 627–646.

Norcross, J.C., & Lambert, M.J. (2011). Evidenced-based therapy relationships. In J.C. Norcross (Ed.), *Psychotherapy relationships that work: Evidence-based responsiveness* (2nd ed., pp. 3–21). New York: Oxford University Press.

O'Hara, M.W., Schiller, C.E., & Stuart, S. (2010). Interpersonal psychotherapy and relapse prevention for depression. In C.S. Richards & M.G. Perry (Eds.), *Relapse prevention for depression* (pp. 77–97). Washington, DC: American Psychological Association.

Oestergaard, S., & Møldrup, C. (2011). Optimal duration of combined psychotherapy and pharmacotherapy for patients with moderate and severe depression: A meta-analysis. *Journal of Affective Disorders, 131*, 24–36.

Olatunji, B.O., Davis, M.L., Powers, M.B., & Smits, J.A.J. (2013). Cognitive-behavioral therapy for obsessive-compulsive disorder: A meta-analysis of treatment outcome and moderators. *Journal of Psychiatric Research, 47*, 33–41.

Olatunji, B.O., Rosenfield, D., Tart, C.D., Cottraux, J., Powers, M.B., & Smits, J.A.J. (2013). Behavioral versus cognitive treatment of obsessive-compulsive disorder: An examination of outcome and mediators of change. *Journal of Consulting and Clinical Psychology, 81*, 415–428.

Olson, M.H., & Hergenhahn, B.R. (2011). *An introduction to theories of personality* (8th ed.). Boston, MA: Prentice-Hall/Pearson.

Otto, M.W., Smits, J.A.J., & Reese, H.E. (2005). Combined psychotherapy and pharmacotherapy for mood and anxiety disorders in adults: Review and analysis. *Clinical Psychology: Science and Practice, 12*, 72–86.

Owen, J., Leach, M.M., Wampold, B., & Rodolfa, E. (2011). Client and therapist variability in clients' perceptions of their therapists' multicultural competencies. *Journal of Counseling Psychology, 58*, 1–9.

Patel, R., Spreng, R.N., Shin, L.M., & Girard, T.A. (2012). Neurocircuitry models of posttraumatic stress disorder and beyond: A meta-analysis of functional neuroimaging studies. *Neuroscience and Biobehavioral Reviews, 36*, 2130–2142.

Piet, J., & Hougaard, E. (2011). The effect of mindfulness-based cognitive therapy for prevention of relapse in recurrent major depressive disorder: A systematic review and meta-analysis. *Clinical Psychology Review, 31*, 1032–1040.

Power, K., McGoldrick, T., Brown, K., Buchanan, R., Sharp, D., Swanson, V., & Karatzias, A. (2002). A controlled comparison of eye movement desensitization and reprocessing versus exposure plus cognitive restructuring versus waiting list in the treatment of posttraumatic stress disorder. *Clinical Psychology and Psychotherapy, 9*, 299–318.

Powers, S.W. (1999). Empirically supported treatments in pediatric psychology: Procedure-related pain. *Journal of Pediatric Psychology, 24*, 131–145.

Ramel, W., Goldin, P.R., Carmona, P.E., & McQuaid, J.R. (2004). The effects of mindfulness meditation on cognitive processes and affect in patients with past depression. *Cognitive Therapy and Research, 28*, 433–455.

Reese, R.J., Toland, M.D., & Hopkins, N.B. (2011). Replicating and extending the good-enough level model of change: Considering session frequency. *Psychotherapy Research, 21*, 608–619.

Reich, W. (1927/1973). *The function of the orgasm*. New York: Farrar, Straus & Giroux.

Reich, W. (1929/1972). *Dialectical materialism and psychoanalysis*. London, England: Socialist Reproduction.

Reich, W. (1949/1972). *Character Analysis* (3rd, enlarged ed.). New York: Farrar, Straus and Giroux.

Renfrey, G., & Spates, C.R. (1994). Eye movement desensitization: A partial dismantling study. *Journal of Behavior Therapy and Experimental Psychiatry, 25*, 231–239.

Resick, P.A., Nisith, P., Weaver, T.L., Astin, M.C., & Feuer, C.A. (2002). A comparison of cognitive-processing therapy with prolonged exposure and a waiting condition for the treatment of chronic posttraumatic stress disorder in female rape victims. *Journal of Consulting and clinical Psychology, 70*, 867–879.

Reynolds, C.F., Dew, M.A., Martire, L.M., Miller, M.D., Cyranowski, J.M., Lenze, E., Whyte, E.M., Mulsant, B.H., Pollock, B.G., Karp, J.F., Gildengers, A., Szanto, K., Dombrovski, A.Y., Andreescu, C., Butters, M.A., Morse, J.Q., Houck, P.R., Bensasi, S., Mazumdar, S., Stack, J.A., & Frank, E. (2010). Treating depression to remission in older adults: A controlled evaluation of combined escitalopram with interpersonal psychotherapy versus escitalopram with depression care management. *International Journal of Geriatric Psychiatry, 25,* 1134–1141.

Reynolds, C.F., Dew, M.A., Pollock, B.G., Mulsant, B.H., Frank, E., Miller, M.D., Houck, P.R., Mazumdar, S., Butters, M.A., Stack, J.A., Schlernitzauer, M.A., Whyte, E.M., Gidengers, A., Karp, J., Lenze, E., Szanto, K., Bansasi, S., & Kupfer, D.J. (2006). Maintenance treatment of major depression in old age. *New England Journal of Medicine, 354,* 1130–1138.

Riemann, D., & Perlis, M.L. (2009). The treatments of chronic insomnia: A review of benzodiazepine receptor agonists and psychological and behavioral therapies. *Sleep Medicine Reviews, 13,* 205–214.

Rutherford, L., & Couturier, J. (2007). A review of psychotherapeutic interventions for children and adolescents with eating disorders. *Journal of the Canadian Academy of Child and Adolescent Psychiatry, 16,* 153–157.

Sacher, J., Neumann, J., Fünfstück, T., Soliman, A., Villringer, A., & Schroeter, M.L. (2012). Mapping the depressed brain: A meta-analysis of structural and functional alterations in major depressive disorder. *Journal of Affective Disorders, 140,* 142–148.

Seidler, G.H., & Wagner, F.E. (2006). Comparing the efficacy of EMDR and trauma-focused cognitive-behavioral therapy in the treatment of PTSD: A meta-analytic study. *Psychological Medicine, 36,* 1515–1522.

Seligman, L.D., & Ollendick, T.H. (2011). Cognitive-behavioral therapy for anxiety disorders in youth. *Child and Adolescent Psychiatric Clinics of North America, 20,* 217–238.

Seligman, M.E.P. (1995). The effectiveness of psychotherapy: The *Consumer Reports* study. *American Psychologist, 50,* 965–974.

Serketich, W.J., & Dumas, J.E. (1996). The effectiveness of behavioral parent training to modify antisocial behavior in children: A meta-analysis. *Behavior Therapy, 27,* 171–186.

Shadish, W.R., Matt, G.E., Navarro, A.M., Siegle, G., Crits-Christoph, P., Hazelrigg, M.D., Jorm, A.F., Lyons, L.C., Nietzel, M.T., Robinson, L., Prout, H.T., Smith, M.L., Svartberg, M., & Weiss, B. (1997). Evidence that therapy works in clinically representative conditions. *Journal of Consulting and Clinical Psychology, 65,* 355–365.

Siev, J., & Chambless, D.L. (2007). Specificity of treatment effects: Cognitive therapy and relaxation for generalized anxiety and panic disorder. *Journal of Consulting and Clinical Psychology, 75,* 513–522.

Sifneos, P. (1992). *Short-term anxiety provoking psychotherapy: A treatment manual.* New York: Basic Books.

Skinner, B.F. (1948). *Walden Two.* Indianapolis, IN: Hackett Publishing Co.

Slade, K., Lambert, M.J., Harmon, S.C., Smart, D.W., & Bailey, R. (2008). Improving psychotherapy outcome: The use of immediate electronic feedback and revised clinical support tools. *Clinical Psychology and Psychotherapy, 15,* 287–303.

Smith, M.L., Glass, G.V., & Miller, T.I. (1980). *The benefits of psychotherapy*. Baltimore, MD: Johns Hopkins University Press.

Spielmans, G.I., Berman, M.I., & Usitalo, A.N. (2011). Psychotherapy versus second-generation antidepressants in the treatment of depression: A meta-analysis. *Journal of Nervous and Mental Disease*, 199, 142–149.

Spielrein, S. (1911/1994). Destruction as the cause of coming into being. *Journal of Analytical Psychology*, 39, 155–186.

Squire, L.R. (1986). Mechanisms of memory. *Science*, 232, 1612–1619.

Stiles, W.B., Barkham, M., Connell, J., & Mellor-Clark, J. (2008). Responsive regulation of treatment duration in routine practice in United Kingdom primary care settings: Replication in a larger sample. *Journal of Consulting and Clinical Psychology*, 76, 298–305.

Stiles, W.B., Glick, M.J., Osatuke, K., Hardy, G.E., Shapiro, D.A., Agnew-Davies, R., Rees, A., & Barkham, M. (2004). Patterns of alliance development and the rupture-repair hypothesis: Are productive relationships U-shaped or V-shaped? *Journal of Counseling Psychology*, 51, 81–92.

Stout, R., Del Boca, F.K., Carbonari, J., Rychtarik, R., Litt, M.D., & Cooney, N.L. (2003). Primary treatment outcomes and matching effects: Outpatient arm. In T.F. Babor & F.K. Del Boca (Eds.), *Treatment matching in alcoholism. International research monographs in the addictions* (pp. 105–134). New York: Cambridge University Press.

Strauss, J.L., Hayes, A.M., Johnson, S.L., Newman, C.F., Brown, G.K., Barber, J.P., Laurenceau, J.-P., & Beck, A.T. (2006). Early alliance, alliance ruptures, and symptom change in a nonrandomized trial of cognitive therapy for avoidant and obsessive-compulsive personality disorders. *Journal of Consulting and Clinical Psychology*, 74, 337–345.

Strupp, H.H. (1996). Some salient lessons from research and practice. *Psychotherapy: Theory, Research, Practice, Training*, 33, 135–138.

Strupp, H.H., & Binder, J.L. (1985). *Psychotherapy in a new key: A guide to time-limited dynamic psychotherapy*. New York: Basic Books.

Sullivan, H.S. (1940). *Conceptions of modern psychiatry*. New York: W.W. Norton.

Svartberg, M., & Stiles, T.C. (1991). Comparative effects of short-term psychodynamic psychotherapy: A meta-analysis. *Journal of Consulting and Clinical Psychology*, 59, 704–714.

Sylvia, L.G., Tilley, C.A., Lund, H.G., & Sachs, G.S. (2008). Psychosocial interventions: Empirically-derived treatments for bipolar disorder. *Current Psychiatry Reviews*, 4, 108–113.

Tang, T.Z., DeRubeis, R.J., Beberman, R., & Pham, T. (2005). Cognitive changes, critical sessions, and sudden gains in cognitive-behavioral therapy for depression. *Journal of Consulting and Clinical Psychology*, 73, 168–172.

Taylor, S., Asmundson, G.J.G., & Coons, M.J. (2005). Current directions in the treatment of hypochondriasis. *Journal of Cognitive Psychotherapy*, 19, 285–304.

Telch, C.F., Agras, W.S., & Linehan, M.M. (2001). Dialectical behavior therapy for binge eating disorder: A promising new treatment. *Journal of Consulting and Clinical Psychology*, 69, 1061–1065.

Tottenham, N., Shapiro, M., Telzer, E.H., & Humphreys, K.L. (2012). Amygdala response to mother. *Developmental Science*, 15, 307–319.

Tsao, J.C.I., Mystkowski, J.L., Zucker, B.G., & Craske, M.G. (2005). Impact of cognitive behavioral therapy for panic disorder on comorbidity: A controlled investigation. *Behaviour Research and Therapy*, 43, 959–970.

Van Oppen, P., de Haan, E., van Balkom, A.J.L.M., Spinhoven, P., Hoogduin, K., & van Dyck, R. (1995). Cognitive therapy and exposure in vivo in the treatment of obsessive compulsive disorder. *Behaviour Research and Therapy*, 33, 379–390.

Vrtička, P., Bondolfi, G., Sander, D., & Vuilleumier, P. (2012). The neural substrates of social emotion perception and regulation are modulated by adult attachment style. *Social Neuroscience*, 7, 473–493.

Vettese, L.C., Toneatto, T., Stea, J.N., Nguyen, L., & Wang, J.J. (2009). Do mindfulness meditation participants do their homework? And does it make a difference? A review of the empirical evidence. *Journal of Cognitive Psychotherapy*, 23, 198–225.

Wampold, B.E., Mondin, G.W., Moody, M., Stich, F., Benson, K., & Ahn, H. (1997). A meta-analysis of outcome studies comparing bona fide psychotherapies: Empirically, "all must have prizes." *Psychological Bulletin*, 122, 203–215.

Warren, S.L., Bost, K.K., Roisman, G.I., Silton, R.L., Spielberg, J.M., Engels, A.S., Choi, E., Sutton, B.P., Miller, G.A., & Heller, W. (2010). Effects of adult attachment and emotional distractors on brain mechanisms of cognitive control. *Psychological Science*, 21, 1818–1826.

Warren, Z., Veenstra-VanderWeele, J., Stone, W., Bruzek, J.L., Nahmias, A.S., Foss-Feig, J.H., Jerome, R.N., Krishnaswami, S., Sathe, N.A., Glasser, A.M., Surawicz, T., & McPheeters, M.L. (2011). *Therapies for children with autism spectrum disorders*. AHRQ Publication No. 11-EHC029-EF, Comparative Effectiveness Reviews, No. 26. Rockville, MD: Agency for Healthcare Research and Quality.

Watson, J.B. (1930). *Behaviorism* (rev. ed.). New York: Norton.

Weisz, J.R., Weiss, B., Han, S.S., Granger, D.A., & Morton, T. (1995). Effects of psychotherapy with children and adolescents revisited: A meta-analysis of treatment outcome studies. *Psychological Bulletin*, 117, 450–468.

Wilfley, D.E., Kolko, R.P., & Kass, A.E. (2011). Cognitive-behavioral therapy for weight management and eating disorders in children and adolescents. *Child and Adolescent Psychiatric Clinics of North America*, 20, 271–285.

Williams, J., Hadjistavropoulos, T., & Sharpe, D. (2006). A meta-analysis of psychological and pharmacological treatments for body dysmorphic disorder. *Behaviour Research and Therapy*, 44, 99–111.

Williams, J.M.G., Crane, C., Barnhofer, T., Brennan, K., Duggan, D.S., Fennell, M.J.V., Hackmann, A., Krusche, A., Muse, K., Von Rohr, I.R., Shah, D., Crane, R.S., Eames, C., Jones, M., Radford, S., Silverton, S., Sun, Y., Weatherley-Jones, E., Whitaker, C.J., Russell, D., & Russell, I.T. (2014). Mindfulness-based cognitive therapy for preventing relapse in recurrent depression: A randomized dismantling trial. *Journal of Consulting and Clinical Psychology*, 82, 275–286.

Wilson, D., Silver, S.M., Covi, W.G., & Foster, S. (1996). Eye movement desensitization and reprocessing: Effectiveness and autonomic correlates. *Journal of Behavior Therapy and Experimental Psychiatry*, 27, 219–229.

Wittels, F. (1924). *Sigmund Freud: His personality, his teaching, & his school*. London, England: Ayer.

Woon, F.L., Sood., S., & Hedges, D.W. (2010). Hippocampal volume deficits associated with exposure to psychological trauma and post-traumatic stress disorder in adults: A meta-analysis. *Progress in Neuro-Psychopharmacology & Biological Psychiatry, 34*, 1181–1188.

Yucha, C., & Montgomery, D. (2008). *Evidence-based practice in biofeedback and neurofeedback*. Wheat Ridge, CO: Association for Applied Psychophysiology and Biofeedback.

Zellner, M.R. (2012). Cognitive and psychodynamic approaches to depression: Surprising similarities, but remaining key differences: Commentary on Aaron T. Beck, Emily A.P. Haigh, and Kari F. Baber's paper. *Psychoanalytic Review, 99*, 539–547.

Zimmermann, G., Favrod, J., Trieu, V.H., & Pomini, V. (2005). The effect of cognitive behavioral treatment on the positive symptoms of schizophrenia spectrum disorders: A meta-analysis. *Schizophrenia Research, 77*, 1–9.

Zuroff, D.C., & Blatt, S.J. (2006). The therapeutic relationship in the brief treatment of depression: Contributions to clinical improvement and enhanced adaptive capacities. *Journal of Consulting and Clinical Psychology, 74*, 130–140.

Glossary

Note that italicized terms are defined elsewhere in the Glossary. The following specific psychotherapeutic techniques are listed and defined in Chapter 4: activity scheduling, analyzing defenses, assertiveness training, assigning homework, behavior monitoring, catharsis, constructing hierarchies, contingent reinforcement, downward arrow, exposure, extinction, feedback, free association, interpretation, journaling, mindfulness, modeling, planning experiments, problem solving, psychoeducation, reframing, rehearsal, relapse prevention, relaxation training, role plays, setting goals, setting time limits for treatment, skill building, stimulus control, and transference work.

Adler, Alfred (1870–1937): He was an Austrian physician who collaborated closely with *Sigmund Freud* between 1902 and 1911. At the time he broke with *Freud*, he was working out a theory of personality that became known as *individual psychology*.

Ainsworth, Mary D.S. (1913–1999): This American-Canadian developmental psychologist contributed heavily to attachment theory, having conducted experiments using the *strange situation*.

Anal stage: According to *psychoanalytic* theory, the *cathexis* of *libido* is normally centered on the anus during the second 18 months of life, and unpleasure is discharged first by expelling and then retaining feces.

Analytical psychology: This is *Jung's* carefully worked-out theory of personality. It describes and relates such concepts as *archetype, complex, collective unconscious*, and many other constructs.

Anima: In *analytical psychology*, this *archetype* is a part-personality complex with female characteristics, for both males and females.

Animus: In *analytical psychology*, this *archetype* is a part-personality complex with male characteristics, for both males and females.

Applied behavior analysis (ABA): This first-wave *behavioral* intervention involves the careful analysis of small segments of behavior, after which basic principles of operant and also classical conditioning are applied to increase or decrease the frequency of specific behaviors.

Archetype: In *analytical psychology* this unconscious, transpersonal structure of the *complex* was originally called a "primordial image." *Jung* described archetypes as "the introspectively recognizable form of a priori psychic orderedness." He viewed them as the structures or tendencies on which humans unconsciously rely to organize their experiences. He enumerated five main archetypes: *persona, shadow, animus, anima,* and *self*.

Attachment: This term refers to the infant's bond to the caregiver that can be observed in humans and other species. There is evidence that successful attachment is required early in life for normal social and cognitive development. Attachment is fairly stable across the lifespan and can be measured in various ways among young children and also among adults. It appears to predict to process and outcome in *psychotherapy* in a manner that is not yet fully understood.

Automatic thought: In cognitive-behavior therapy, automatic thoughts are very quick appraisals of one's situation. They are said to arise spontaneously and to coexist with the more manifest stream of thoughts. Automatic thoughts are not based on reflection or deliberation, and they are accepted as true, without any real evaluation. In particular, automatic *negative* thoughts are those that lead to emotional distress. Conceivably, they may be accurate and useful, or they may lack accuracy and/or utility. Such automatic negative thoughts represent one focus of the work in cognitive-behavior therapy.

Bandura, Albert (1925–): This Canadian-born psychologist who has lived most of his life in the United States contributed heavily to early applications of cognitive-behavioral theory. He is particularly known for his ideas regarding observational learning and self-efficacy.

Beck, Aaron T. (1921–): This American psychiatrist is known for his seminal contributions to the application of *cognitive-behavioral* principles to psychotherapeutic treatment.

Behaviorism: This is an approach to *psychotherapy* that relies heavily on behavior theory and involves the use of learning principles to change problematic behavior. Behaviorism is often divided into three "waves," corresponding to radical behaviorism, *cognitive-behavioral* approaches, and *mindfulness*-based approaches.

Bernheim, Hippolyte (1840–1919): This French neurologist was very interested in hypnosis. *Freud* studied with him in 1889.

Biofeedback: This technique involves the provision of real-time information about a body process of which the individual is not normally much aware.

Body armor: This is the term *Reich* used to refer to an individual's characteristic muscular tone, which is intended to prevent the individual from behaving inappropriately, especially in relationship to others. *Reich* believed that a particular body armor reflects one's *defense* structure.

Bowlby, John (1907–1990): This psychoanalytically trained English physician wrote extensively about infant *attachment* and maternal deprivation.

Breuer, Josef (1842–1925): A neurologist and early colleague of *Sigmund Freud*, he contributed to the early development of *Freud's* ideas about hysteria.

Brief Cognitive Therapy for Panic Disorder: This *cognitive-behavioral* intervention involves the modification of thoughts and behaviors in the treatment of panic disorder.

Cathexis: In *psychoanalytic* theory, cathexis describes the investment of an amount of psychic "energy" in a mental *object* or the self. The "energy" referenced here corresponds to *Freud's* concept of psychic energy distribution in his *economic theory*.

Character disorder: This *psychoanalytic* term refers to the condition that results when an individual makes nearly exclusive use of a very narrow range of *defenses*. In more modern terms, character disorder is approximately equivalent to the concept of personality disorder.

Charcot, Jean-Martin (1825–1893): This French neurologist experimented extensively with the treatment of hysteria. *Freud* studied with him for five months in 1885.

Classical conditioning: Also referred to as "respondent conditioning," this term describes how a specific response can be elicited following a neutral stimulus. Starting with an old stimulus-response pattern, a new stimulus can come to elicit the old response if the old and new stimuli are repeatedly paired. In view of the temporal contiguity between the old and new stimuli, which are consistently followed by the response (to the old stimulus), the organism learns that the new stimulus is associated with the response. Following multiple trials, the organism displays the response each time the new stimulus is presented, even when the old stimulus is not presented.

Client-centered therapy: This model of *psychotherapy*, developed by *Rogers*, is sometimes referred to as the "third force" in American *psychotherapy* (after *behaviorism* and *psychoanalysis*).

Cognitive-behavioral therapy (CBT): Broadly speaking, this term refers to any second-wave *behavioral* intervention in which the therapist sets out to modify cognitions and behaviors that may be causing problems for the patient. Probably the best-known version of CBT is the one described by *Beck*.

Collaborative empiricism: This term describes a fundamental value or stance of the cognitive-behavior therapist. The therapist doesn't know in advance whether a patient's particular automatic thought is valid or invalid, nor is its utility indisputable. Therefore, patient and therapist collaborate in designing an experiment to evaluate the consequence of acting (or not acting) on the patient's thought. Only when empirical data have been gathered can therapist and patient decide whether to modify the automatic thought, to leave it alone, or to learn new skills that permit a change in the patient's behavior. The concept of collaborative empiricism reflects the emphasis in cognitive-behavior therapy that is placed on the development of a mutually respectful, reasonably egalitarian relationship between patient and therapist, who together work out how to gather and then analyze data about the patient's problems.

Collective unconscious: In *analytical psychology* the *unconscious* is divided into two parts. The collective unconscious contains material reflecting universals shared by all humans. It is distinguished from the *personal unconscious*.

Complex: According to *analytical psychology*, mental activity is organized around groups of ideas with a particular emotional tone. The outer shell of a complex is related to immediate personal experiences and associations, while the nuclear element contains *archetypes*.

Condensation: This *psychoanalytic* term refers to the process by which psychic elements associated by some commonality are distilled into a single representation, giving a result that is a compromise between censorship and expression. The use of this term is most commonly associated with dreams, but the mechanism is not confined to dreaming. For instance, condensation is evident in slips of the tongue. In dreams, condensation is the mechanism by which elements may have more than one meaning.

Conscious: This *psychoanalytic* term refers to the ideas and memories of which the individual is currently aware. It is to be distinguished from *preconscious* and *unconscious*. This term can also be used an adjective that describes what a person is directly aware of.

Constructive alternativism: This is the term *Kelly* used to refer to his idea that people construct their views of the world from among a number of choices.

Conversion: This ego psychological *defense* involves the expression of emotional distress in the form of physical symptoms, such as the paralysis of a limb, certain pain phenomena, and so forth.

Core belief: In *cognitive-behavior therapy*, this term refers to the rigid, global idea one has about oneself, the world, or one's future. Three common core beliefs of depressed people are the ideas that one is worthless, helpless, or fundamentally unlovable. Anxious people may harbor the core belief that they cannot respond effectively to surprising or threatening events. The core beliefs of individuals with personality disorders represent the cognitive equivalent of fundamental diagnostic criteria. For example, individuals with histrionic personality disorder believe that they are only worthwhile to the extent that they entertain others, while those with avoidant personality disorder believe that they are incapable of tolerating awareness of painful thoughts, feelings, and situations. By contrast, people without mental disorders usually have the core belief that they are fundamentally worthwhile, able to do many things, and capable of being loved by others.

Countercathexis: This *psychoanalytic* term refers to the process by which the psychic "energy" that might have been attached to or focused on a certain mental *object* is redirected to another *object* deemed by the ego to present less risk if such energy were immediately discharged. For example, the ego prevents sexual desire from being attached to the mental image of a parent. Instead, through the process of countercathexis such instinctually based energy is displaced to another mental *object*, such as a peer, one's schoolwork, or the value one attaches to orderliness.

Counterconditioning: This is a form of *classical conditioning*, according to which an individual learns a new conditional response that is inconsistent with the old conditional response. For example, in the treatment of phobia, patients are taught to achieve a deep state of relaxation, which they then pair with increasingly disturbing mental images of or physical proximity to the phobic stimulus. In time, patients learn to associate the phobic stimulus with a new response (relaxation) that is inconsistent with the old response (anxiety).

Countertransference: This is originally a *psychoanalytic* term but has since been appropriated by other models of *psychotherapy*. It reflects the idea that a psychotherapist responds to patients in a way that reflects earlier experiences in the therapist's life. *Freud* thought of countertransference as an unconscious process, but more recent definitions also include the therapist's conscious awareness of his or her distorted perception. There is consistent evidence that unmanaged countertransference has an adverse effect on outcome from psychotherapy, while managed countertransference serves as a useful source of information about what is occurring in treatment.

Creative self: This term describes the belief in *individual psychology* that one is free to act on and combine early influences as one wishes. In other words, no one is bound, based on early experience, to develop in a particular way.

Defense/Defense Mechanism: This *psychoanalytic* term refers to any strategy employed by the ego to control and regulate "unacceptable" material projected by the id. *Freud* wrote extensively about *repression*, while various ego psychologists have described more specific defenses, including *conversion, denial, displacement, dissociation, identification, isolation of affect, projection, rationalization, reaction formation, regression, splitting, sublimation, suppression, undoing*, and others.

Denial: This ego psychological *defense* involves a refusal to accept external reality because it is too threatening. People with addiction are likely to engage in denial about their addiction, but the defense is seen at some level in everyone.

Depressive position: A term invented by *Melanie Klein*, this refers to a period in the second three months of life when the infant fears that aggressive or greedy impulses will destroy external *objects*. Klein believed that successful resolution of the depressive position permits the infant to begin to combine good and bad *objects* and thus to decrease reliance on the *defense* of *splitting*. Thus, the ego becomes better integrated, and rudimentary development of the superego begins.

Dialectical behavior therapy (DBT): Developed by *Linehan*, DBT is a third-wave *behavioral* treatment that specifically aims to decrease self-injurious behaviors. It is most often utilized with individuals diagnosed with borderline personality disorder.

Discrimination: In learning theory, this refers to the extent to which an individual's response depends on the precise details of a situation. When, based on previous learning, an organism is highly discriminant, a given response will be elicited only in very specific situations. Discrimination is contrasted with *generalization*.

Displacement: This ego psychological *defense* involves shifting an emotion from its real target to a target that is less threatening. For example, one might become angry at a family member rather than to experience anger toward a superior at work.

Dissociation: This ego psychological *defense* involves the development of a profound separation of a group of mental processes from the rest of one's integrated consciousness, memory, perception, and sensorimotor behavior. The dissociating individual cannot consciously attend to the separated processes and other integrated functions at the same time.

Dodo bird hypothesis: In its extreme form, this hypothesis asserts that all forms of *psychotherapy* are equally effective. In its more nuanced version, it asserts that the difference in *efficacy* among various forms of *psychotherapy* is much less than the overall *efficacy* of psychotherapeutic treatment. The Dodo bird hypothesis stands in opposition to the hypothesis that certain kinds of *psychotherapy* are much more effective than others.

Drive derivative: This term from *psychoanalysis* refers to the various obscure ways that repressed drives manifest themselves, including as symptoms and fantasies.

Dynamic theory: This proposition describes *Freud*'s understanding of how conscious mental life is affected by unconscious factors. *Freud* believed that every conscious thought or act is caused by prior mental events, many of which are not accessible to conscious awareness. This idea is sometimes referred to as *psychic determinism*.

Eclecticism: This is a treatment strategy in which interventions based on a range of psychotherapies are used in an idiosyncratic (and often rapidly shifting) manner to treat the patient's symptoms. It is to be distinguished from (dogmatic) *consistency* and also *pluralism*.

Economic theory: This proposition describes *Freud*'s understanding of how energy is transferred within the mind. He stated that when an instinctual drive arises, it creates a hypothetical central stimulation. Because the central nervous system functions so as to minimize incoming stimulation, the discharge of such psychic energy is desirable. However, the psychic energy may be attached to or focused on an *object* with characteristics such that a discharge of the energy might be perceived by the ego as "dangerous." Therefore, the energy is moved to another *object* through the process of *countercathexis*.

Effect size: This is a general statistical term with particular application to *meta-analyses*, where it represents the amount by which two conditions differ from one another. For example, an effect size might describe the change from pretreatment to posttreatment of a typical *psychotherapy* patient. Effect sizes, including the mathematically very similar d and g, are often expressed in units basically equivalent to standard deviations. In other words, an effect size of $d = .5$ implies that the means of two groups or conditions differ from one another by half a standard deviation. The use of effect sizes permits one to compare the relative sizes of various interventions, such as the overall effect on outcome of being in *psychotherapy* ($d = .87$) versus the effect on outcome of a strong or weak *therapeutic alliance* ($d = .57$). Another kind of effect size is the *odds ratio*.

Effectiveness: This term refers to the degree to which *psychotherapy* has beneficial results, as measured in routine clinical situations. It is distinguished from the concept of *efficacy*.

Efficacy: This term refers to the degree to which *psychotherapy* has beneficial results, as measured in *randomized controlled trials* (i.e., "in the lab"). It is distinguished from the concept of *effectiveness*.

Ego psychology: This is a *psychodynamic* school that largely postdates *Freud*. Rather than viewing the ego's *defenses* as essentially reactive, ego psychologists shift the focus of attention to the coherent organization of the ego itself. Mental phenomena are understood in terms of optimal ego functioning, rather than as the efficiency with which id impulses are dispatched or neutralized. Much more attention is devoted to the details of ego *defenses*, which are thought to be useful coping strategies that help one to live in the world.

Eight stages of development: *Erikson* expanded *Freud*'s developmental scheme and identified eight stages, each associated with specific conflicts, virtues, and *ritualizations/ritualisms*. The stages are infancy, early childhood, preschool age, school age, adolescence, young adulthood, adulthood, and old age.

Ellis, Albert (1913–2007): This American psychologist developed a *cognitive-behavioral* psychotherapy called rational-emotive behavior therapy.

Empirically supported treatment: This refers to a health intervention that has been shown in several studies to be more efficacious than waitlist control. There is no universal agreement on exactly how many or what sorts of studies are required, but in most cases *randomized controlled trials* demonstrating efficacy in at least two laboratories are considered to be sufficient evidence of efficacy.

Erikson, Erik H. (1902–1994): This German-born man lived in the United States for many years. He contributed heavily to the theory of *ego psychology* and is particularly known for his *eight stages of development*.

Eros: This *psychoanalytic* term refers to the life-directed instinct. Associated with eros is the psychic energy referred to as *libido*.

Expectancy: This learning theory term describes an individual's subjective belief that one particular event will follow another particular event. The term is used in many contexts, including to describe an individual's estimate of the likelihood that a given behavior will lead to a certain reinforcement. It is also used to describe a patient's prediction regarding the outcome of treatment.

Exposure and response prevention (ERP): This *cognitive-behavioral* model of treatment is applied specifically to symptoms of obsessive-compulsive disorder. More generally, principles of ERP are helpful in the treatment of most anxiety disorders.

External validity: This term refers to the degree to which the conclusions of a particular study can be generalized beyond the study sample itself. External validity is distinguished from *internal validity*.

Extinction: After an individual performs a target behavior, an expected reinforcer is not delivered, thus decreasing the likelihood that the target behavior will be performed again.

Eye movement desensitization and reprocessing (EMDR): In this novel *psychotherapeutic* technique developed by *Shapiro*, principles of *cognitive-behavioral* treatment are supplemented by special eye movements to ameliorate symptoms of posttraumatic stress disorder.

False self: *Winnicott* used this term to describe a child's façade that is designed to please others (in order to feel safer in the world), as a consequence of which the child does not experience spontaneity or the sense of being fully alive. *Winnicott* contrasted false self with *true self*.

Ferenczi, Sándor (1873–1933): A long-time friend and colleague of *Freud*, Ferenczi collaborated with *Rank* in efforts to shorten the course of *psychoanalysis*. He also treated many prominent early *psychoanalytic* writers and is sometimes referred to as "the mother of psychoanalysis."

Fictional finalism: This *individual psychology* term describes the cognitive structures and goals a child develops in response to his or her particular *Weltanschauung*.

Fixation: According to *psychoanalytic* theory, an individual can become "stuck" at a particular stage of psychosexual development, which results in stunted emotional growth and the probable development of a *character disorder*.

Fonagy, Peter (1952–): This Hungarian-born psychologist, who has lived for many years in London, has contributed heavily to the development of a model of *psychotherapy* known as *mentalization-based treatment*.

Freud, Anna (1895–1982): The youngest child of *Sigmund Freud*, she lived for many years in London and contributed to the development of child *psychotherapy* and wrote extensively on the topic of *ego psychology*, with a particular focus on ego *defenses*.

Freud, Sigmund (1856–1939): A physician born in the Austro-Hungarian Empire and residing in Vienna for most of his life, he was primarily responsible for developing the theory of *psychoanalysis*. He is rightly referred to as "the father of psychoanalysis."

Generalization: In learning theory, this refers to the extent to which a behavior learned in one situation is likely to be emitted in other situations. Generalization is contrasted with *discrimination*.

Genetic theory: This proposition describes *Freud's* understanding of developmental shifts in the *cathexis* of *libido* during childhood. *Freud* believed that in normal development *libido* is focused first in one body area and then another, until at last *libido* is genitally focused. *Freud* believed that each developmental stage is associated with specific psychological tasks. For example, he believed that the *Oedipus complex* is normally worked out during the *phallic stage*.

Genital stage: According to *psychoanalytic* theory, this stage begins at the time of puberty and involves the individual's amorous involvement with peers.

Grief problem area: In the *interpersonal psychotherapy* treatment of depression, patients are assigned the grief problem area if they have not fully mourned the death of someone very close to them.

Hayes, Steven C. (1948–): This American psychologist developed Acceptance and Commitment Therapy, a third-wave *behavioral* intervention.

Identification: This ego psychological *defense* involves improving one's self-esteem by affiliating with someone who has more power. More specifically, identification with the aggressor involves the adoption of the values and mannerisms of a feared person, while altruistic surrender provides vicarious satisfaction of one's own ambitions by identifying with the satisfactions and frustrations of another person.

Individual psychology: This is *Adler's* theory of personality, in which primary emphasis is given to the idea of *striving for superiority*. The theory relates early childhood experiences to the development of a *Weltanschauung* and each individual's resulting *style of life*.

Individuation: In *analytical psychology*, this term refers to the discovery and integration of the various parts of an individual's personality.

Instinct: In *psychoanalysis* instincts are said to have four characteristics. They correspond to body deficiency of some kind, they aim to eliminate the deficiency, they seek an *object* that will accomplish this, and their magnitude depends on the degree of the body deficiency. When an instinctual drive arises, it creates a hypothetical central stimulation. Consistent with *Freud's* view that the central nervous system functions so as to minimize stimulation, the discharge of instinctually derived energy is desirable.

Intermediate belief: In *cognitive-behavior therapy*, intermediate beliefs are cognitions that exist at a level between *automatic thoughts* and *core beliefs*. These cognitions consist of the rules, attitudes, and assumptions that individuals develop in order to get through life, given their fundamental ideas about the world. People typically don't view their intermediate beliefs as assumptions about the world. Instead, they simply accept them as true and usually don't even recognize that they have them. Intermediate beliefs often take the form of if/then statements, such as the following: "If I try to act on my own, I will fail; if I submit myself to the will of another person, he or she will protect me and will make decisions for me."

Internal validity: This term refers to the logical accuracy with which particular conclusions can be drawn for the sample within a given study, given the design and data analysis. Internal validity is distinguished from *external validity*.

Interoceptive exposure: In the *cognitive-behavioral* treatment of panic, the therapist encourages the patient to act in such a way as to induce feared internal experiences, such as tachycardia, dyspnea, or dizziness, in order to show the patient after a number of trials that such experiences are not dangerous and do not need to be avoided.

Interpersonal deficits problem area: In the *interpersonal psychotherapy* treatment of depression, patients are assigned the interpersonal deficits problem area when they have limited social contacts and skills.

Interpersonal inventory: In the first few sessions of *interpersonal psychotherapy*, part of the conceptualization process involves the collection by the therapist of extensive information regarding important relationships in the patient's life, past and present.

Interpersonal psychotherapy (IPT): This model of treatment relates psychopathological symptoms to disturbances in social functioning. It was developed in the late 1960s by *Klerman* and *Weissman*.

Isolation of affect: This ego psychological *defense* involves separating the feelings from one's thoughts and actions.

Jung, Carl G. (1875–1961): This Swiss psychiatrist collaborated with *Freud* between 1907 and 1913. He later developed a theory of personality and treatment that is now known as *analytical psychology*. He wrote extensively and worked out the details of *archetypes, complexes, collective unconscious*, and many other ideas.

Kabat-Zinn, Jon (1944–): This American psychologist developed one of the first manualized third-wave *behavioral* interventions, which he applied to individuals with chronic pain. The intervention is called mindfulness-based stress reduction.

Kelly, George (1905–1967): This American psychologist developed a model of psychopathology called personal construct theory, which he further developed into an unusual approach to psychotherapy.

Kernberg, Otto F. (1928–): This Austrian psychiatrist, who grew up in Chile but has lived for many years in the United States, has written extensively on borderline personality organization and is responsible for the development of *transference-based psychotherapy*.

Klerman, Gerald L. (1928–1992): This American psychiatrist, together with his future wife, *Myrna M. Weissman*, developed *interpersonal psychotherapy*.

Klein, Melanie (1882–1960): Originally from Vienna, she spent the largest part of her working life in London, where she contributed heavily to the theory of *object relations*.

Kohut, Heinz (1913–1981): A physician who grew up in Vienna but spent most of his adult life in Chicago, Kohut is responsible for the development of *self psychology*.

Latency stage: According to *psychoanalytic* theory, after resolution of the *phallic stage*, there follows a period of relative quiescence in which sexual matters are less prepotent.

Libido: In *psychoanalysis*, this term refers to the psychic energy associated with the life-directed *instinct*, which is called *eros*. *Freud* believed that much of normal and pathological development can be traced to the (mis)direction of libido in the psyche.

Linehan, Marsha M. (1943–): This American psychologist developed *dialectical behavior therapy*, an intervention designed to decrease self-injurious behavior among patients, many of whom are diagnosed with borderline personality disorder.

Mahler, Margaret S. (1897–1985): This Hungarian psychoanalyst contributed heavily to *attachment* theory and maintained a particular interest in separation-individuation.

Mentalization-based Treatment (MBT): Developed by *Fonagy* and others, this *psychodynamic* treatment aims to increase patients' awareness of thoughts and feelings, both in themselves and in others, thus increasing their psychological-mindedness.

Meta-analysis: This is a statistical technique in which the statistical findings from several studies are combined to draw conclusions from all the studies at once, rather than to consider the conclusions of each study individually.

Mindfulness-based cognitive therapy (MBCT): This third-wave, manualized *behavioral* intervention employs a group format to decrease patients' risk for relapse in the treatment of recurrent depression.

Motivational Interviewing (MI): This brief *psychotherapeutic* technique is designed to help individuals struggling with ambivalence to make a decision. MI is based on techniques from *client-centered therapy* but adds specific verbal strategies that have the effect of moving the individual toward a decision—not infrequently one that is consistent with the therapist's intention.

Multidetermination: In *psychoanalysis*, this term refers to the process by which all psychic phenomena arise as a convergence or compromise among multiple factors or causes. Therefore, a single phenomenon has multiple origins and may serve multiple purposes.

Negative reinforcement: After an individual performs a target behavior, the expected punishment does not occur, thus increasing the likelihood that the target behavior will be performed again.

Neuroplasticity: This term refers to the fact that neurons change, sometimes quite fundamentally, in response to external stimuli, thus facilitating learning and general adaptation.

Number needed to treat (NNT): This statistic permits one to compare the effects of several treatments. For a given condition, treatment, and criterion of improvement, NNT equals the average number of patients who would need to receive the treatment before at least one more patient reaches the improvement criterion, in comparison with the number of patients who would have reached criterion without treatment.

Object: This *psychoanalytic* term refers to a person, a part of a person, or a mental representation of the same. A distinction is made between objects that are internal (mental representations) and those that are external or real. The self is a particular object that consists of an internal image of one's own person.

Object relations: This is a *psychodynamic* school that largely postdates *Freud*, in which the primary interest is in the structural and dynamic interactions between internal *objects* and the *self object* (not to be confused with *selfobject*, *Kohut's* term for a different construct).

Observing ego: In *psychoanalysis* this term refers to the ability to observe one's own psychological processes and the ability to construct a working alliance with the therapist for the purpose of treatment.

Odds ratio (OR): This is a kind of *effect size*. The odds ratio compares the likelihood that something will happen in one group against the likelihood that it will happen in another group. For example, if the odds of recovery in one treatment are twice as high as the odds of recovery in another treatment, this is expressed as $OR = 2.0$.

Oedipus complex: According to *Freud*, this universal developmental crisis permits young boys to negotiate three-person relationships and sets the stage for the development of superego. The three- or four-year-old boy desires his mother sexually but fears castration by his father. The boy ultimately abandons his desire for his mother and comes to identify with the feared aggressor, his father, in the process introjecting his father's values. However, *Freud* was unable to work out a detailed version of this process for females.

Operant conditioning: This term describes the relationship between a behavior that acts on the environment and its associated reinforcement schedule. Essentially, the frequency with which one continues to perform a behavior depends on one's experience with the previous consequences of performing the behavior.

Optimal frustration: This is *Kohut's* term that describes how the therapist responds to a patient in a manner that slightly lacks empathy, with the consequence that the patient gradually develops the capacity to self-soothe.

Oral stage: According to *psychoanalytic* theory, the *cathexis* of *libido* in the first 18 months is normally centered on the mouth, lips, and tongue, and unpleasure is discharged by sucking, biting, and chewing.

Organ inferiority: This *individual psychology* term refers to the idea that humans are aware of their somatic weaknesses, and they naturally strive to overcome them.

Organismic valuing system: In *Rogers' client-centered therapy*, this refers to one's internal "felt sense" about the best course of action, based on one's particular needs and goals. To the extent that one loses contact with one's organismic valuing system, one is at increased risk for the development of psychopathology.

Paranoid-schizoid position: *Klein* used this term to refer to a period in the first three months of life during which the infant is fearful regarding self-preservation. *Splitting* and *projection* are particularly common at this time. If the infant is dominated by positive fantasies, it can project the negative *instincts* outward and maintain some degree of stability. If not, the infant may be overwhelmed by anxiety and may reject all real experience.

Paratactic mode: *Sullivan* used this term to describe one's moment-by-moment experience of the world using private symbols.

Pavlov, Ivan P. (1849–1936): This Russian Nobel prize winner demonstrated the operation of *classical conditioning* in dogs.

Persona: In *analytical psychology* this *complex* is said to mediate between the ego and the external world. It is a sort of mask that people wear in their everyday lives. The persona is distinguished from the *shadow*.

Personal unconscious: In *analytical psychology* the *unconscious* is divided into two parts. The personal unconscious contains material reflecting only one's own personal history. It is distinguished from the *collective unconscious*.

Personality type: In *analytical psychology* personality is represented along three orthogonal axes: the interpersonal attitudes of extraversion versus introversion, the perceptual functions of sensation versus intuition, and the judgment functions of thinking versus feeling. In *psychotherapy* based on *analytical psychology*, the patient is given feedback about his or her personality type, sometimes with the encouragement to discover whether other personality characteristics may be operative below the surface.

Phallic stage: According to *psychoanalytic* theory, the *cathexis* of *libido* is normally centered on the genitalia from about age three to age five. The *Oedipus complex* normally arises during this period.

Play therapy: This *psychodynamic* technique is used in the treatment of younger children. The child and therapist play together, and in the context of the developing relationship, the therapist uses the data arising from the play and the structure of the play itself to perform the same functions as those accomplished in psychodynamic psychotherapy with older patients.

Pleasure principle: In *psychoanalysis*, the immediate discharge of instinctual energy is said to be pleasurable, because the central nervous system is understood to function so as to minimize stimulation. However, when the psyche immediately discharges energy in accordance with the pleasure principle, adverse consequences may ensue, which would be inconsistent with the *reality principle*.

Pluralism: This is a treatment strategy in which interventions based on a range of *psychotherapies* are applied sequentially and intentionally, addressing first one symptom or condition and then another, based on research showing a link between the *psychotherapy* model and the particular symptom or condition. It is to be distinguished from (dogmatic) consistency and also *eclecticism*.

Positive reinforcement: After an individual performs a target behavior, a desirable consequence is provided, thus increasing the likelihood that the target behavior will be performed again.

Preconscious: This *psychoanalytic* term refers to the hypothesized system of the psyche that operates between the *conscious* and the *unconscious*. Although preconscious content is not currently available to awareness, with effort one can bring such material to awareness. The preconscious functions as a censor by pushing back "dangerous" images or impulses that bubble up from the *unconscious*.

Primary process: In *psychoanalysis*, the *unconscious* is said to operate on the basis of the primary process, which is alogical, lacks negatives but permits contradictions, has no time sense, and utilizes *displacement, condensation*, and symbolization. The primary process is distinguished from the *secondary process*, which is more consistent with the concept of "common sense."

Projection: This ego psychological *defense* involves shifting unacceptable thoughts, feelings, and impulses to someone else. This permits the troubling material to be expressed, although one doesn't assume any responsibility for it. In *psychotherapy* projection is sometimes evident when the patient suggests that the therapist might be thinking or feeling something that in fact originates from the patient himself or herself.

Prolonged Exposure for Posttraumatic Stress Disorder (PE-PTSD): This *cognitive-behavioral* intervention involves the modification of thoughts and behaviors, with a particular emphasis on exposure, as a means to treat PTSD.

Prototaxic mode: *Sullivan* used this term to describe the infant's experience of the world in an asymbolic and prelinguistic way.

Psychic determinism: Forming a central part of the *dynamic theory*, psychic determinism asserts that every thought or act is caused by prior mental events, many not accessible to *conscious* awareness.

Psychoanalysis: *Freud* spoke of psychoanalysis as a theory of personality, a method of inquiry, and a type of psychological treatment. He insisted that psychoanalytic theory depends upon the assumption that there are *unconscious* mental processes, that *resistance* and *repression* play important roles in psychic life, and that sexuality and the *Oedipus complex* are also central features. Psychoanalysis as a treatment technique rests on the idea that improved insight equals improved mental health. *Freud* proposed a series of techniques to promote insight into ego *defenses*, including particularly analysis of *resistance* and of the *transference*.

Psychodynamic psychotherapy: Psychodynamic therapists generally accept the idea that much of psychopathology results from ego *defenses* gone awry. However, psychodynamic treatments may differ from one another because of different theoretical perspectives on the question of what it is that fundamentally drives human development. Some psychodynamic treatments are based on *Freud's* notion that sexual *instinct* is the prime mover in development, while others are based on different mechanisms, such as *striving for superiority*, the need to self-realize, or the tension between union and separation, among others. Notwithstanding these differences, psychodynamic treatments make use of many quintessentially *psychoanalytic* techniques.

Psychotherapy: Each model of psychotherapy consists of a set of primarily verbal techniques delivered in the context of a personal relationship between therapist and patient over the course of one or many sessions. The techniques associated with each treatment model are based, at least in part, on an explicit theory of psychopathology that permits the therapist to conceptualize the patient's mental disorder in such a way that the verbal techniques might reasonably lead to symptom amelioration. Change may result from the verbal interaction between therapist and patient and their relationship with one another. It may also arise from changes in behavior that the patient makes during or between sessions. Models of psychotherapy may emphasize individual approaches, group approaches, or a combination of both. Psychotherapy can also be offered to smaller or larger groups within a family.

Punishment: After an individual performs a target behavior, an aversive consequence is provided, thus decreasing the likelihood that the target behavior will be performed again.

Randomized controlled trial (RCT): In this experimental design two or more groups of participants receive different treatments, and measurements are taken to determine whether the different treatments yield different results. However, prior to initiation of the treatments, substantial effort is devoted to ensure that important demographic and other variables do not distinguish the means of groups in each arm of the study. Further, the design minimizes any differences in participants' relevant experience over the course of the study, other than such experience as naturally results from the differing treatments. RCTs are said to have high *internal validity*, in that they are designed so as to ensure that any differences after treatment are likely to be due to the treatments themselves, rather than to other variables.

Rank, Otto (1884–1939): A member of *Freud's* circle who studied philosophy at university, Rank became the first nonmedical analyst. He is remembered for his ideas about union and separation, as well as for recommendations regarding shorter, more accessible treatment.

Rationalization: This ego psychological *defense* involves the use of faulty logic or reasoning to convince oneself that one has not done something wrong. For example, one might excuse shoplifting by pointing out that merchants figure such losses into their prices.

Reaction formation: This ego psychological *defense* involves converting unconscious impulses that might be very threatening into their opposites. In *psychotherapy* this sometimes manifests itself when the patient expresses anger toward the therapist, in response to an *unconscious* wish for intimacy.

Reality principle: This *psychoanalytic* term describes the ego's strategy of reducing tension in a manner that is as adaptive as possible to external reality. More emphasis is placed on the attainment of pleasure in the future than at present. Such a strategy of deferring gratification and considering the constraints of reality stands in opposition to the *pleasure principle*.

Regression: This ego psychological *defense* involves behaving immaturely rather than dealing with a scary situation in a more adult manner.

Reich, Wilhelm (1897–1957): A physician born in Poland, he was for a time in *Freud's* circle in Vienna but broke away in part due to his convictions about Marxism and sex. His more mainstream contributions to *psychoanalytic* theory include commentary on the relationship between character pathology and musculature.

Reinforcement schedule: This *behavioral* term refers to the rate of reinforcement in response to a particular operant behavior. Under a fixed-interval schedule, the individual is reinforced for the behavior only after a certain period of time has passed since the last reinforcement. Under a fixed-ratio schedule, the reinforcement is given only after the behavior is performed a certain number of times. Under a variable-interval schedule, the individual is reinforced only if the target behavior occurs after a varying interval following the last reinforcement. Under a variable-ratio schedule, reinforcement is provided only after the behavior is performed a varying number of times. In general, variable reinforcement schedules yield more consistent behavior change than fixed schedules.

Repression: This psychoanalytic *defense* involves the ego preventing conscious awareness of threatening thoughts and feelings, either by keeping the threatening material in the *unconscious* or by moving it from the *conscious* to the *unconscious*. It may be evident from memory lapses, naïveté, a failure to understand one's situation, or the ability to recall a feeling but not the associated thoughts. Repression does not involve conscious intent, and repressed material cannot normally be recalled with effort. In this way repression differs from *suppression*.

Resistance: This *psychoanalytic* term refers to the fact that patients wish to change but not infrequently fail to follow the therapist's directives, even though doing so would help to resolve their symptoms. Resistance is universally recognized in all models of *psychotherapy*, but in some models it is understood differently than it is in *psychoanalysis*, where it is said to reflect operation of the ego's *defenses* in the face of threatening material that might become *conscious* if the patient does as the therapist asks. It is as if the ego is trapped between wanting to feel better and the cost of doing what is required to accomplish that goal.

Ritualism: *Erikson* used this term to describe exaggerated culturally sanctioned transactions that humans use to help in moving through developmental stages. In contrast to *ritualizations*, ritualisms may lead to poor adjustment. For example, the school-age child learns how to accomplish a range of tasks in various settings, using the *ritualization* of formality.

However, if exaggerated, formality becomes formalism, and the child falls into the habit of focusing more on technique than on the intent of the task.

Ritualization: *Erikson* used this term to describe the normal, culturally sanctioned transactions that humans use to help in moving through developmental stages. If ritualizations are exaggerated, they become *ritualisms*, with negative consequences for the individual.

Rogers, Carl R. (1902–1987): This American psychologist is primarily responsible for the development of *client-centered therapy*, sometimes referred to as the "third force" in American *psychotherapy* (after *behaviorism* and *psychoanalysis*).

Role disputes problem area: In the *interpersonal psychotherapy* treatment of depression, patients are assigned the role disputes problem area if they are struggling to deal with major conflict in an important interpersonal relationship.

Role transitions problem area: In the *interpersonal psychotherapy* treatment of depression, patients are assigned the role transitions problem area if they are experiencing distress as a consequence of a significant role change, including marrying or divorcing, beginning to work or retiring, becoming a parent or coping with "empty nest syndrome," and so forth.

Rotter, Julian B. (1916–2014): This American psychologist made early contributions to *cognitive-behavioral* theories of personality and laid out the tenets of social learning theory.

Secondary process: In *psychoanalysis*, the *conscious* is said to operate on the basis of the secondary process, which involves delay of *instinctual* discharge, binding of mental energy in accordance with external reality, and avoidance of unpleasure. The secondary process is distinguished from the *primary process*.

Self: This term has many distinct meanings within the field of *psychotherapy*. In *analytical psychology*, self is the *archetype* that provides unity, organization, and stability in personality functioning. In *self psychology*, the development of a coherent self is a central psychological principle. *Kohut* related the nuclear, virtual, grandiose, and cohesive selves to one another. *Freud* actually had little to say about the concept of self.

Self-efficacy: This is *Bandura's* term for the belief that one can respond effectively, either to a particular problem or to life problems in general.

Self psychology: Often viewed as the fourth *psychodynamic* school, self psychology postdates *Freud*, having been developed by *Kohut* to show how psychopathology can result from the failure to develop a coherent *self*. *Kohut* applied *object relations* theory to understand individuals with narcissistic personality disturbance. He proposed that the *self* develops as a consequence of important relationships, mostly early in life. In particular, he identified a special kind of *object*, which he called the *selfobject*, that he believed contributed to the development of a coherent *self*, but he also emphasized the value of small empathic failures in early relationships. *Kohut* tied kinds of psychopathology to characteristic failures in the development of a *self*.

Selfobject: This is the term used in *self psychology* that describes the functions that other people perform, such as mirroring and idealizing, to help the child to develop appropriately. Selfobjects are distinguished from other *objects*, in that selfobjects are experienced by the individual as part of the *self*.

Self-dynamism: *Sullivan* described these specific behavior patterns that protect against anxiety. They include dissociation, selective inattention, and others.

Sexual seduction hypothesis: In 1896 *Freud* proposed that patients with hysteria had been sexually victimized earlier in life. However, in 1897 and subsequently he largely repudiated this hypothesis.

Shadow: In *analytical psychology* this *complex* is an alter ego filled with repressed or primitive feelings. The shadow is distinguished from the *persona*.

Shaping: To teach a complex new behavior, a *behaviorist* may start with a behavior already in the individual's repertoire and may then move toward the target behavior in small steps, sequentially reinforcing successive approximations to the new behavior.

Shapiro, Francine (1948–): This American psychologist developed *eye movement reprocessing and desensitization*, a novel treatment for post-traumatic stress disorder.

Skinner, Burrhus F. (1904–1990): This American psychologist experimented extensively in the area of *operant conditioning*.

Spielrein, Sabina N. (1885–1942): This Russian psychoanalyst was an early patient of *Jung*. She later worked in Zurich, Munich, and Vienna before returning to Russia. She published theoretical pieces pertaining to schizophrenia and *thanatos*.

Splitting: This ego psychological *defense* involves the failure to integrate the negative and positive aspects of other people or of oneself. In splitting, the individual perceives others or the *self* as all negative, as all positive, or as alternating between negative and positive. It is often suggested that individuals with borderline personality disorder are particularly likely to engage in splitting, and this assumption forms an important basis for *transference-focused psychotherapy*.

Spontaneous recovery: This *behavioral* term refers to the fact that at some point following *extinction*, the conditional stimulus in question may again begin to elicit the extinguished response.

Stern, Daniel N. (1934–2012): This American psychiatrist wrote about the relationship between *attachment* and the young child's developing sense of *self*.

Strange situation: This is an experimental paradigm used by *Ainsworth* and others to assess the *attachment* pattern of a young child. Patterns identified by the strange situation include secure, anxious-resistant, anxious-avoidant, and disorganized *attachment*.

Striving for superiority: This central concept in *individual psychology* states that humans are innately programmed to seek superiority or perfection. *Adler* believed that this, rather than the sexual *instinct*, was the force that drives human development. He subsequently modified his view a little to state that humans strive not for personal superiority but for a superior or perfect society.

Structural theory: This proposition describes *Freud's* final understanding of the psyche, which he divided into three agents: id, ego, and superego. The id is entirely *unconscious*, while ego and superego are partially conscious and partially *unconscious*. The id contains all the *instinctual* drives, as well as the wishes reflecting memories of earlier gratifications. The ego includes all the mental elements that regulate the interaction between the id and the demands of both the superego and external reality. The superego has the functions of critical self-observation, conscience, and maintenance of the ego ideal. The superego also contains this ego ideal, which has arisen from internalized idealized parental images and is a separate counterfunction to that of the superego.

Style of life: This *individual psychology* term refers to a way of living, including profession and other major features of one's life, that flows directly from one's *fictional finalism*, which is in turn a result of the *Weltanschauung* one developed early in life. A style of life can be either effective or mistaken, a distinction that directly reflects the associated level of social involvement.

Sublimation: This ego psychological *defense* involves the transformation of sexual or aggressive impulses into more socially acceptable actions, behavior, or emotion. In psychoanalytic thinking, sublimation is viewed as the basis of all culture.

Sudden early gain: This refers to significant improvement in a patient that occurs earlier in treatment than is generally expected according to the theory underlying the treatment being offered.

Sullivan, Harry Stack (1892–1949): An American psychiatrist, he was the first major exponent of the interpersonal school and described *self-dynamisms*, modes of communication, and other ideas.

Supportive psychotherapy: This term is used in a variety of ways, generally referring to those *psychotherapeutic* interventions that aim to shore up an individual's functioning without making changes in basic *defenses*.

Suppression: This ego psychological *defense* involves the displacement of threatening thoughts and feelings from the *conscious* into the *preconscious*. Unlike *repression*, in which the threatening material is simply unavailable to awareness, suppression permits one to move scary material out of awareness temporarily, with the ability to return to it later, as one wishes.

Syntaxic mode: *Sullivan* used this term to refer to one's experience of the world using spoken language, which permits symbolization.

Systems theory: Based on concepts from the field of cybernetics, systems theory posits that that families function as self-correcting systems, with built-in servomechanisms to prevent change. Individual symptoms, family structure, and communication patterns are each seen as indicators of one another. Psychotherapeutic treatments based on systems theory analyze family relationships in terms of the structure of the participants' communication with one another. Symptoms are modified through modification of family structure or communication patterns.

Thanatos: In *psychoanalysis*, this is the aggressive or death-directed instinct. Although other theorists had earlier mentioned thanatos, *Freud* didn't begin to write about it until the early 1920s.

Therapeutic alliance: This term refers to the quality of the working relationship between therapist and patient. There are several definitions and several measures of therapeutic alliance, but the best known is the Working Alliance Inventory, which measures alliance based on agreement on the tasks and goals of therapy, as well as the strength of the affective bond between therapist and patient. Therapeutic alliance is known to predict relatively strongly to outcome from *psychotherapy*.

Thorndike, Edward L. (1874–1949): This prolific American psychologist conducted some early experiments that established a foundation for the theory of *operant conditioning*.

Topographic theory: This proposition, first enunciated in *The Interpretation of Dreams*, describes *Freud's* understanding of the psyche according to the interrelationships among three systems: *conscious, preconscious*, and *unconscious*.

Training analysis: Individuals wishing to become psychoanalysts are expected to undertake a training analysis, which is a course of *psychoanalytic* treatment slightly modified for educational purposes.

Transference: This *psychoanalytic* term, now used more broadly, asserts that people perceive one another partly based on interpersonal templates that are established early in life. *Freud* urged that the psychotherapist pay careful attention to patients' transference errors that lead to misperception of the therapist, because such errors might signal the presence of earlier problems in relationships, as well as to point to the development of particular ego *defenses* and thus symptoms of psychopathology.

Transference-focused psychotherapy: Developed by *Kernberg*, this manualized adaptation of *psychoanalytic* treatment aims primarily to help individuals with borderline personality disorder overcome *splitting*.

Transitional object: This is a term coined by *Winnicott* to describe a special object, such as a particular blanket, that helps a young child move from *self* as center of the universe to *self* among many selves in the universe.

True self: *Winnicott* used this term to describe the child's complete access to emotions and to a sense of being fully alive. He believed the true self results when the caregiver deals supportively with the child while at the same time limiting the child's fear resulting from feelings of helplessness in the world. *Winnicott* contrasted true self with *false self*.

Twelve-Step facilitation: This model of *psychotherapy* involves the provision of support for an individual newly recovering from addiction. The patient is strongly encouraged to attend groups like Alcoholics Anonymous, and therapist and patient work through the first five Steps of the AA program.

Unconscious: This *psychoanalytic* term refers to the repository of all the unacceptable desires, memories, thoughts, and feelings pushed out of conscious awareness by *repression*. It is to be distinguished from *preconscious* and *conscious*. This term can also be used an adjective that describes what a person is not aware of.

Undoing: This ego psychological *defense* involves ritualistic activities that atone for unacceptable thoughts or actions.

Watson, John B. (1878–1958): This American psychologist was a prominent *behaviorist* in the first wave.

***Weltanschauung*:** This German word is used in *individual psychology* to describe an individual's view of life or of the world, as influenced by early life experiences.

Weissman, Myrna M. (1935–): Employed as a social worker at the time, this American woman (together with her future husband, *Gerald L. Klerman*) is primarily responsible for the development of *interpersonal psychotherapy*.

Winnicott, Donald W. (1896–1971): This English physician contributed heavily to the theory of *object relations* and is responsible for terms like *transitional object* and good-enough mothering, among others.

Wish fulfillment: In *psychoanalysis*, this is a strategy used by the id to achieve gratification in the face of an unresolved drive. Specifically, the id conjures up an image, which, if real, would be able to satisfy the drive.

Wolpe, Joseph (1915–1997): This South African psychiatrist contributed heavily to the use of *behavioral* techniques in the treatment of anxiety disorders. He is credited with having developed systematic desensitization.

Working through: In *psychoanalysis* this refers to technique of addressing psychological material repeatedly and in depth to overcome the patient's *resistance*.

Index

f denotes figure; t denotes table

A

AA (Alcoholics Anonymous), 223–224
ABA (applied behavior analysis)
  case example, 212–213
  definition, 273
  model of psychopathology, 211
  research findings, 212
  treatment strategies, 211–212
  use of shaping in, 63
A-B-C model of emotional disturbance, 65
Abraham, K., 44
Academy of Cognitive Therapy, 140
acceptance and commitment therapy (ACT), 69
Ackerman, S. J., 94
active imagination, 33
activity scheduling, 124, 175
actual relationship, between child and caregiver, 46, 92
ADHD (attention-deficit/hyperactivity disorder), 77, 232
Adler, A., 12f, 28–30, 33, 35, 36, 49, 273
Adler, V., 29
adolescence stage of development, 41t, 42
adult attachment, 96f
adulthood stage of development, 41–42, 41t, 47, 163
affiliation, 42
aggression, 22, 29, 31, 48, 50, 66, 124
aggressive impulses, 38, 39, 44
agoraphobia, 179, 197–199
Ainsworth, M. D. S., 12f, 53, 273
Alcoholics Anonymous (AA), 223–224
alcohol use disorder
  motivational interviewing (MI) treatment of, case example, 221–223
  twelve-step facilitation treatment of, case example, 225–227
alliance rupture, 93, 94, 98, 151
alter-ego/twinship, 51
altruistic surrender, 38
ambivalence, 110, 118, 219, 220–222
Ametrano, R. M., 96
amygdala, 76, 78, 81
anal characters, 48
anal expulsive, 48
anal retentive, 48
anal stage of development, 40, 273
analysis of resistance, 11, 143
analysis of the transference, 11, 26
analytical psychology, 32, 34–35, 273
analyzing defenses, 124, 143, 151
animus/anima, 34, 273
anterior cingulate cortex, 77, 78, 81
antidepressants, 100, 104
anxiety
  about ending treatment, 143
  attachment-based family therapy and, 245
  Barlow on, 109
  behavioral treatments for, 67
  biofeedback and, 231, 232
  CBT for treatment of children with, 180
  core beliefs and, 176
  counterconditioning and, 60
  diagnostic criteria for, 250
  ERPs and, 193
  exposures and, 126, 234, 255
  hierarchy items and, 193, 201
  H. S. Sullivan on, 47
  implicit memory and, 75
  MBCT and, 241
  M. Klein on, 44, 45
  M. S. Mahler on, 53
  relationship conflicts and, 79
  relaxation training and, 128, 196
  role of avoidance in, 254
  safety behaviors and, 197
  S. C. Hayes on, 69
  S. Freud on, 24, 25, 48
  of therapist, 97
anxiety disorders, 4, 66, 68, 75, 77, 103, 179, 180, 197, 216
anxious-avoidant child, 53
anxious-resistant child, 53
applied behavior analysis (ABA)
  case example, 212–213
  definition, 273
  model of psychopathology, 211
  research findings, 212
  treatment strategies, 211–212
  use of shaping in, 63
approach-approach conflicts, 219
approach-avoidance conflicts, 219
archetypes, 34, 35, 273
Arnkoff, D. B., 96
The Art of Becoming an Original Writer in Three Days (Börne), 15
assertiveness training, 124, 175, 206
assigning homework, 124
attachment, 52, 53, 54, 55, 77–78, 79, 82, 94, 95, 96, 96f, 161, 252, 254, 274
attachment-based family therapy, 243, 245
attachment theory, 214
attending and listening (as basic skills), 114, 116–117, 119, 130, 131, 233, 256
attention
  as one of four processes of observational learning, 64
  as psychological construct, 74, 77, 78
attention and meditative states, 252

INDEX

attention-deficit/hyperactivity disorder (ADHD), 77, 232
augmenting treatments, 234
authenticity, 42
authoritism, 43
autism spectrum disorder, 169, 170, 212, 232
  applied behavior analysis (ABA) treatment of, case example, 212–213
automatic negative thoughts, 65, 66, 175, 177, 178
automatic thought, 175, 176f, 177, 274
autonomy, 40
avoidance, 79, 81–82, 94, 95, 96, 121, 175, 180, 196, 200, 244, 252, 254–255
avoidance-avoidance conflicts, 219
avoidant type of personality, 30
Ayllon, T. J., 59t, 60, 61
Azrin, N. H., 59t, 60, 61

B

Bandura, A., 59t, 63–64, 274
Barlow, D. H., 109, 180, 252
basal ganglia, 76
basic mistrust, 40
basic trust, 40
Beck, A. T., 58, 59t, 64, 65, 66, 79, 174, 175, 274
behavioral experiments, conducted by patients, 66
behavioral tasks, 65, 244
behavioral theorists, list of, 59t
behavioral theory/behaviorism
  contrasted with psychodynamic theory, 4
  definition, 274
  first wave, 58–63
  historical context of, 4–5, 8
  second wave, 63–67
  third wave, 67–69
behavior monitoring, 125, 243
benign cycle, 252

Berman, M. I., 100
Bernays, M., 17
Bernecker, S. L., 96
Bernheim, H., 17, 274
Beyond the Pleasure Principle (S. Freud), 23
Binder, J. L., 151
binge-eating disorder, 208, 216
biofeedback
  case example, 232–233
  definition, 274
  model of psychopathology, 231
  research findings, 232
  treatment strategies, 231–232
bipolar disorder, 67, 102, 103, 214, 216
birth order, 30
Blais, M. A., 86
Bleuler, E., 31
blissful union, 51
Blomberg, J., 144
body armor, 49, 274
boot camp interventions, 91
borderline personality disorder (BPD), 50, 51, 54, 55, 68, 156, 157, 162, 205–206, 207–208
  dialectical behavior therapy (DBT) treatment of, case example, 208–211
  transference-focused psychotherapy (TFP) treatment of, case example, 157–161
Börne, L., 15, 18
Bowlby, J., 12f, 53, 214, 274
brain imaging studies, 77, 80, 81
Brambilla, P., 77
Bratton, S. C., 169
Breuer, J., 12f, 15, 16, 17, 274
brief cognitive therapy for panic disorder
  case example, 198–200
  definition, 274
  mentioned, 110
  model of psychopathology, 196
  research findings, 197
  treatment strategies, 196–197
British Psychoanalytic Society, 45
Bronstein, L., 29
Buchheim, A., 79

Buddhism, 67
bulimia, 216
Burlingame, G. M., 237
Butler, A. J., 81

C

care, virtue of, 43
case examples
  Alan and Dr. Reilly (psychoanalysis), 145–150
  Barbara and Dr. Thompson (psychodynamic psychotherapy), 152–156
  Charlene and Dr. Underwood (transference-focused psychotherapy), 157–161
  Dave and Dr. Vanderzee (mentalization-based treatment), 162–164
  Ella and Dr. Wilson (supportive psychotherapy), 166–168
  Federico and Dr. Yao (play therapy), 170–172
  George and Dr. Brown (cognitive-behavior therapy), 180–185
  Helene and Dr. Brown (cognitive-behavior therapy), 185–187
  Ian and Dr. Brown (cognitive-behavior therapy), 187–189
  Juanita and Dr. Brown (cognitive-behavior therapy), 189–192
  Kevin and Dr. Chu (exposure and response prevention), 193–196
  Lou Ann and Dr. Dennison (brief cognitive therapy for panic disorder), 198–200
  Mark and Dr. Evans (prolonged exposure for posttraumatic stress disorder), 201–204
  Nancy and Dr. Fratelli (dialectical behavior therapy), 208–211

Oleg and Dr. Gaston (applied behavior analysis), 212–213
Paula and Dr. Heller (interpersonal psychotherapy), 217–219
Quinn and Dr. Ito (motivational interviewing), 221–223
Rona and Dr. Johnson (twelve-step facilitation), 225–227
Sam and Dr. Knowles (eye movement desensitization and reprocessing), 229–231
Tina and Dr. Landon (biofeedback), 232–233
Ulrich and Dr. Morris (group psychotherapy), 238–240
Valerie and Dr. Newell (mindfulness-based cognitive therapy), 241–242
Walt, Xenia, and Dr. Philips (family therapy), 245–247
catharsis, 125
cathected, energy as, 22
cathexis, 22, 23, 275
cats, Thorndike's research on, 58, 60, 64
CBASP (Cognitive-Behavioral Analysis System of Psychotherapy), 102
CBT (cognitive-behavior therapy)
beginnings of, 64–65
case examples, 180–192
compared to EMDR, 227, 228
definition, 275
evolution of, 58–63
levels of cognition in, 176*f*
mentioned, 78, 79, 100, 101, 102, 104, 110, 140
model of psychopathology, 174–175, 174*f*
research findings, 179–180
treatment strategies, 175–179

use of in group therapy, 237
cerebellum, 74, 76
certifications, 140
challenges, delivery of (as basic skill), 114, 122–123, 130, 132
change talk, 220
character, psychodynamic approaches to, 48–52
Character Analysis(Reich), 49
character disorders, 48, 275
character disturbances, 49
Charcot, J.-M., 17, 275
checklists
 symptom checklists, 110
 therapist compliance checklists, 133, 256
cheerleading, 216
Chiesa, A., 77, 79
child analysis, and developmental theory, 52–54
child-management skills/training, 243, 245
chronicity, 254
chronic major depression, 101
Clark, D. A., 79
classical conditioning, 59, 60, 61, 64, 275
client-centered psychotherapy, 37, 114–115, 120, 220, 275
clomipramine, 103
closed questions, 119, 120, 131
cocaine, 15–16
cognition(s), 45, 61, 64, 65, 66, 67, 80, 174, 175, 176, 177, 179, 180, 201, 211, 214, 228, 243, 244, 252
Cognitive-Behavioral Analysis System of Psychotherapy (CBASP), 102
cognitive-behavior therapy (CBT)
beginnings of, 64–65
case examples, 180–192
compared to EMDR, 227, 228
definition, 275
evolution of, 58–63
levels of cognition in, 176*f*
mentioned, 78, 79, 100, 101, 102, 104, 110, 140
model of psychopathology, 174–175, 174*f*
research findings, 179–180
treatment strategies, 175–179

use of in group therapy, 237
cognitive therapy, 66, 104, 174, 193
See also brief cognitive therapy for panic disorder
See also mindfulness-based cognitive therapy (MBCT)
cognitive variables, 63
cohesive self, 51
collaboration, 2, 28, 33
collaborative empiricism, 178, 275
collective psychology, 34
collective unconscious, 34, 275
Columbo, 123
combined treatment, 86, 100–103
competence, virtue, 42
complementary and alternative medicine therapies, 233–235
complexes, 34, 276
See also Oedipus complex
condensation, 20, 21, 276
conduct disorder, 91, 238, 245
conscience, 25
conscious, 20, 21, 23, 24, 25, 38, 276
Constantino, M. J., 96
constructing hierarchies, 125
constructive alternativism, 66, 276
Consumer Reports, 86
contingent reinforcement, 125–126, 212
continuation and maintenance psychotherapy, 103–105
conversion, 38, 276
core beliefs, 66, 175, 176, 177, 179, 200, 201, 276
core mindfulness, 206
core self, 53
core-self-with-another, 53
cortical mapping, 74

cortical remapping, 74
cortico-limbic integration, 78, 81
cortico-limbic pathways, 78, 79
countercathexis, 22, 276
counterconditioning, 60, 276–277
countertransference, 10, 11, 26, 28, 31, 32, 36, 47, 54, 96, 97, 98, 106, 130, 133, 162, 277
couples therapy, 243–244
creative self, 30, 277
critical incident stress debriefing, 91
A critical review of the Freudian sexual theory of psychic life(Adler), 28
Cuijpers, P., 101, 166
cultural challenges/issues/ implications, 28, 117, 122

D

DBT (dialectical behavior therapy)
 case example, 208–211
 definition, 277
 mentioned, 68, 69, 157, 236
 model of psychopathology, 205
 research findings, 207–208
 treatment strategies, 206–207
death instinct, 22, 31, 44, 292
decision analysis, 216
defenses, analyzing of, 124
defenses/defense mechanisms, 10, 24, 37, 38–39, 45, 277
defense structure, 10, 26, 88, 129, 143, 144, 165, 168
De Jonghe, F., 103, 151
Dekker, J., 103, 151
Del Re, A. C., 93
De Maat, S., 103, 151, 166
demands, 65
denial, 39, 277
dependency issues, 48
depressed perfectionistic patients, 95, 98
depression
 A.T. Beck on, 66
 Barlow on, 109
 behavioral treatments for, 67

biofeedback and, 232
CBASP and, 102
CBT and, 179, 180
combined treatment of, 100
cortico-limbic integration and, 81
exposures and, 82, 234
IPT and, 214, 215, 216
MBCT and, 68, 69, 104, 240, 241, 254
meditation for, 68
mentalized-based treatment for, 55
M. Klein on, 44
neurobiology and psychotherapy of, 78–80
non-directive supportive therapy and, 166
S. Freud on, 65
symptomatic level of patient and, 94
depressive position of development, 45, 277
despair, 43
developing discrepancy, 220
development, Erikson's eight stages of, 41t, 279
developmental positions, as compared to stages, 44
development theory, child analysis and, 52–54
dialectical behavior therapy (DBT)
 case example, 208–211
 definition, 277
 mentioned, 68, 69, 157, 236
 model of psychopathology, 205
 research findings, 207–208
 treatment strategies, 206–207
Dialectical Materialism and Psychoanalysis(Reich), 49
differential effectiveness (of psychotherapy), 89–90
direct disputation, 65
discrepancy, development of, 220
discrimination, 63, 277
disorder-specific, versus principle-driven treatment, 254
disorganized attachment, 53

displacement, 20–21, 22, 38, 278
dissociation, 39, 47, 278
dissociative identity disorder, 91
distress tolerance, 206
diversity issues, 117
Dodo bird hypothesis, 5, 6, 90, 92, 114, 233, 250, 278
dogmatic consistency, as therapeutic stance, 6, 110
dogs, Pavlov's research on, 58, 59
dorsolateral prefrontal cortex, 77
dorsomedial frontal cortex, 78
dose-response issues, 84, 87–89
downward arrow, 126, 177
Dr. Bob, 223
dream analysis/ interpretation, 20, 143, 151
dreams, 19, 20, 21, 22, 24, 65
Driessen, E., 166
drive derivatives, 21, 278
Drug Abuse and Resistance Education programs, 90
DSM-5, 80, 101, 232, 250
DSM-IV, 80, 101, 103, 216, 250
dynamic theory, 19, 21, 278
dysphoric thoughts, 240
dysthymia, 101, 103, 216
D'Zurilla, T. J., 59t, 66

E

early attachment experiences, 52
early childhood experiences, 10, 11, 40, 43, 47, 54, 95
early childhood stage of development, 40, 41t
Eastern philosophy, 33
eating disorders, 55, 66, 180, 208, 216
eclecticism, 6, 110, 278
economic theory, 19, 21–22, 278
effectiveness
 definition, 279
 versus efficacy, 85–87, 100

effect size, 85t, 101, 144, 166, 221, 278–279
efficacy
 definition, 279
 versus effectiveness, 85–87, 100
efficacy studies, 85, 86, 91, 100, 250
ego, 10, 23, 24, 26, 40, 44
ego defenses, 10, 22, 24, 37, 38, 43, 48, 165
ego development, 40
ego ideal, 25
ego integrity, 43
ego psychology, 10, 37–43, 50, 51, 252, 279
either-or views, 68
elitism, 42
Ellis, A., 59t, 64, 65, 66, 279
Ellison, W. D., 96
EMDR (eye movement desensitization and reprocessing)
 case example, 229–231
 compared to CBT, 227, 228
 definition, 280
 model of psychopathology, 227
 research findings, 228
 treatment strategies, 228
emotional disturbance, A-B-C model of, 65
emotional release, 52
emotion regulation, 206
empathic therapist, 52
empathy, showing of (as basic skill), 54, 114, 120–121, 130, 131–132
empirically supported treatment, 2, 6, 84, 90–91, 92, 109, 110, 151, 179–180, 234, 250, 279
encoding, 75, 76, 81
encounter groups, 108
energy transfer theory, 21
environmental conditioning, 60
Erikson, E. H., 12f, 37, 39–43, 279
eros, 22, 279
erotic countertransference, 31
erotic transference, 28, 31
ERP (exposure and response prevention)
 case example, 193–196
 definition, 279
 mentioned, 61
 model of psychopathology, 192
 research findings, 193
 treatment strategies, 192–193
ethnicity, 94, 95, 98
expectancy, 2, 64, 94, 96, 109, 279
experiencing, Sullivan's three modes of, 47
experiments, planning of, 127
explicit memory, 75, 76, 80
exposure, 126
exposure and response prevention (ERP)
 case example, 193–196
 definition, 279
 mentioned, 61
 model of psychopathology, 192
 research findings, 193
 treatment strategies, 192–193
external ("real") anxiety, 25
external reinforcement, 64
external validity, 86, 280
extinction, 61–62, 62f, 63, 77, 81–82, 102, 126, 211, 243, 280
extraversion (as dominant attitude in Jung's theory of personality types), 34, 36f
eye movement desensitization and reprocessing (EMDR)
 case example, 229–231
 compared to CBT, 227, 228
 definition, 280
 model of psychopathology, 227
 research findings, 228
 treatment strategies, 228
Eysenck, H. J., 84, 85

F

Falk, P., 123
fallback rule, 118, 120, 131
false self, 46, 280
family therapy
 case example, 245–247
 mentioned, 144
 model of psychopathology, 242–243
 research findings, 245
 treatment strategies, 243–244
father–child relationship, 36
Fava, G. A., 104
Fava, M., 104
feedback, 126, 234
feeling (as rational function in Jung's theory of personality types), 34, 36f
feeling understood, 114
Ferenczi, S., 12f, 28, 35, 36, 37, 44, 54, 150, 280
fictional finalisms, 30, 280
fidelity, 42
fixation, 23, 48, 280
fixed-interval reinforcement schedule, 62
fixed-ratio reinforcement schedule, 62
flight into health, 88
Floortime, 169, 170
Flückiger, C., 93
Foa, E. B., 103
Fonagy, P., 12f, 54, 280
formalism, 42
formality, 42, 288–289
Forman, E. M., 87
free association, 11, 15, 17, 18, 31, 65, 126, 142–143, 151, 168
Freud, A., 12f, 17, 24, 27, 37–39, 40, 44, 45, 52, 169, 280
Freud, E., 12
Freud, J. (Jakob), 12, 14, 19
Freud, J. (Johann), 13, 16
Freud, J. (Julius), 13
Freud, S.
 and Adler, 28, 30
 case of Little Hans, 169
 on character disorders, 48
 childhood and family, 11–15
 on countertransference, 97
 described, 280
 on ego, 37
 and Ferenczi, 35
 ideas about psychoanalytic treatment, 25–26
 and Jung, 31, 32–33
 and Klein, 44
 medical training and early career, 15–17
 on nature of therapeutic relationship, 92

Freud, S. (*Cont.*)
old age, 26–27
as one of major psychodynamic theorists, 12*f*
overview, 10–11
and primary process thinking, 143
private practice in Vienna, 17–19
psychoanalysis model, 142
and Rank, 35, 36
and Reich, 49
understanding of psychopathology, 25
understanding of the psyche, 19–25
Freudians, 45
Friedman, M. A., 101
frontal cortex, 78, 79
functional behavior assessment, 212
functional family therapy, 244, 245
The Function of the Orgasm(Reich), 49
fusiform gyrus, 81

G

generalization, 63, 280
General Medical Society of Psychotherapy, 33–34
generalized anxiety disorder
biofeedback treatment of, case example, 232–233
psychodynamic psychotherapy treatment of, case example, 152–156
generationalism, 43
generativity, 42–43
genetic theory, 19, 22–23, 280–281
genital characters, 48
genital stage of development, 23, 42, 281
Gestalt psychotherapy, 85, 108
getting-leaning type of personality, 30
gist memory, 81
Glass, C. R., 96
Glass, G. V., 84
goals, setting of, 128
Goldfried, M. R., 59*t*, 66

good-enough mothering, 46
grandiose self, 51, 52
Greenberg, L. S., 93
gregariousness/isolation poles, 48
grief problem area, 281
group cohesion, 236
group psychotherapy
case example, 238–240
model of psychopathology, 236–237
research findings, 237–238
treatment strategies, 237
guided imagery, 234
Guidi, J., 104
guilt, 14, 25, 39, 42, 215

H

Hansen, N. B., 87
Hassidic Jews, 14
Hayes, S. C., 59*t*, 69, 281
hierarchies, construction of, 125
Hilsenroth, M. J., 94
Hoag, M. J., 237
hobby analysis, 108
Hofmann, S. G., 102
holding (by mother of infant), 46
Homburger, Dr., 39, 40
Homburger, E.
See Erikson, Erik H.
homework, assignment of, 124–125
hope, 2, 40, 88
Horvath, A. O., 93
human development, Erikson's tripartite model of, 40, 41*t*
Hungarian Society of Psychoanalysis, 44
hydraulic theory, 21
hypnosis, 15, 16, 17, 18, 234
hysteria, 16, 17, 18, 19, 22

I

id, 19, 23–24, 25, 26, 37, 44
idealized parent imago, 51
idealized selfobject, 52
identification, 38, 45, 281
identification with the aggressor, 38

identity crisis, 39, 42
ideology, 42
idolism, 40
id psychology, 37
imaginal exposure, 82, 200, 201
imipramine, 78, 101
impersonation, 42
implicit memory, 75, 76, 252
Independents, 45
individual psychology, 29–30, 281
individuation, 33, 52, 281
industry, 42
infancy stage of development, 40, 41*t*, 45, 47
infants, application of psychoanalysis to, 44
inferiority, 11, 29, 30, 36, 42
initiative, 41
instincts, 20, 21, 22, 28, 32, 44, 45, 150, 281
See also death instinct
See also sexual instincts
insula, 81
integralism, 43
intermediate beliefs, 175, 176*f*, 177, 281
intermittent reinforcement, 62
internal objects, 43, 45
internal validity, 85, 281
interoceptive exposure, 197, 282
Interpersonal and Social Rhythm Therapy (IPSRT), 214
interpersonal deficits problem area, 215, 282
interpersonal effectiveness, 206
interpersonal inventory, 215, 282
interpersonal psychotherapy (IPT)
case example, 217–219
definition, 282
mentioned, 77, 101, 102, 104
model of psychopathology, 214
research findings, 216
treatment strategies, 214–216
interpersonal relationships, 5, 47, 55, 215, 252
interpersonal school, 46–48, 214

interpretation, 126
The Interpretation of Dreams (S. Freud), 19, 20, 28, 58
intersubjective perspective, 54
intersubjectivity, 54
intimacy, 42, 77, 95, 96, 96f, 106, 243, 244
intrapsychic conflict, 25, 214
introjection, 45, 48
introversion (as dominant attitude in Jung's theory of personality types), 34, 36f
intuition (as irrational function in Jung's theory of personality types), 34, 36f
invalidating environment, 205
in vivo exposure, 82, 192, 193, 197, 200
IPSRT (Interpersonal and Social Rhythm Therapy), 214
IPT (interpersonal psychotherapy)
 case example, 217–219
 definition, 282
 mentioned, 77, 101, 102, 104
 model of psychopathology, 214
 research findings, 216
 treatment strategies, 214–216
isolation, 42, 236
isolation of affect/dissociation, 39, 282

J

James, K. H., 81
Jewishness, of S. Freud, 14–15, 27, 32–33
Jews
 in Central Europe, 12, 27, 28, 31, 32, 36, 37, 39, 48, 51
 and General Medical Society of Psychotherapy, 33–34
Jones, E., 27, 28, 44
Jones, L., 169
journaling, 126
judiciousness, 42
Jung, C. G., 12f, 28, 30–35, 223, 282
Jungian analysis, 32, 33, 34

K

Kabat-Zinn, J., 59t, 68, 126, 282
Keller, M. B., 103
Kelly, G., 59t, 66–67, 282
Kennedy, S. H., 78
Kernberg, O. F., 12f, 48, 50, 52, 156, 282
Klein, M., 12f, 43–45, 46, 52, 53, 169, 282
Kleinians, 45
Klerman, G. L., 214, 282
Knekt, P., 144
Kohut, H., 12f, 48, 51–52, 54, 282
Korte, K. J., 102

L

Lambert, M. J., 87, 92
latency period of development, 23, 42, 282
Lazar, A., 144
learning, as psychological construct, 74–75
legalism, 42
Leichsenring, F., 144
Levy, K. N., 96
libido, 20, 22, 23, 28, 32, 44, 50, 283
Lilienfeld, S. O., 90, 234
limbic system, 79
Linehan, M. M., 59t, 68, 205–206, 207, 283
Little Hans (case of), 169
London, as hotbed of psychoanalytic thinking, 37, 43
long-term potentiation, 76, 78
Luborsky, L., 89

M

Mahler, M. S., 12f, 52–53, 283
maintenance IPT, 104, 216
major depressive disorder, 79, 101, 103
 cognitive-behavior therapy (CBT) treatment of, case example, 180–185
 interpersonal psychotherapy (IPT) treatment of, case example, 217–219
 mindfulness-based cognitive therapy (MBCT) treatment of, case example, 241–242

Manber, R., 102
manualized treatments, 6, 133, 157, 256
marital counseling, 242
massage, 50
MBCT (mindfulness-based cognitive therapy)
 case example, 241–242
 definition, 283
 development of, 68
 mentioned, 179
 model of psychopathology, 240
 and relapse, 104, 254
 research findings, 240–241
 treatment strategies, 240
MBT (mentalization-based treatment)
 case example, 162–164
 as current trend in psychodynamic psychotherapy, 54, 55
 definition, 283
 mentioned, 151
 model of psychopathology, 161
 research findings, 162
 treatment strategies, 161–162
McRoberts, C., 237
medial prefrontal regions, 81
meditation, 67–69, 77, 127, 206, 223, 224, 240
meditation training, 77, 79
Meichenbaum, D. H., 59t, 66
melancholia, 44
memory
 explicit, 75, 76, 80
 gist, 81
 implicit, 75, 76
 procedural, 76
 as psychological construct, 75–77
 retaining of, 76
 working, 75–76, 80
memory reconsolidation, 76
mentalism, 60
mentalization, 54, 55
mentalization-based treatment (MBT)
 case example, 162–164
 as current trend in psychodynamic psychotherapy, 54, 55
 definition, 283

mentalization-based treatment (MBT) (Cont.)
mentioned, 151
model of psychopathology, 161
research findings, 162
treatment strategies, 161–162
mental life, S. Freud's approaches to/theory of, 19, 21, 22, 23, 37
meta-analysis, 78, 84, 85, 86, 89, 90, 93, 96, 100, 101, 102, 104, 144, 151, 169, 221, 237, 241, 283
MI (motivational interviewing)
case example, 221–223
definition, 283
mentioned, 110, 118, 122
model of psychopathology, 219–220
research findings, 221
treatment strategies, 220–221
Mikulincer, M., 77
Miller, T. I., 84
Miller, W. R., 219
Minami, T., 86
mindfulness, 126–127, 179, 205, 206
mindfulness-based cognitive therapy (MBCT)
case example, 241–242
definition, 283
development of, 68
mentioned, 179
model of psychopathology, 240
and relapse, 104, 254
research findings, 240–241
treatment strategies, 240
mindfulness-based stress reduction, 68
mindfulness meditation studies, 77
mirroring selfobjects, 51
mirror neurons, 252
mixed-model theorist, Kernberg as, 50
modeling, 127, 128, 236
Møldrup, C., 104
monotherapy, 5, 100–103, 216
mood disorders, 66, 68, 75, 77, 102, 197, 214, 215, 216

moral anxiety, 25
Moses and Monotheism(S. Freud), 27
mother–child relationship, 30, 36
motivation, as one of four processes of observational learning, 64
motivational enhancement therapy, 220–221, 225
motivational interviewing (MI)
case example, 221–223
definition, 283
mentioned, 110, 118, 122
model of psychopathology, 219–220
research findings, 221
treatment strategies, 220–221
motor reproduction, as one of four processes of observational learning, 64
Mowrer, O. H., 59t, 60
Mowrer, W. M., 59t, 60
multidetermination (overdetermination), 21, 283
Munder, T., 89
Muran, J. C., 93
muscle tension, 50, 231
muscle tone, 49, 50

N

narcissism, 50, 51, 52
Narcotics Anonymous, 223
National Institute of Mental Health (NIMH), 90
nefazodone, 102
negative identity, 42
negative reinforcement, 61, 62f, 192, 200, 212, 283
neurobiological correlates, overview, 5
neurobiology
and psychotherapy of depression, 78–80
and psychotherapy of PTSD, 80–82
neurogenesis, 74, 76
neuroplasticity, 74–78, 80, 82, 283
neuroscience, anticipations in, 252–253

neurotransmitters, 76
neutrality (of therapist), 143
New Introductory Lectures(S. Freud), 25
NIMH (National Institute of Mental Health), 90
non-directive supportive therapy, 166
Norcross, J. C., 92
nuclear self, 51
nucleus accumbens, 79
number needed to treat (NNT), 87, 283
numinous, 40

O

O., Anna (case of), 15, 16, 18
object
according to S. Freud, 22
definition, 43, 284
relationship with self, 50
objectivity, 46
object relations couples therapy, 243
object relations/object relations theory, 10, 37, 43–46, 47, 50, 51, 52, 54, 168, 284
observational learning, 64
observing ego, 24, 26, 142, 284
obsessive-compulsive disorder (OCD), 38, 61, 77, 90, 103, 179, 192, 193, 254, 255
exposure and response prevention (ERP) treatment of, case example, 194–196
obsessive-compulsive personality disorder, cognitive-behavior therapy (CBT) treatment of, case example, 186–189
occipital cortex, 79
odds ratio (OR), 284
Oedipal phase of development, 23
Oedipus complex, 11, 13–14, 19, 20, 25, 26, 28, 30, 42, 44, 151, 169, 284
Oestergaard, S., 104
old age stage of development, 41t, 43
one-person psychology, 11, 54

open questions, 119, 120, 131, 220
operant conditioning, 58, 59–60, 61, 125, 211, 284
optimal frustration, 52, 284
oral characters, 48
oral stage of development, 23, 40, 48, 284
orbitofrontal cortex, 77
organ inferiority, 29, 284
organismic valuing system, 114–115, 284
overdetermination (multidetermination), 21
Oxford Group, 223

P

panic disorder, 90, 110, 196–198
 brief cognitive therapy for panic disorder treatment of, case example, 198–200
Papakostas, G. I., 104
paranoid-schizoid position of development, 45, 285
paraphrasing, 116, 117, 118
parataxic mode of experience, 47, 48, 285
parent-child interactions, 40
parent-child interaction therapy, 243, 245
paroxetine, 102, 104
parroting, 118
participant-observer, 48
patient factors predicting to outcome, 94–96
Pavlov, I. P., 58, 59t, 60, 62, 285
PE-PTSD (prolonged exposure for posttraumatic stress disorder)
 case example, 201–204
 definition, 286
 model of psychopathology, 200
 research findings, 201
 treatment strategies, 200–201
perception, 10, 26, 36f, 43, 46, 60, 97, 121, 156, 157

persistent depressive disorder, 101
persona, 34, 285
personal construct theory of psychopathology, 66
personality
 according to Sullivan, 47–48
 sexual instincts as prime mover in development of, 19
 theory of, 25, 29
personality development, theories of, 19
personality disorders, 24, 48, 66, 75, 77, 95, 144, 157, 176, 177, 236
personality integration techniques, 33
personality type(s)
 definition, 285
 theory of, 34, 36f
personal unconscious, 34, 285
phallic phase of development, 23, 42, 48, 285
pharmacotherapy, 6, 80, 86, 88, 100, 101, 102, 103, 104, 105–106
pharmacotherapy alliance, 105
phobias, 25, 60, 64, 125, 126, 127, 128, 179, 197, 216
placebo, 85, 102, 103, 105, 109, 193, 252
planning experiments, 127
play therapy
 case example, 170–172
 definition, 285
 mentioned, 52
 model of psychopathology, 168–169
 research findings, 169–170
 treatment strategies, 169
pleasure principle, 21, 22, 285
pluralism, 6, 110, 285–286
positive reinforcement, 61, 62f, 211, 243, 286
posthypnotic amnesia, 17
posttraumatic stress disorder (PTSD), 55, 74, 75, 80–82, 89, 179, 216, 227, 228, 232
 eye movement desensitization and reprocessing (EMDR) treatment of, case example, 229–231

prolonged exposure for post-traumatic stress disorder (PE-PTSD) treatment of, case example, 202–204
prayer, 197, 223, 224
preconscious, 20, 23, 24, 38, 286
precuneus, 81
prefrontal cortex, 76, 77, 78, 80, 81–82
pregenual anterior cingular cortex, 78
preschool stage of development, 41t, 42
pride/humility poles, 48
primal repression, 81
primary maternal preoccupation, 46
primary process, 20, 21, 23, 45, 143, 286
priming, 75, 76
problem solving, 127
procedural memories, 75, 76
process note, 133
projection, 39, 45, 286
"The Project" (S. Freud), 19
prolonged exposure for posttraumatic stress disorder (PE-PTSD)
 case example, 201–204
 definition, 286
 model of psychopathology, 200
 research findings, 201
 treatment strategies, 200–201
promiscuity/chastity poles, 48
proposed learning sequence
 for basic skills, 130–132
 for methods of psychotherapy, 132–133
prototaxic mode of experience, 47, 286
psyche, S. Freud's understanding of, 19–25
psychiatric treatment studies, overview of, 5
psychiatry, psychotherapy within, 108–111
psychic conflict, 44
psychic determinism, 21, 286
psychic energy, 21, 22
psychic structures, theories of, 19

psychoanalysis
case example, 145–150
definition, 286
model of psychopathology, 142
phases of, 143
psychodynamic psychotherapy, as distinct from, 10
research findings, 144
treatment strategies, 142–143
psychoanalytic treatment, S. Freud's ideas about, 25–26
psychodynamic psychotherapy
case example, 152–156
definition, 286–287
model of psychopathology, 150
research findings, 151
treatment strategies, 150–151
psychodynamic theory
contrasted with behavioral theory, 4
current trends in, 54–55
evolution of, 10–55
historical context of, 4–5, 8
major psychodynamic theorists, 12f
psychoeducation, 127, 128, 165, 177, 192, 196, 201, 215, 244, 245, 252
psychological-mindedness, 54, 161
psychological theory, anticipations in, 254–255
psychology
for neurologists, 19
research findings in, 84–99
psychoneuroses, sexual etiology of, 19
psychopathology
occurrence of, 54
S. Freud's understanding of, 25
psychosexual development, theory of, 22
psychosis, 25, 31, 32, 45, 50, 51, 178, 250
psychosocial treatments, 234
psychotherapists
list of, 59t
Strupp's ten desiderata for, 98–99

psychotherapy
basic skills of, 114, 116–123, 130
bringing psychotherapeutic understanding to pharmacotherapy, 105–106
common techniques of, 124–129
continuation and maintenance, 103–105
definition, 287
differential effectiveness of, 89–90
dose-response issues, 87–89
efficacy versus effectiveness, 85–87
empirically supported treatment, 90–91
group psychotherapy See group psychotherapy
how it works, 92–99
log-linear relationship between symptomatic relief and time in treatment, 87f
mean effect sizes of various types of, 85t
overall effectiveness of, 84–85
patient factors predicting to outcome, 94–96
within psychiatry, 108–111
rate of recovery in, 84–92
relationship factors in, 92–94
therapist factors predicting outcome of, 96–98
training, 140
psychotropic medications, 5, 67, 89, 91, 100, 103, 215
PTSD (posttraumatic stress disorder), 55, 74, 75, 80–82, 89, 179, 216, 227, 228, 232
See also prolonged exposure for posttraumatic stress disorder (PE-PTSD)
punishment, 25, 42, 61, 62, 62f, 205, 287
purpose, virtue of, 42
purposeful misattunements, 54

Q

questions (as basic skills), 114, 119–120, 130, 131
See also closed questions
See also open questions

R

Rabung, S., 144
radical environmentalism, 60
randomized controlled trial (RCT), 85, 86, 87, 88, 89, 90, 101, 144, 151, 162, 180, 193, 221, 224, 240, 287
random walk, 88
Rank, O., 12f, 28, 35–37, 150, 287
rational-emotive behavior therapy (REBT), 65
rationalization, 39, 287
Ray, D., 169
reaction formation, 38, 39, 48, 287
reality principle, 23–24, 288
reconsolidation, 76–77, 81
recording, of sessions with supervisor, 132
recovered memory techniques, 91
recurrence, 5, 68, 103, 104, 214, 216, 240, 241
reframing, 127
regression, 23, 38, 44, 288
rehearsal, 127
Reich, W., 12f, 23, 48–50, 288
reinforcement
contingent, 125–126, 212
external, 64
negative, 61, 192, 200, 212, 283
positive, 61, 211, 243, 286
self-reinforcement, 64
types of, 62f
vicarious, 64
reinforcement schedules, 60, 62–63, 211, 212, 288
rejection, 45, 77, 78, 96, 196, 254
relapse, 5, 68, 103, 104, 214, 216, 240, 241
relapse prevention, 5, 127–128, 175, 193, 197, 201, 216

relational approaches, 54
relational psychoanalysis, 54
relationship factors, 92–94, 96, 98
relaxation training, 128, 196, 201, 234
religion, S. Freud's ideas about, 11, 14, 15, 26
remission, 5, 88, 100, 102, 103, 104, 165, 193, 236, 240, 244, 245, 254
REM sleep, 227
repression, 20, 22, 24, 26, 28, 38, 44, 48, 288
resistance, 10, 18, 24, 26, 104, 109, 110, 142, 143, 151, 179, 219, 220, 221, 288
restatements, 114, 117–119, 121, 130, 131
retention, as one of four processes of observational learning, 64
Reynolds, C. F., 101
Rhine, T., 169
right paracingulate cortex, 78
Rita (case of), 44
ritualisms, 40, 42, 288–289
ritualizations, 40, 42, 43, 289
Rogers, C. R., 36, 37, 114, 120, 289
role confusion, 41
role disputes problem area, 215, 289
role plays
  as common psychotherapy technique, 128, 178, 216
  for learning psychotherapy skills, 130–132, 256
role transitions problem area, 215, 289
rolling with resistance, 220
Rotter, J. B., 59t, 64, 289
ruling-dominant type of personality, 30
rumination, 77, 252, 254–255
Russian Psychoanalytic Association, 32

S

Sacher, J., 78
safety behaviors, 192, 197, 255

Sandell, R., 144
sapientism, 43
Sawyer, A. T., 102
Scared Straight interventions, 91
schema-focused therapy, 157
schizoaffective disorder, cognitive-behavior therapy (CBT) treatment of, case example, 189–192
schizophrenia, 31, 32, 47, 67, 140, 180, 244, 245
Schoevers, R., 103, 151
school-age stage of development, 41
Schur, M., 27
Scott, L. N., 96
secondary elaboration, 21
secondary process, 20, 289
secure attachment, 53, 77, 78, 79, 94, 95, 96f, 98, 162, 169
secure base, 53, 252
selective inattention, 47
self
  as archetype, 34, 35
  cohesive self, 51
  concept of, 54
  creative self, 277
  definition, 289
  grandiose self, 51, 52
  as internal object, 43
  and interpersonal context, 51
  nuclear self, 51
  psychodynamic approaches to, 48–52
  relationship with object, 50
  subjective self, 54
  true self, 293
  verbal self, 54
  virtual self, 51
self-analysis, 11, 13, 33
self-cohesion, 51
self-correcting systems, 242
self-dynamisms, 47, 290
self-efficacy, 64, 220, 221, 289
self-esteem, 38, 50, 51, 52, 219
self-injury, 68, 157, 206, 207
self-knowledge, 26, 32, 142
selfobjects, 51–52, 290
self-observation, 18, 25
self-preservation, 45

self psychology, 51, 54, 289–290
self-realization, 35
self-regulation, 180, 252
self-reinforcement, 64
self-talk, 66
sensation (as irrational function in Jung's theory of personality types), 34, 36f
separation, 36, 39, 51, 74, 150, 151, 287
separation-individuation, 52–53
sequential treatment, 104
Serretti, A., 77
setting goals, 128
setting time limits for treatment, 128
sex
  conflict about, 48
  and dreams, 22
sexual identity, 48
sexual instincts/sexual instinctual drives, 19, 21, 23, 36
sexual matters
  child's experience at school affected by, 45
  in genital stage, 23
  and hysteria, 17, 18, 22
sexual ontogeny and phylogeny, 36
sexual seduction hypothesis, 18, 19, 21, 290
sexual theory, 20, 28
Shadish, W. R., 86
shadow, 34, 290
sham psychotherapy, 85
shaping, 63, 290
Shapiro, F., 227, 290
Shaver, P. R., 77
short psychodynamic supportive psychotherapy, 166
short-term treatment methods, 30
sick role, 215
skill building, 128, 133, 207
Skinner, B. F., 59t, 60, 61, 290
Smith, J. Z., 96
Smith, M. L., 84, 85, 89
Smits, J. A. J., 102
social anxiety disorder, cognitive-behavior therapy (CBT) treatment of, case example, 185–187
social-cognitive theory, 63–64

social interest, 30
socially useful type of personality, 30
socioenvironmental circumstances, 49
Socratic questioning, 128–129, 178
somatic interventions, 2, 5, 67, 74, 252, 254
Spielmans, G. I., 100
Spielrein, S., 31–32, 290
Spivack, G., 59t, 66
splitting, 39, 45, 50, 156, 290
spontaneous recovery, 62, 290
stagnation, 41, 43
Stern, D. N., 12f, 53–54, 290
Stiles, T. C., 151
stimulus control, 129, 212
strange situation, 53, 291
stress hormones, 76
structural theory, 19, 23–25, 291
Strupp, H. H., 98, 151
Studies on Hysteria (Breuer and Freud), 16
style of life, 30, 291
subgenual anterior cingulate cortex/subgenual cingulate, 78, 79
subjective early experience, 10, 11
subjective self, 54
subjectivity, 46
sublimation, 38, 48, 291
substance abuse, 66, 110, 208, 216, 220, 221, 223, 232, 236
sudden early gains, 5, 88, 92, 291
Sullivan, H. S., 12f, 46–48, 54, 291
summaries, 221
summary statement, 117, 118
superego, 19, 23, 25, 38, 44, 45, 50
superiority, striving for, 29, 35, 150, 165, 291
supervision, 114, 120, 121, 130, 132, 133
supportive psychotherapy
case example, 166–168
definition, 291
model of psychopathology, 165
research findings, 166
treatment strategies, 165
suppression, 38, 80, 81, 291

sustain talk, 219, 220, 221
Svartberg, M., 151
Symonds, D., 93
symptomatic relief, 87f, 142
symptom checklists, 110
synaptic consolidation, 76
syntaxic mode of experience, 47, 48, 292
systematic desensitization, 60, 61, 64, 85
systems consolidation, 76
systems theory, 245, 292
systems therapies, 242

T

tactical silence, 116
talk therapy, 2, 5, 165
Taoist philosophy, 33
teaching tales, 16–17
tenderness, 47
TFP (transference-focused psychotherapy)
case example, 157–161
definition, 292
as developed by Kernberg, 50
mentioned, 151
model of psychopathology, 156–157
research findings, 157
treatment strategies, 157
thalamus, 79, 81
thanatos (death instinct), 22, 31, 44, 292
theory of instincts, 20, 28
therapeutic alliance, 78, 84, 91, 93–94, 98, 101, 114, 179, 216, 221, 233, 234, 236, 254, 292
therapist compliance checklists, 133, 256
therapist factors predicting outcome, 5, 84, 92, 96–98
therapist motor habits, 116
therapist neutrality, 143
therapist regrets, 98
therapist's attachment style, 97, 254
thinking (as rational function in Jung's theory of personality types), 34, 36f
Thorndike, E. L., 58, 59t, 60, 64, 292
thought-action fusion, 192
thoughts

automatic negative thoughts, 65, 66, 175, 177, 178
automatic thoughts, 176, 176f, 177, 274
dysphoric thoughts, 240
as transient mental phenomena, 66
Three Essays on the Theory of Sexuality (S. Freud), 22
time limits for treatment, setting of, 128
titles, of professionals working in psychotherapy, 140
token economy, 60, 61
topographic theory, 19, 20–21, 292
totalism, 41
training
assertiveness training, 124, 138, 175, 206
child-management skills/ training, 243, 245
meditation training, 77, 79
psychotherapy training, 140
relaxation training, 128, 196, 201, 234
training analysis, 26, 32, 45, 292
transdiagnostic variant (of CBT), 180
transference, 10, 11, 22, 26, 28, 31, 32, 36, 45, 51, 52, 92, 94, 133, 142, 143, 162, 236, 292
transference-focused psychotherapy (TFP)
case example, 157–161
definition, 292
as developed by Kernberg, 50
mentioned, 151
model of psychopathology, 156–157
research findings, 157
treatment strategies, 157
transference work, 129, 143, 151, 157, 161
transient mental phenomena, 67, 69
transitional objects, 46, 51, 292
treatment manuals, 109, 179, 180, 256

Treatment of Depression Collaborative Research Program (NIMH), 100
Treatments That Work, 179
treatment studies, research findings from, overview, 100–106
tricyclic antidepressants, 104
Trotsky, L., 29, 32
true self, 46, 293
trunk lean, 116
twelve-step facilitation
  case example, 225–227
  as decreasing relapse, 104
  definition, 293
  model of psychopathology, 223–224
  research findings, 224–225
  for substance abuse, 110
  treatment strategies, 224
two-person psychology, 11, 47, 54

U

unconscious, 10, 15, 17–18, 20, 21, 22, 23, 24, 25, 26, 28, 33, 34, 37, 38, 39, 293
unconscious conflict, 165
unconscious material, 142, 143
undoing, 38, 39, 48, 293

unified protocols, 109, 180, 255
union, 36, 150, 287
unlearn, 75
unpleasure, 20, 21, 23
Usitalo, A. N., 100

V

validity
  external, 86, 280
  internal, 85, 281
vanity/self-hatred poles, 48
variable-interval reinforcement, 62
variable-ratio reinforcement schedule, 63
venlafaxine, 79
verbal self, 54
vicarious introspection, 52
vicarious reinforcement, 64
videotaping, of role plays, 132, 133, 256
Vienna Psychoanalytic Society, 28, 40
virtual self, 51
von N., Emmy (case of), 18
von R., Elisabeth (case of), 18

W

W., Bill, 223
Walden Two (Skinner), 60

Wampold, B. E., 89
Watson, J. B., 59t, 60, 61, 293
Weissman, M. M., 214, 293
Weltanschauung (worldview), 30, 293
will, 36, 40–42
Winnicott, D. W., 12f, 43, 45–46, 293
wisdom, 43
wish fulfillment, 20, 23, 293
Wolpe, J., 59t, 60, 293
word association tests, 31, 32
Working Alliance Inventory, 93
working memory, 75–76, 80, 81–82
working through, 17, 18, 24, 26, 42, 142, 293
worldview (*Weltanschauung*), 30, 293

Y

young adulthood stage of development, 41t, 42

Z

Zellner, M. R., 80